Atlas of Salivary Gland Pathology

Joaquín J. García

Atlas of Salivary Gland Pathology

Springer

Joaquín J. García, MD
Mayo Clinic School of Medicine
Department of Laboratory Medicine & Pathology
Mayo Clinic Rochester
Rochester, MN
USA

ISBN 978-3-319-09020-7 ISBN 978-3-319-09021-4 (eBook)
https://doi.org/10.1007/978-3-319-09021-4

Library of Congress Control Number: 2018950422

This Springer imprint is published by the registered company Springer Nature Switzerland AG
The registered company address is: Gewerbestrasse 11, 6330 Cham, Switzerland

Dedicated to Qwest, Arolyn, & the Queen Bee . . .

Preface

The incidence of salivary gland cancer is relatively low, affecting approximately 8 per 100,000 persons in the United States each year. Since benign and malignant salivary gland neoplasms commonly share overlapping clinical, radiologic, and pathologic features, a subset of cases continues to pose diagnostic challenges to head and neck specialists. Misclassification may pose patient care challenges, including undertreatment or overtreatment. The *Atlas of Salivary Gland Pathology* represents a gross and microscopic visual tour of salivary gland neoplasms for aspiring and practicing diagnosticians.

Rochester, MN, USA   Joaquín J. García, MD

Contents

Contributors

Tiffany Y. Chen, MD Mayo Clinic School of Medicine, Mayo Clinic Rochester, Rochester, MN, USA

Joaquín J. García, MD Mayo Clinic School of Medicine, Department of Laboratory Medicine & Pathology, Mayo Clinic Rochester, Rochester, MN, USA

Jeffrey R. Janus, MD Mayo Clinic School of Medicine, Department of Otorhinolaryngology, Mayo Clinic Rochester, Rochester, MN, USA

Nirusha Lachman, PhD Mayo Clinic School of Medicine, Department of Anatomy, Mayo Clinic Rochester, Rochester, MN, USA

Luke D. Wilson, PA (ASCP) Mayo Clinic School of Medicine, Department of Laboratory Medicine & Pathology, Mayo Clinic Rochester, Rochester, MN, USA

1 Gross Anatomy

Major salivary glands are visible as three paired organs: *parotid*, *submandibular*, and *sublingual glands*. The parotid gland is, for practical purposes, divided into superficial and deep lobes. The facial nerve courses between the superficial and deep lobes, serving as a surgical landmark. *Stensen's duct*, formed by the convergence of several excretory ducts within the parotid gland, empties into oral cavity buccal mucosa opposite the maxillary second molar. The submandibular gland is located in the submandibular triangle and empties glandular secretions into the anterior floor of mouth by way of *Wharton's duct*. Lastly, the sublingual gland is situated in the lingual sulcus of the floor of mouth and empties into the oral cavity via *Bartholin's duct*.

Minor salivary glands, distributed widely throughout the mucosa and submucosa of the upper aerodigestive tract, are typically grossly inapparent (Figs. 1.1–1.8).

J. J. García, *Atlas of Salivary Gland Pathology*, https://doi.org/10.1007/978-3-319-09021-4_1

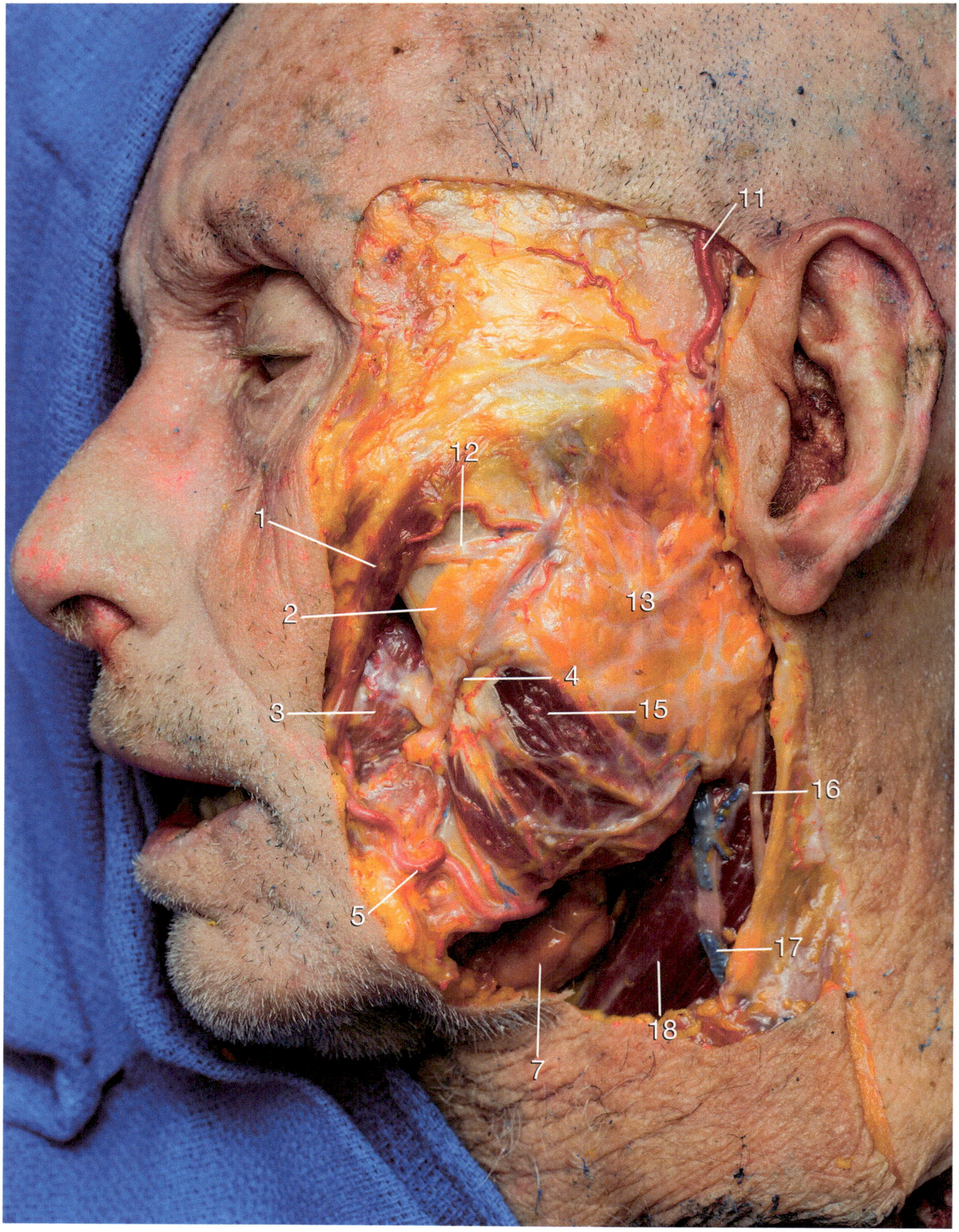

Fig. 1.1 (Gross Anatomy) Anatomic relationships of parotid and submandibular glands. 1—Zygomaticus major muscle, 2—Accessory parotid gland, 3—Buccinator muscle, 4—Stensen's duct, 5—Facial artery, 7—Submandibular gland, 11—Superficial temporal artery, 12—Zygomatic branch of facial nerve, 13—Parotid gland, superficial lobe, 15—Masseter muscle, 16—Great auricular nerve, 17—External jugular vein, 18—Sternoclediomastoid muscle

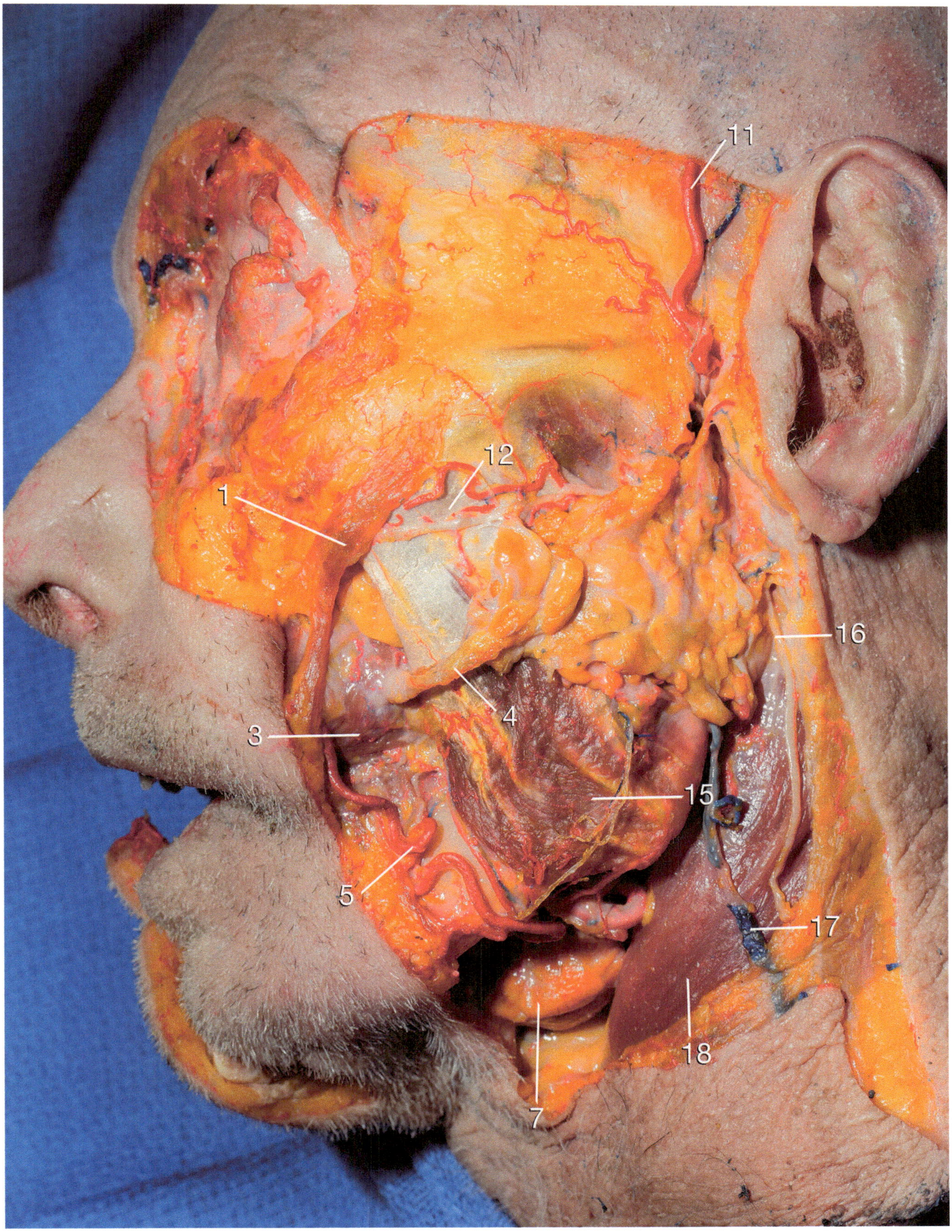

Fig. 1.2 (Gross Anatomy) Anatomic relationships of parotid and submandibular glands. 1—Zygomaticus major muscle, 3—Buccinator muscle, 4—Stensen's duct, 5—Facial artery, 7—Submandibular gland, 11—Superficial temporal artery, 12—Zygomatic branch of facial nerve, 15—Masseter muscle, 16—Great auricular nerve, 17—External jugular vein, 18—Sternoclediomastoid muscle

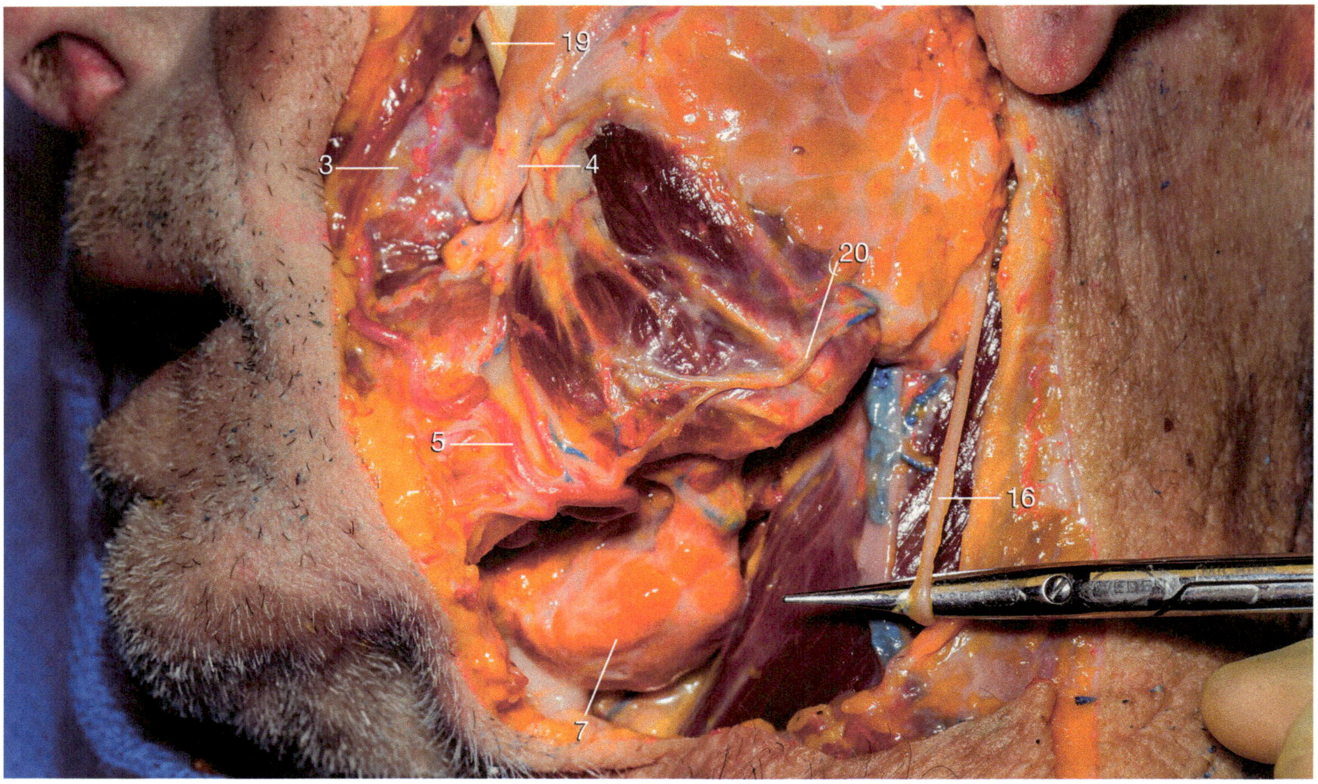

Fig. 1.3 (Gross Anatomy) Anatomic relationships of parotid and submandibular glands. 3—Buccinator muscle, 4—Stensen's duct, 5—Facial artery, 7—Submandibular gland, 16—Great auricular nerve, 19—Tendon of masseter muscle, 20—Marginal mandibular branch of facial nerve

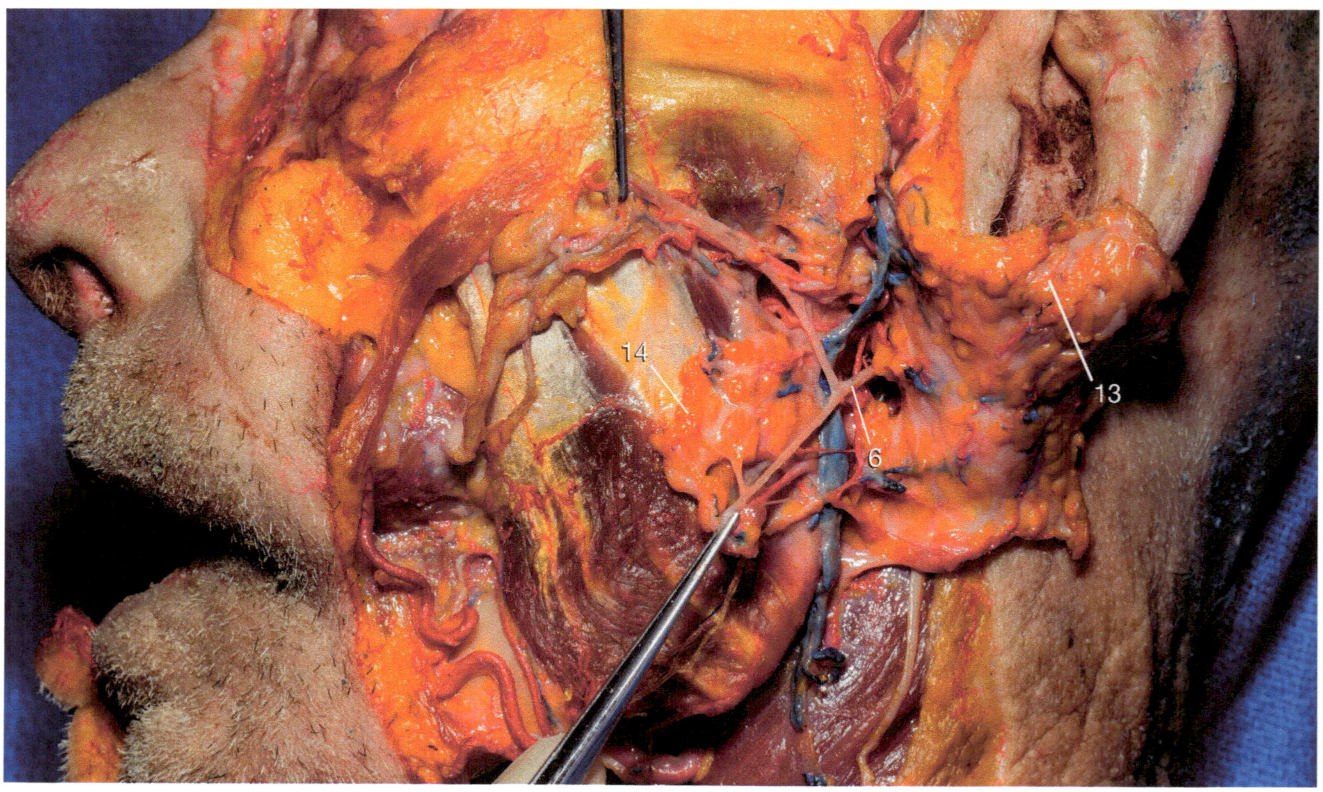

Fig. 1.4 (Gross Anatomy) Anatomic relationships of parotid and submandibular glands. 6—Buccal branch of facial nerve, 13—Parotid gland, superficial lobe, 14—Parotid gland, deep lobe

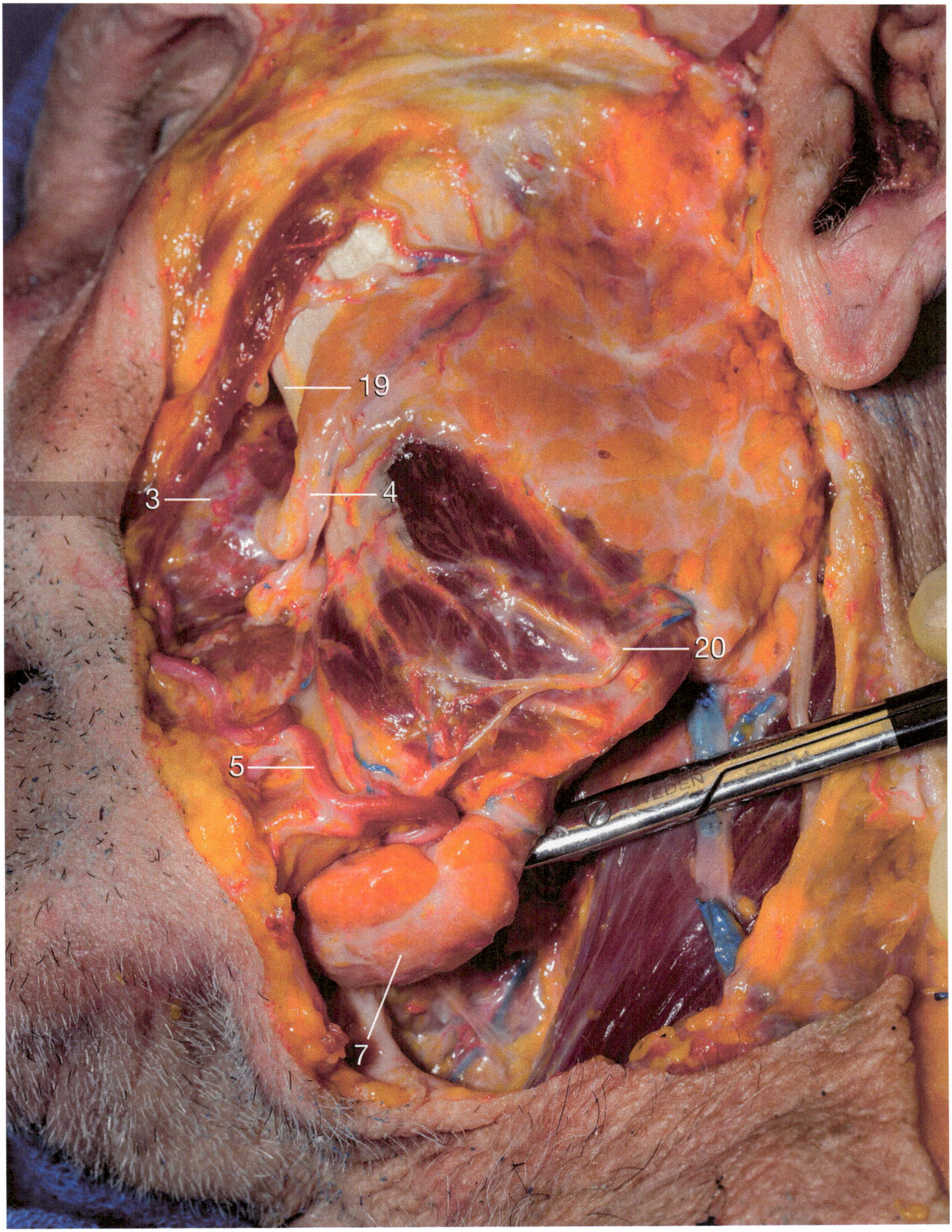

Fig. 1.5 (Gross Anatomy) Anatomic relationships of parotid and submandibular glands. 3—Buccinator muscle, 4—Stensen's duct, 5—Facial artery, 7—Submandibular gland, 19—Tendon of masseter muscle, 20—Marginal mandibular branch of facial nerve

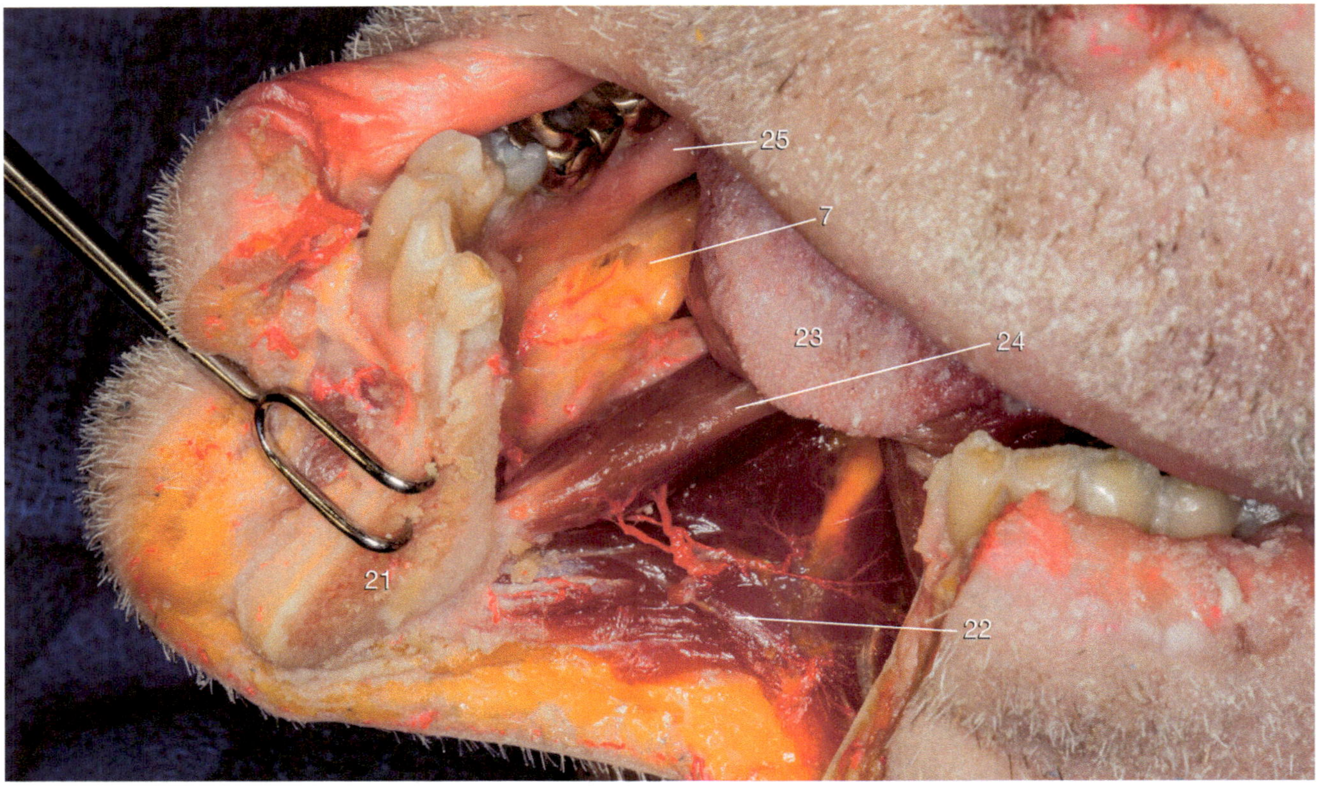

Fig. 1.6 (Gross Anatomy) Anatomic relationships of submandibular gland. 7—Submandibular gland, 21—Mandible, 22—Mylohyoid muscle, 23—Tongue, 24—Geniohyoid muscle, 25—Gingival mucosa

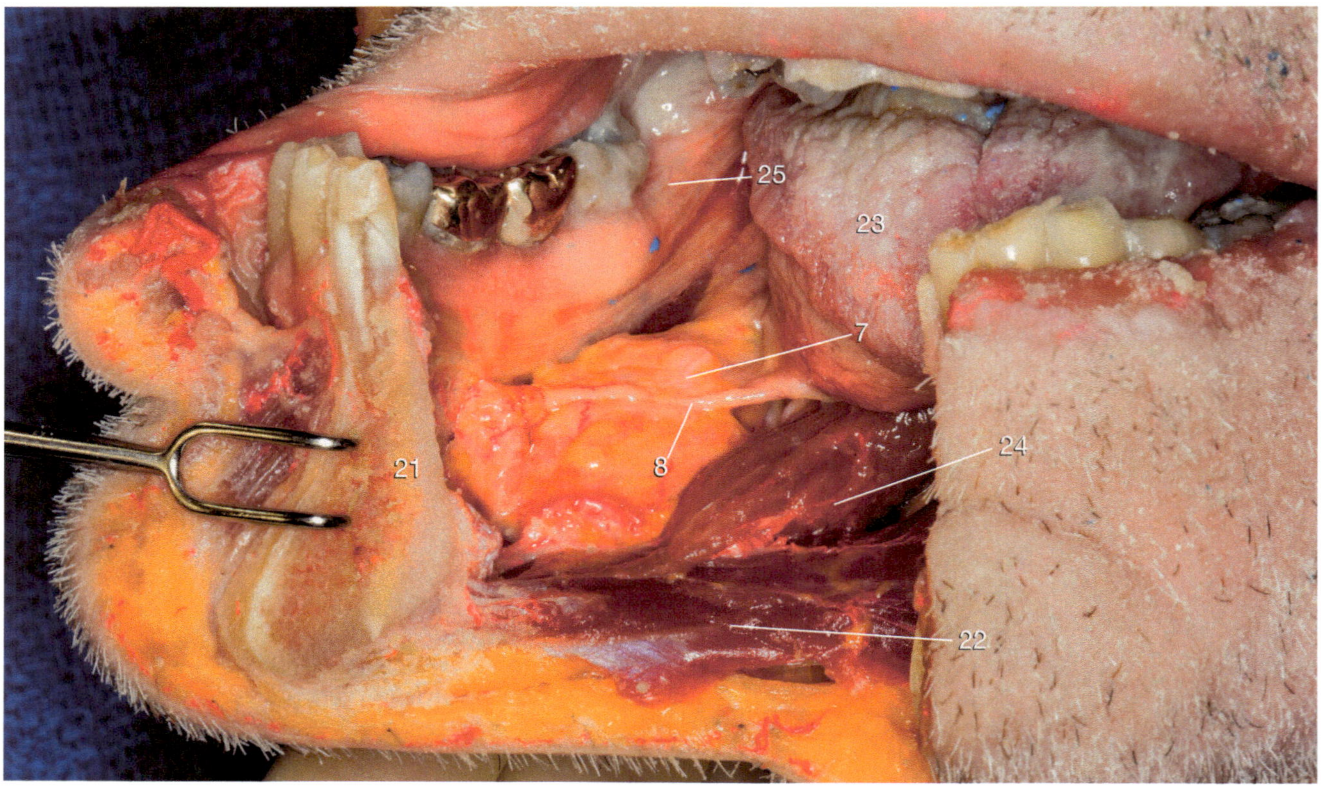

Fig. 1.7 (Gross Anatomy) Anatomic relationships of submandibular gland. 7—Submandibular gland, 8—Wharton's duct, 21—Mandible, 22—Mylohyoid muscle, 23—Tongue, 24—Geniohyoid muscle, 25—Gingival mucosa

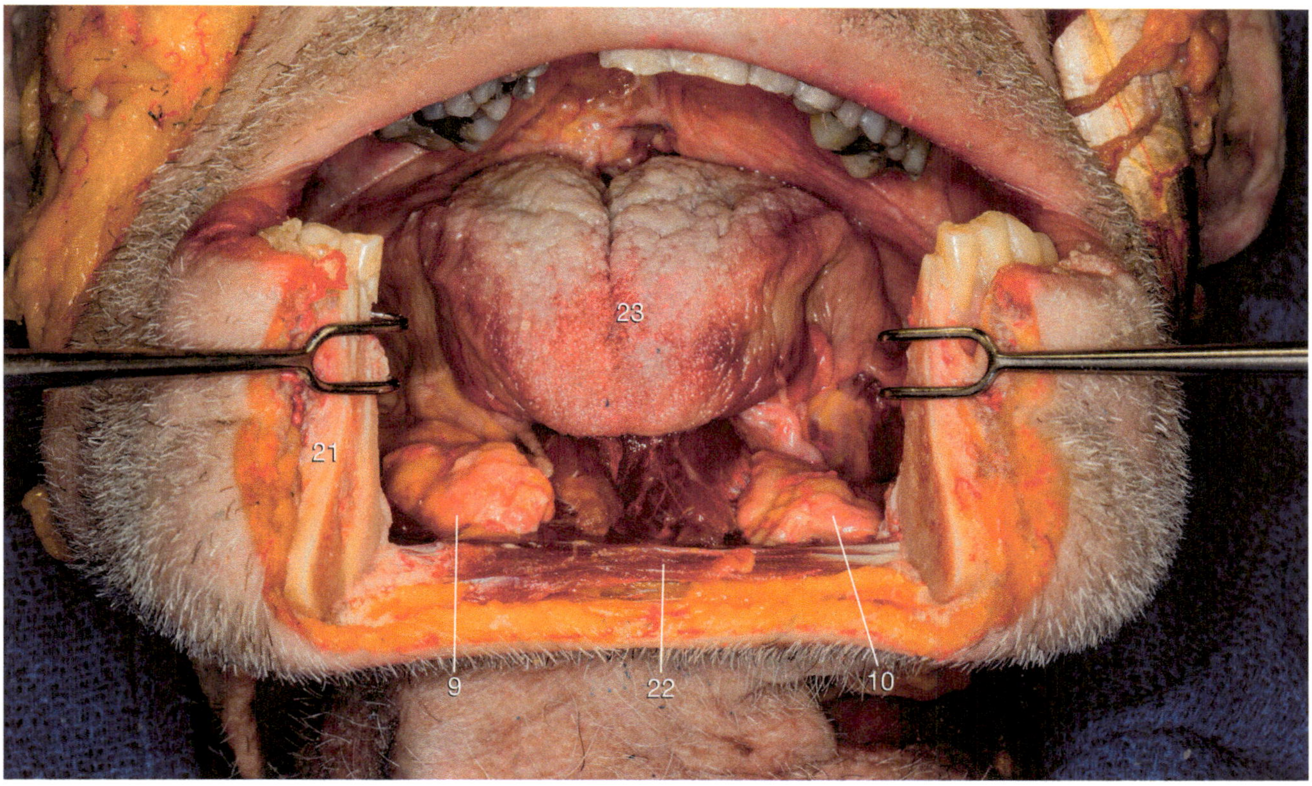

Fig. 1.8 (Gross Anatomy) Anatomic relationships of sublingual glands. 9—Sublingual gland, right, 10—Sublingual gland, left, 21—Mandible, 22—Mylohyoid muscle, 23—Tongue

Suggested Reading

Standring S. Section 4: head and neck. In: Standring S, editor. Gray's anatomy: the anatomical basis of clinical practice. 40th ed. Edinburgh: Churchill Livingstone/Elsevier; 2008. p. 467–95.

2 Microscopic Anatomy

Salivary gland tissue contains two types of secretory cells: *serous* and *mucous*. The relative distribution of serous and mucous cells varies tremendously between parotid, submandibular, and sublingual glands. Parotid gland secretory units are lined primarily by serous cells and produce a watery secretion. Submandibular gland secretory units have a higher density of mucous cells and produce a secretion of intermediate consistency. Sublingual gland secretory units have the highest density of mucous cells and produce a viscous secretion. *Myoepithelial cells* circumferentially envelop secretory acini and intercalated ducts to aid in secretion.

Terminal secretory units lead into a series of ducts with diverse histomorphologic and physiologic attributes. *Intercalated ducts* are most proximal to the secretory unit and lined by cuboidal cells. Intercalated ducts lead to *striated ducts,* lined by eosinophilic columnar cells and named after the striated appearance caused by prominent basal plasma membrane folds and mitochondria. Lastly, interlobular and extraglandular *excretory ducts* are lined by pseudostratified columnar cells and converge upon one another before leading to Stensen's, Wharton's, or Bartholin's ducts.

Minor salivary glands are composed of serous and mucous cells arranged in lobules within the mucosa and submucosa of the upper aerodigestive tract. Given that most of these glands contribute little, if anything, to saliva, the term *submcuosal seromucinous glands* is also used (Figs. 2.1–2.15).

J. J. García, *Atlas of Salivary Gland Pathology*, https://doi.org/10.1007/978-3-319-09021-4_2

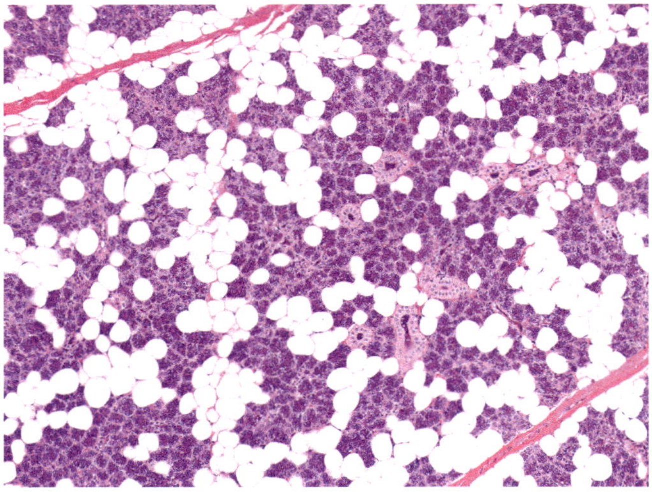

Fig. 2.1 (H&E, 100×) Parotid gland, lobules

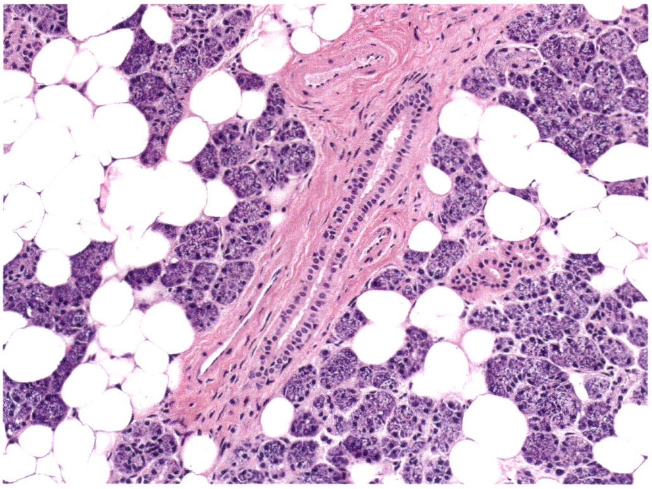

Fig. 2.2 (H&E, 200×) Parotid gland, excretory duct

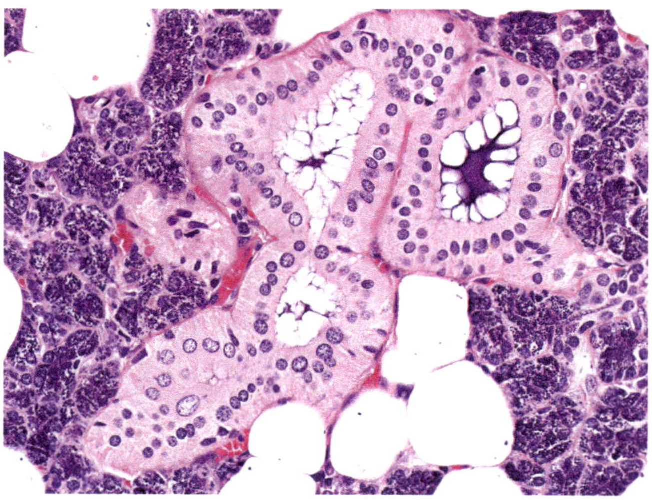

Fig. 2.3 (H&E, 400×) Parotid gland, striated ducts

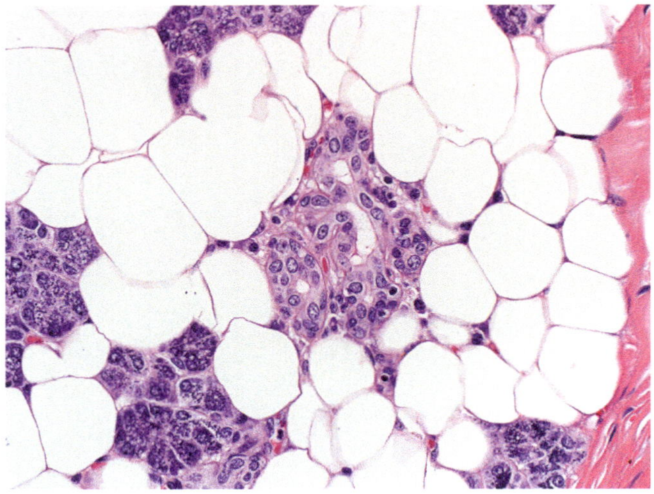

Fig. 2.4 (H&E, 400×) Parotid gland, intercalated ducts

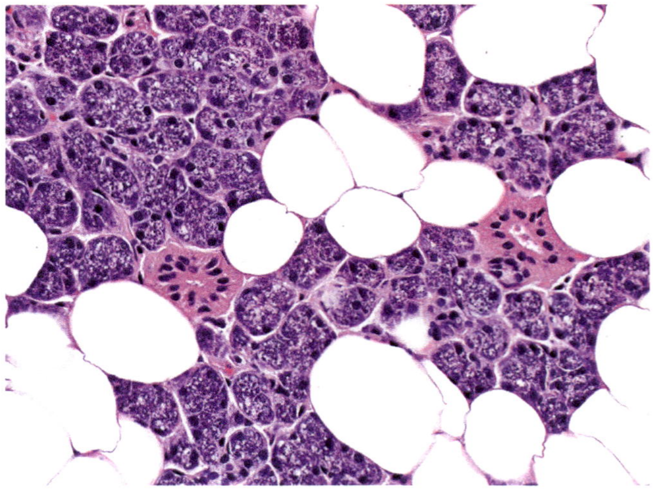

Fig. 2.5 (H&E, 400×) Parotid gland, serous acini

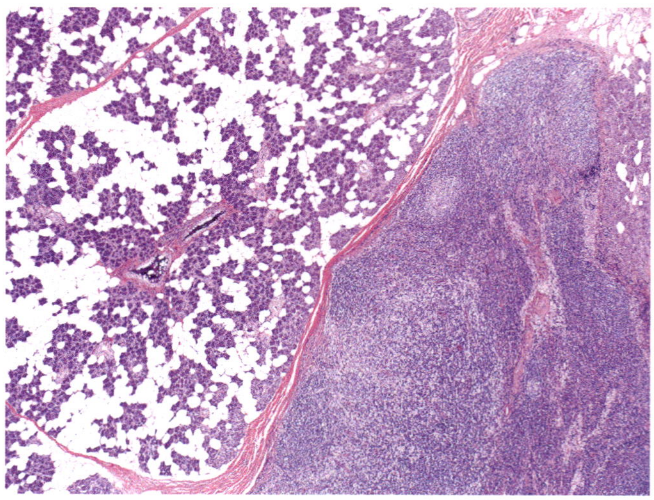

Fig. 2.6 (H&E, 40×) Parotid gland, intraparotid lymph node

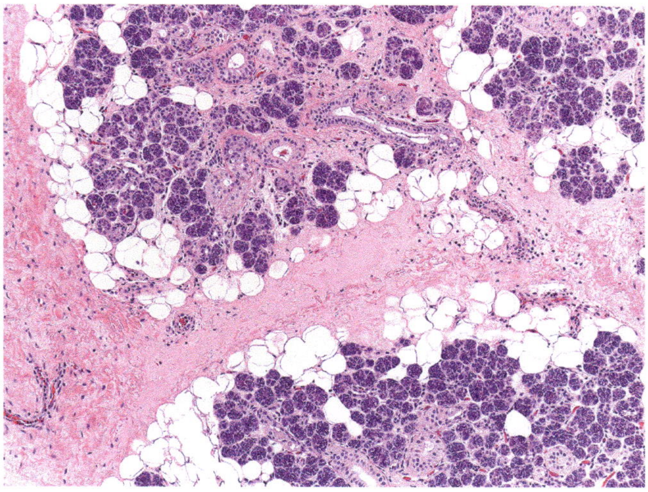

Fig. 2.7 (H&E, 100×) Submandibular gland, lobules

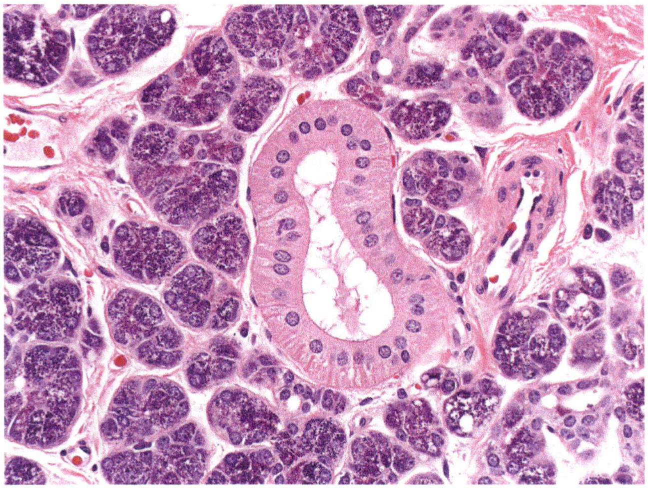

Fig. 2.8 (H&E, 400×) Submandibular gland, striated duct

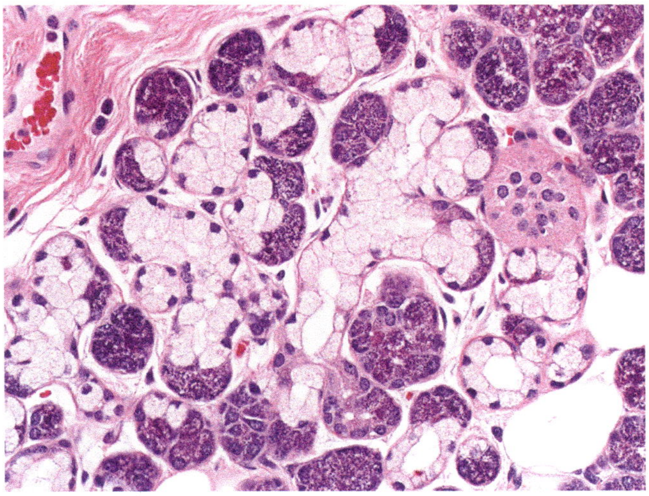

Fig. 2.9 (H&E, 400×) Submandibular gland, seromucinous acini (serous demilunes)

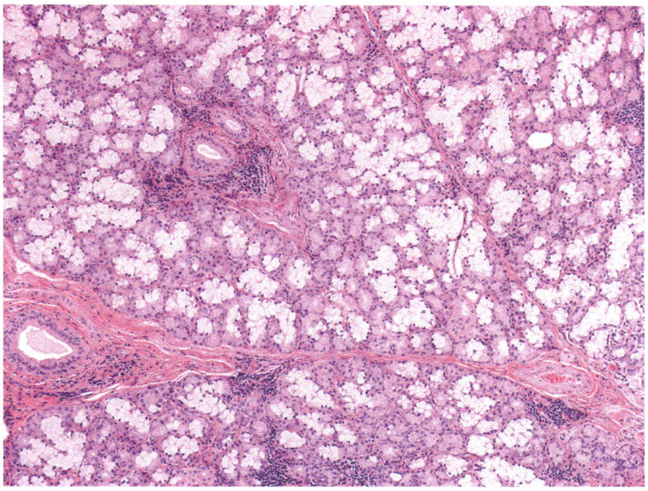

Fig. 2.10 (H&E, 100×) Sublingual gland, lobules

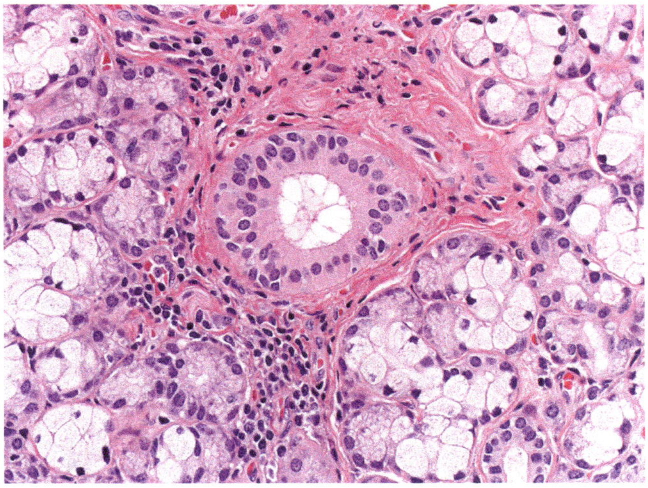

Fig. 2.11 (H&E, 400×) Sublingual gland, striated duct

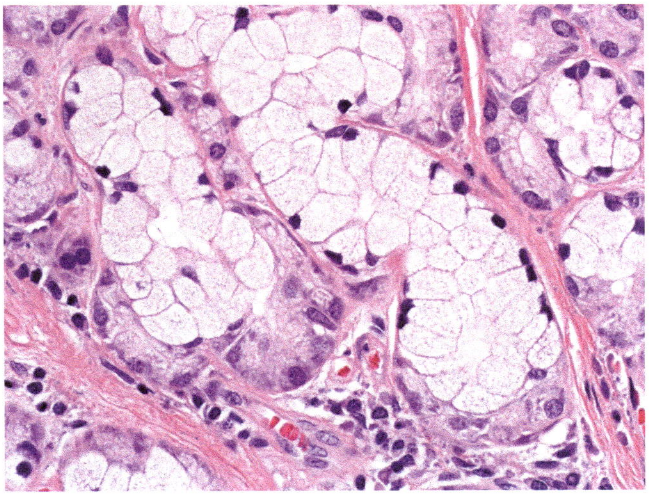

Fig. 2.12 (H&E, 600×) Sublingual gland, mucinous acini

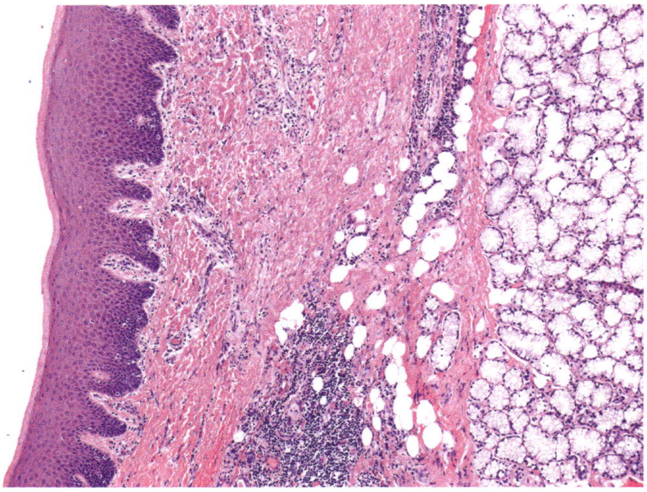

Fig. 2.13 (H&E, 100×) Palate, lobules

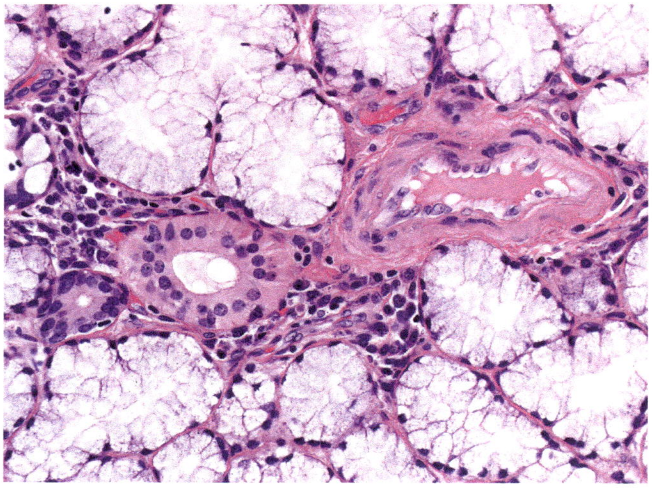

Fig. 2.14 (H&E, 200×) Palate, striated duct

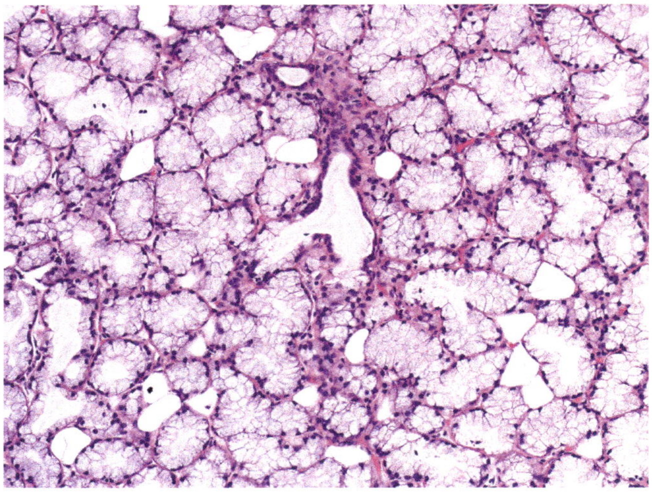

Fig. 2.15 (H&E, 400×) Palate, mucinous acini

Suggested Reading

Mill SE. Histology for Pathologists. 4th ed. Philadelphia: Lippincott Williams & Wilkins; 2012. p. 477–502.

Young B, Lowe JS, Stevens A, Heath JW. Wheater's functional histology: a text and colour atlas. 5th ed. Edinburgh: Churchill Livingstone/Elsevier; 2006. p. 251–62.

3 Intraoperative Examination

The complexity of head and neck anatomy and biologic heterogeneity of salivary gland neoplasms present several challenges to surgeons. Surgical management may be further complicated by the need to preserve function and meet cosmetic expectations. In the setting of clear surgical margins, benign salivary gland parenchyma or capsule surround the neoplasm (Figs. 3.1–3.7).

J. J. García, *Atlas of Salivary Gland Pathology*, https://doi.org/10.1007/978-3-319-09021-4_3

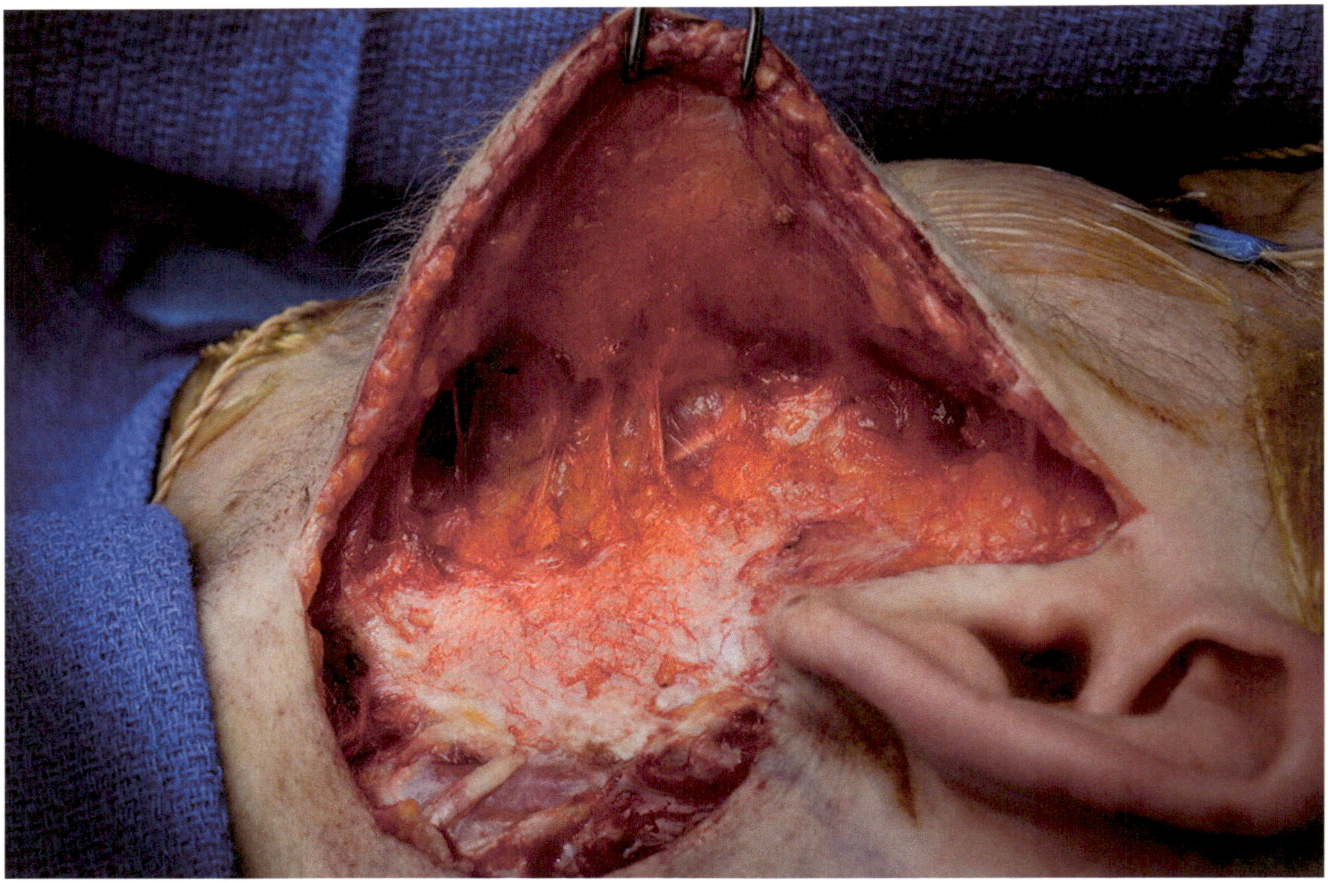

Fig. 3.1 (Intraoperative examination) Parotid gland, fascia intact

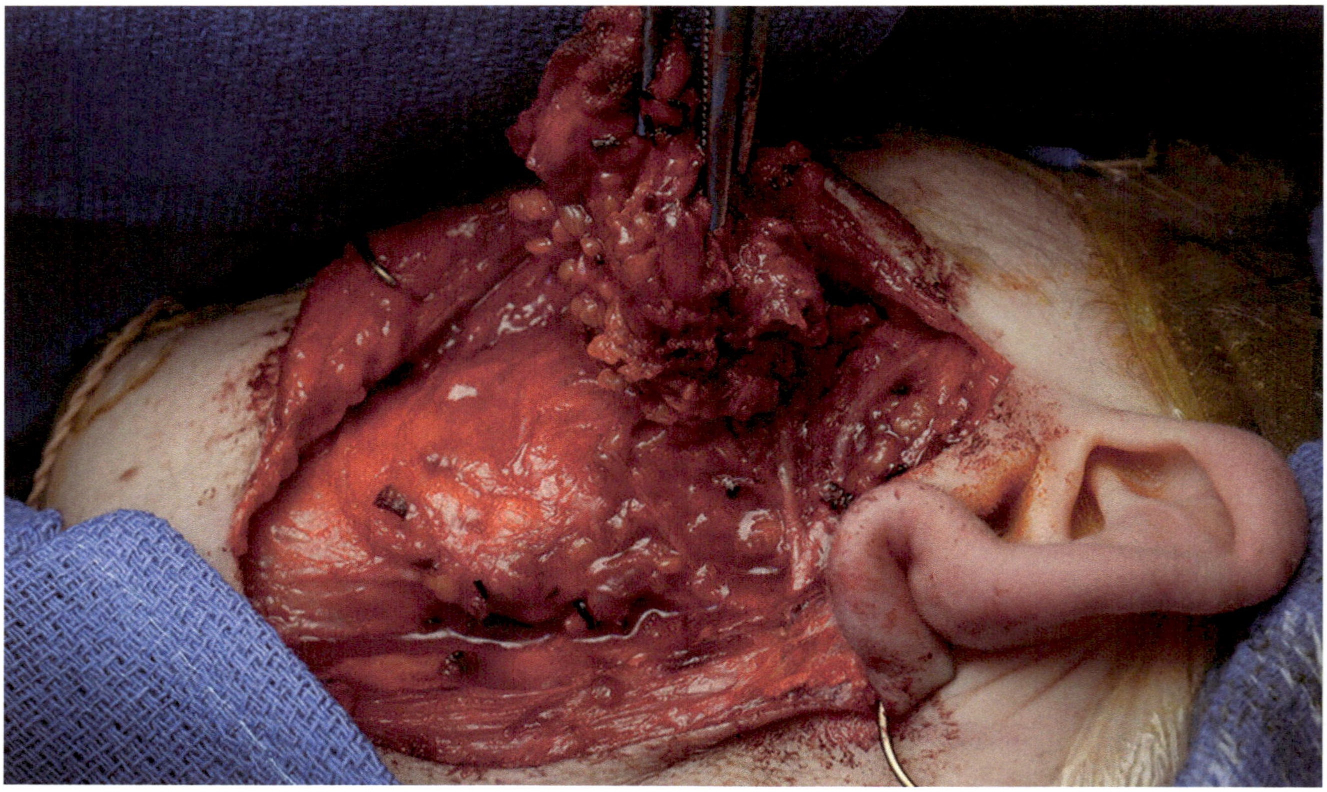

Fig. 3.2 (Intraoperative examination) Parotid gland, superficial lobe reflected

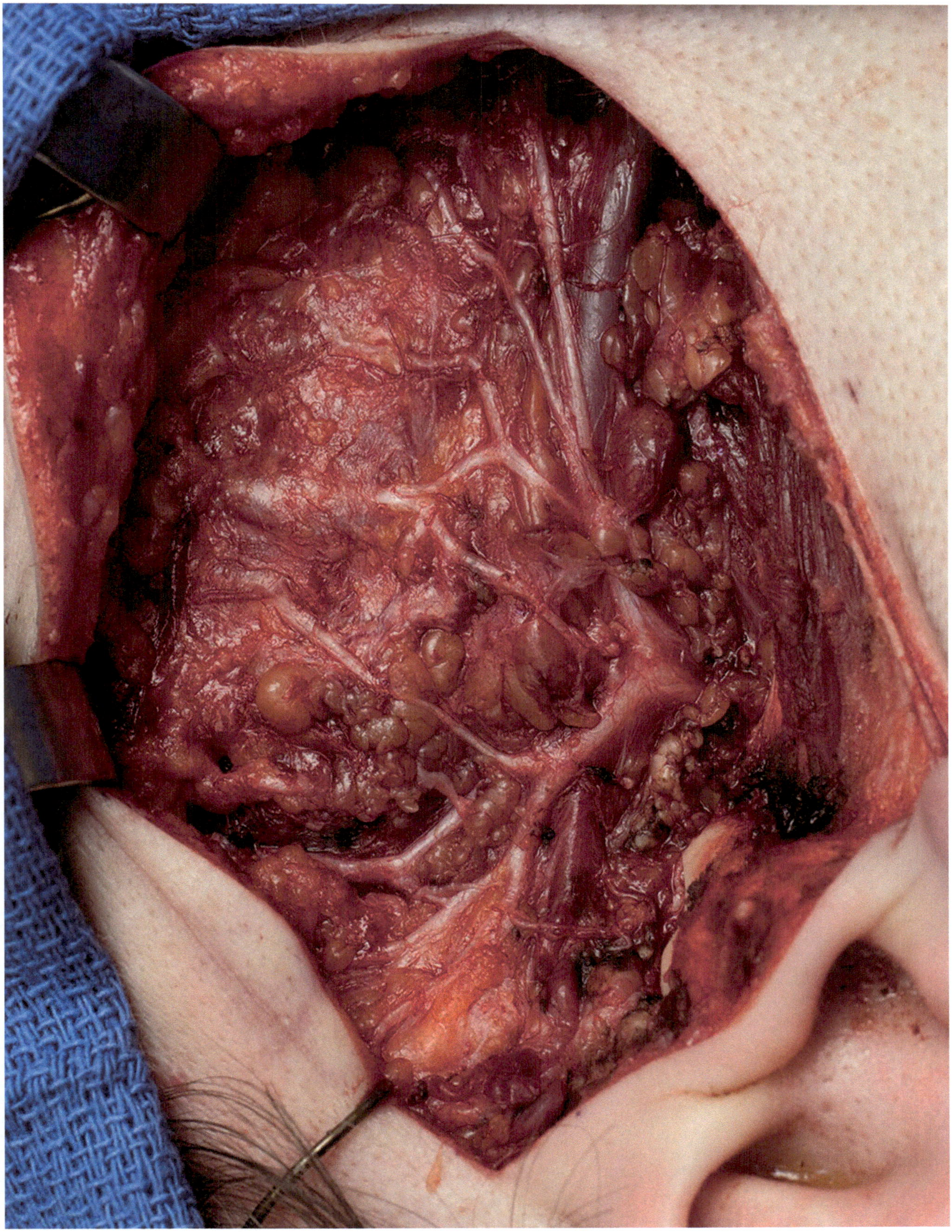

Fig. 3.3 (Intraoperative examination) Parotid gland, superficial lobe removed

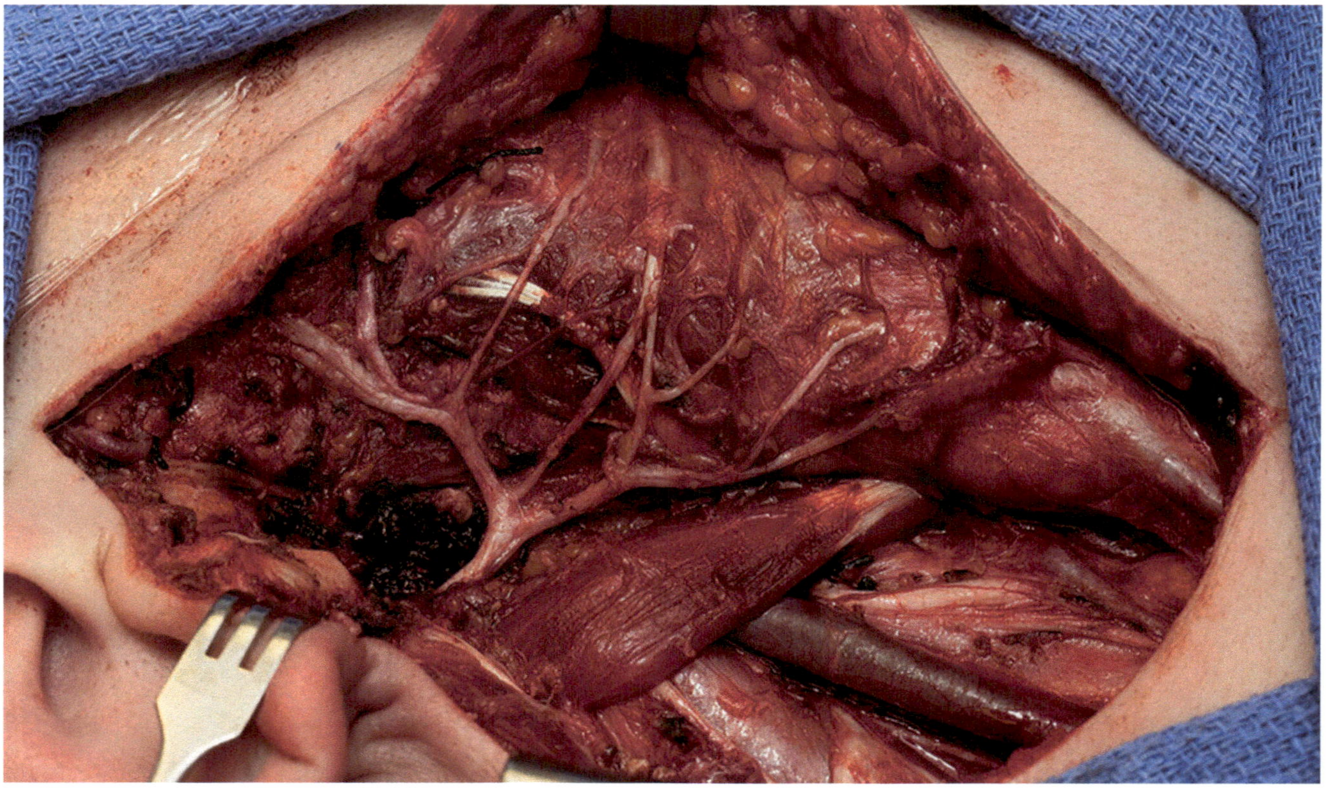

Fig. 3.4 (Intraoperative examination) Parotid gland, deep lobe removed

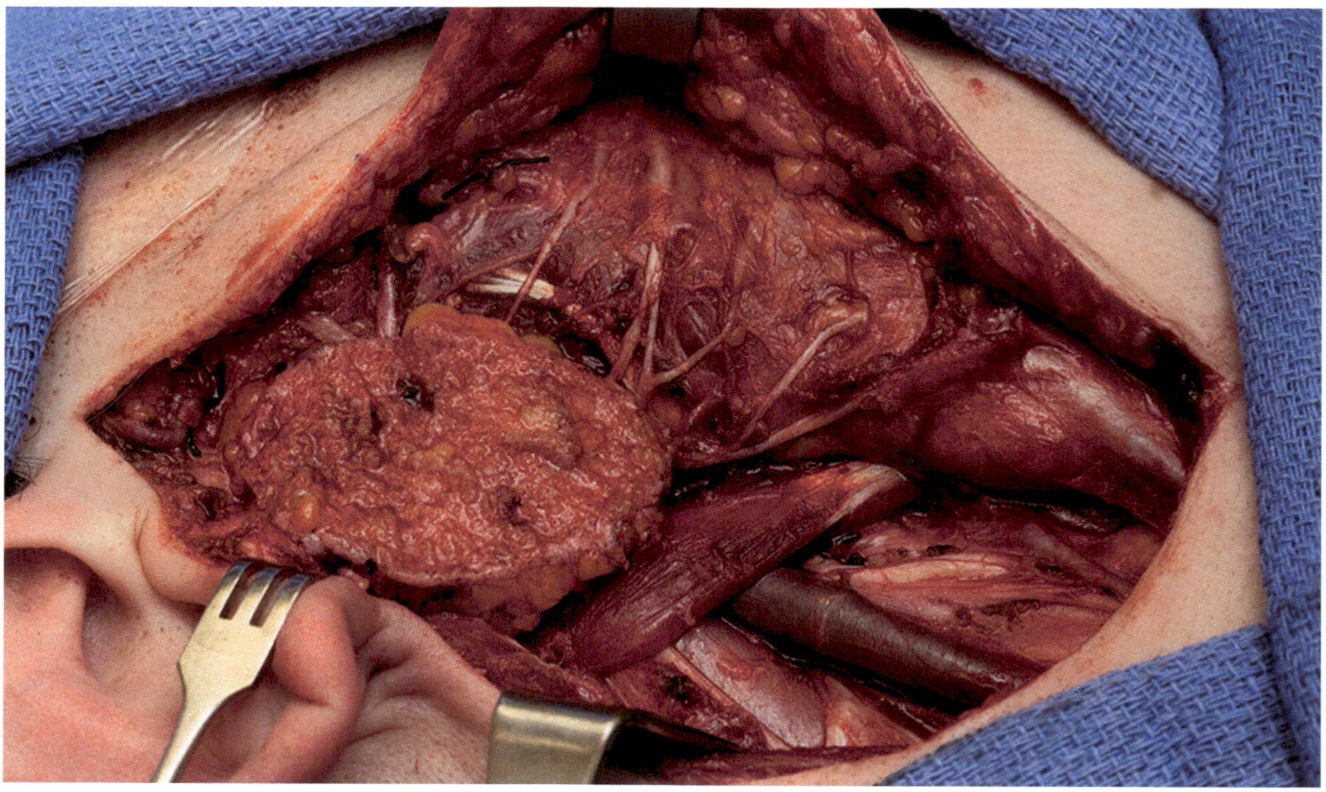

Fig. 3.5 (Intraoperative examination) Parotid gland, abdominal dermal fat graft

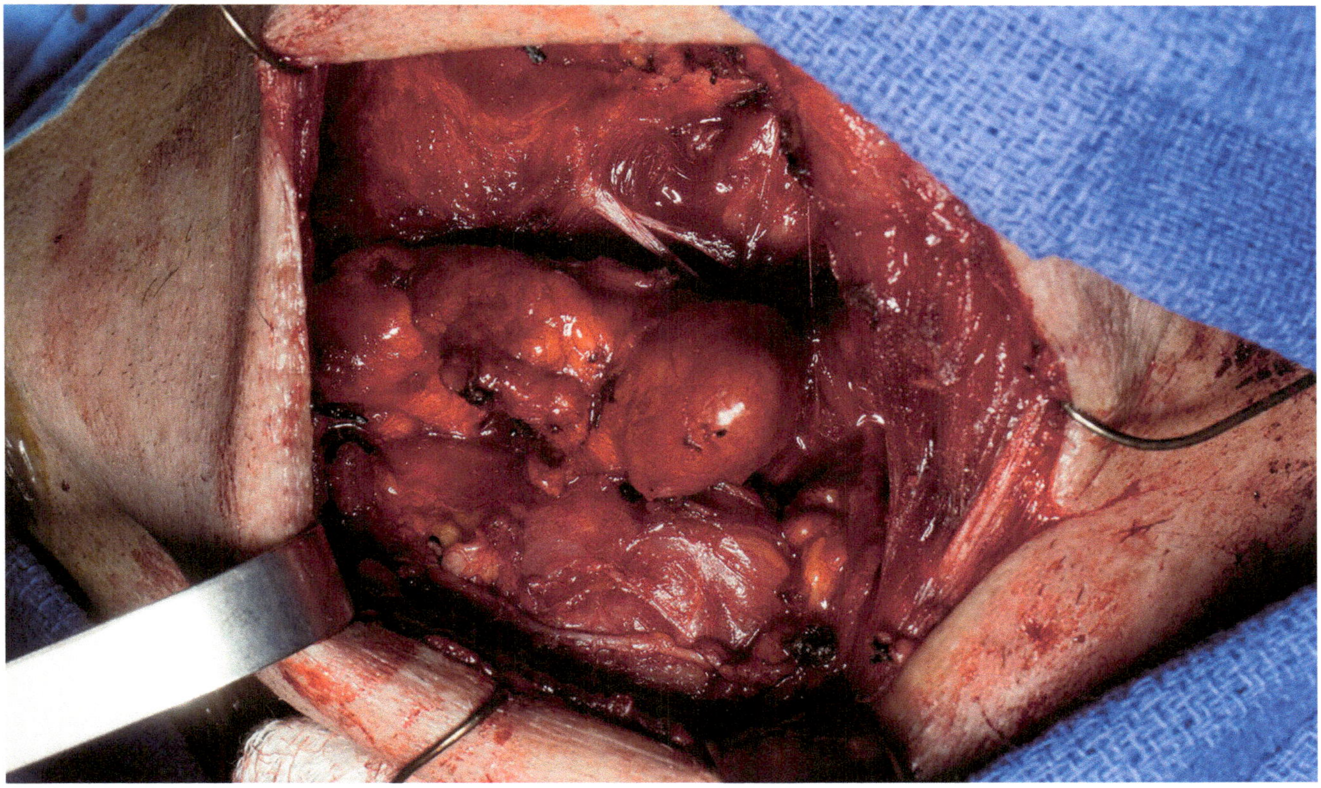

Fig. 3.6 (Intraoperative examination) Submandibular gland, submandibular triangle

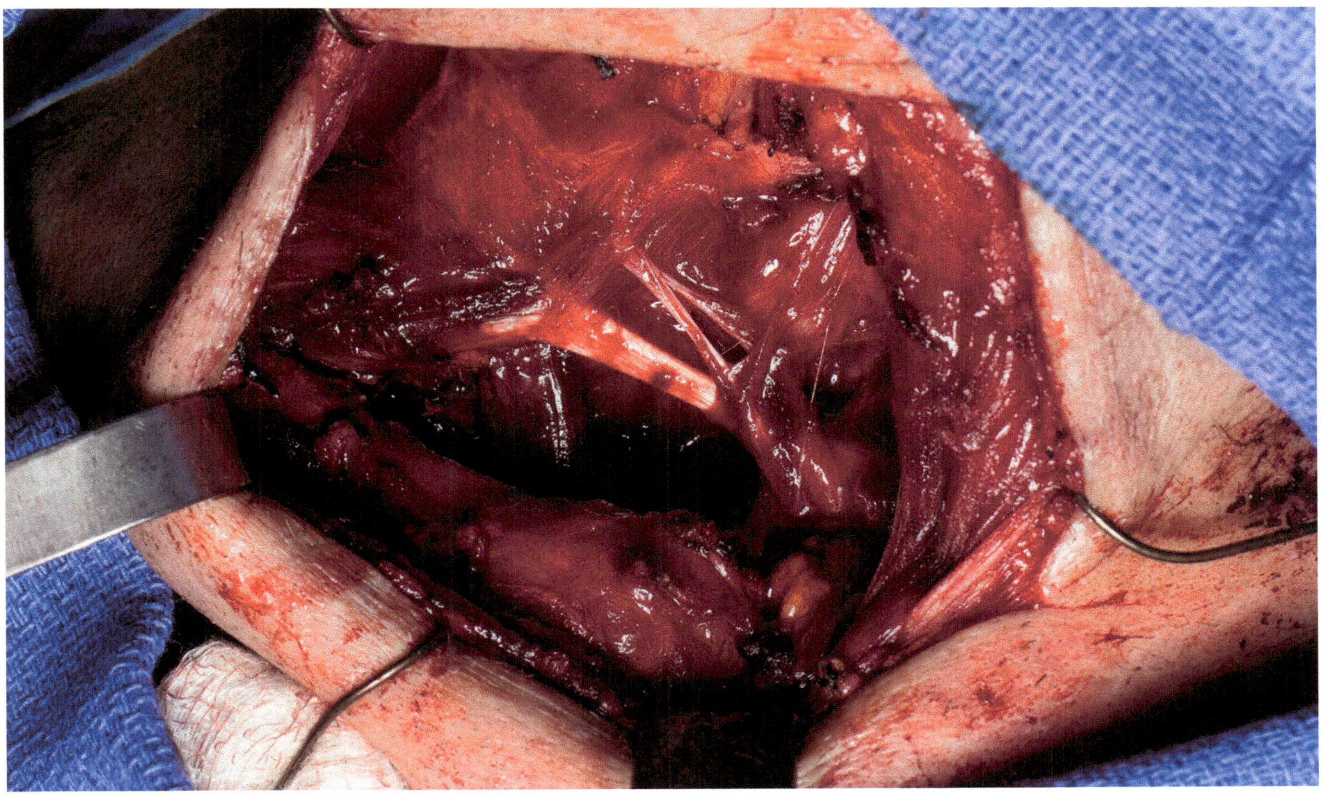

Fig. 3.7 (Intraoperative examination) Submandibular gland, removed

4 Gross Examination

Comprehensive gross examination of a salivary gland neoplasm is often requisite to its accurate classification. Although benign and malignant neoplasms routinely mimic one another grossly, visual inspection directs appropriate tissue sampling for microscopic examination. Some of the commonly encountered gross appearances include the following (Figs. 4.1–4.36):

- *Encapsulated*
- *Circumscribed*
- *Nodular*
- *Infiltrative*
- *Chondroid*
- *Oncocytic*
- *Hemorrhagic*
- *Cystic*
- *Necrotic*

J. J. García, *Atlas of Salivary Gland Pathology*, https://doi.org/10.1007/978-3-319-09021-4_4

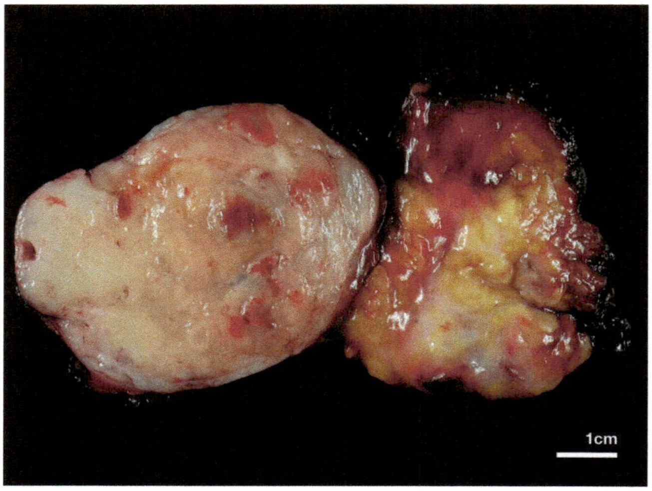

Fig. 4.1 (Gross examination) Encapsulated, pleomorphic adenoma

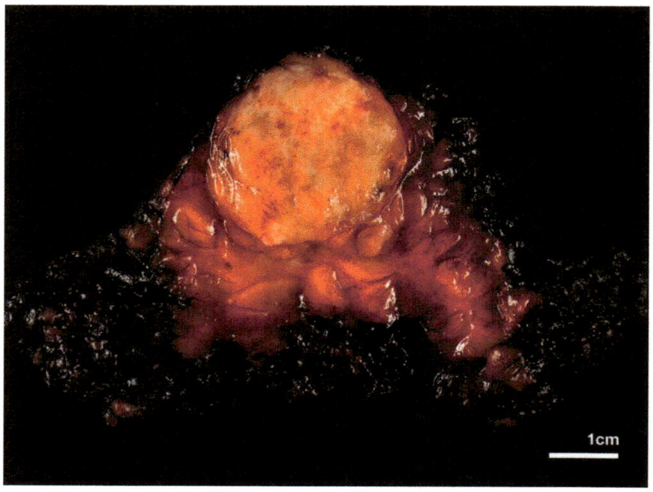

Fig. 4.2 (Gross examination) Encapsulated, carcinoma ex pleomorphic adenoma

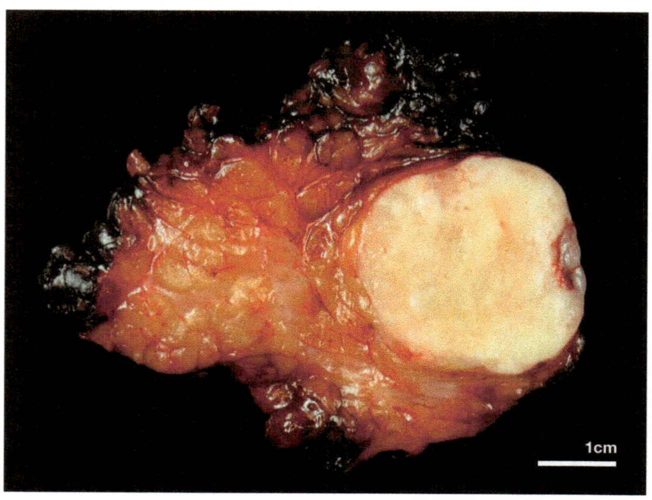

Fig. 4.3 (Gross examination) Circumscribed, pleomorphic adenoma

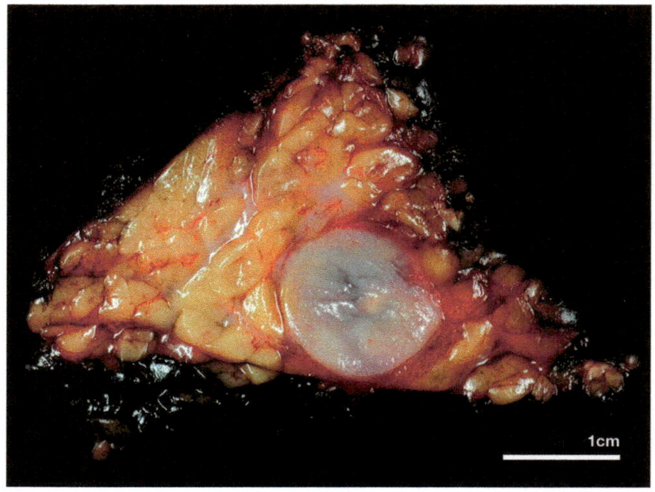

Fig. 4.4 (Gross examination) Circumscribed, basal cell adenoma

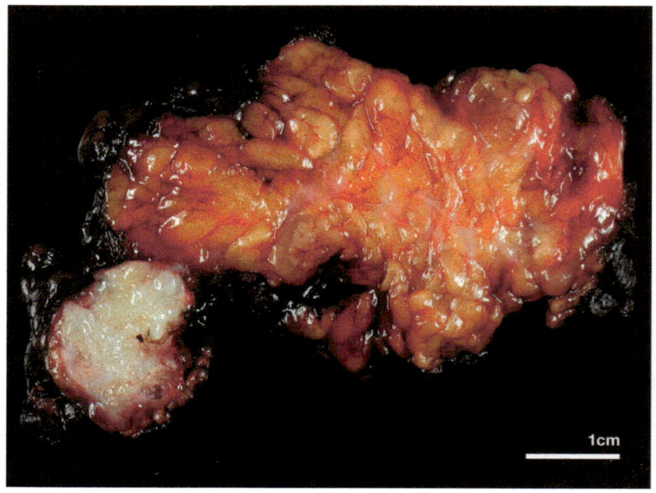

Fig. 4.5 (Gross examination) Circumscribed, mucoepidermoid carcinoma

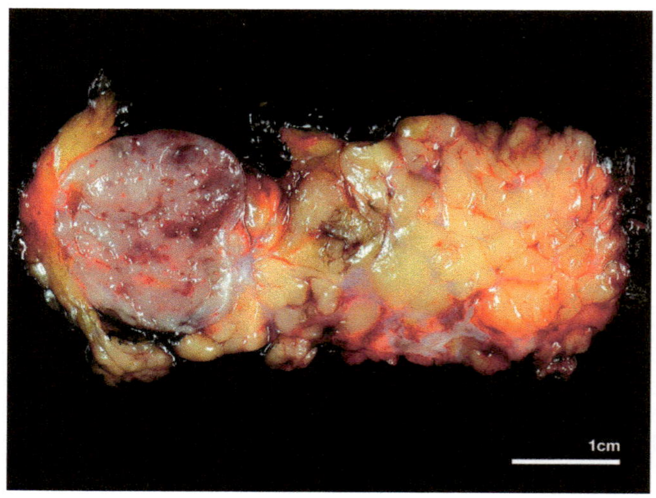

Fig. 4.6 (Gross examination) Circumscribed, acinic cell carcinoma

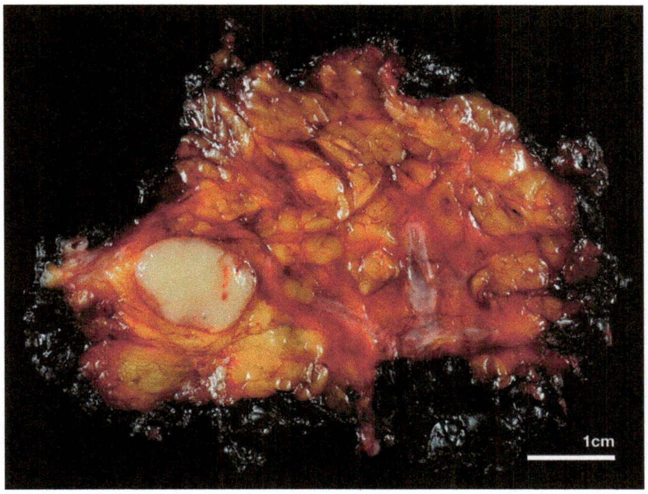

Fig. 4.7 (Gross examination) Circumscribed, lymphoepithelial carcinoma

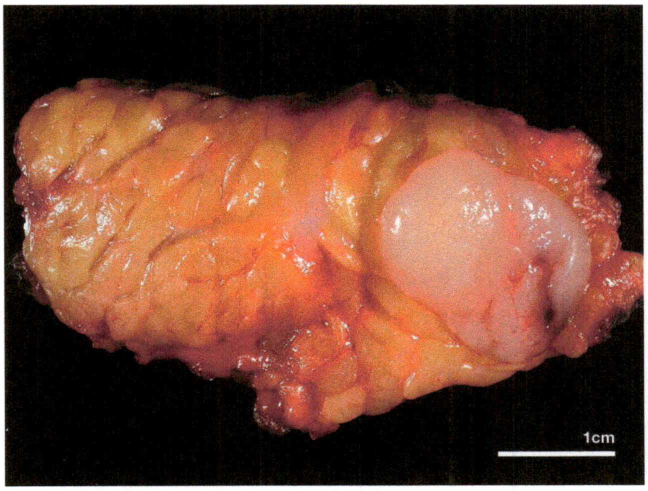

Fig. 4.8 (Gross examination) Circumscribed, lymphoma

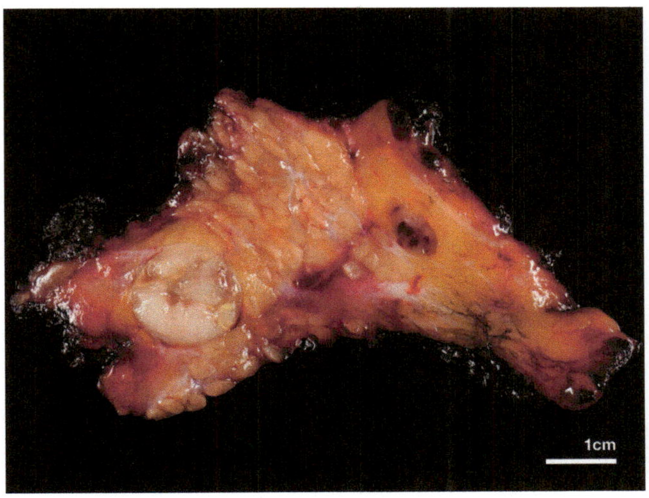

Fig. 4.9 (Gross examination) Circumscribed, metastatic oropharyngeal cancer

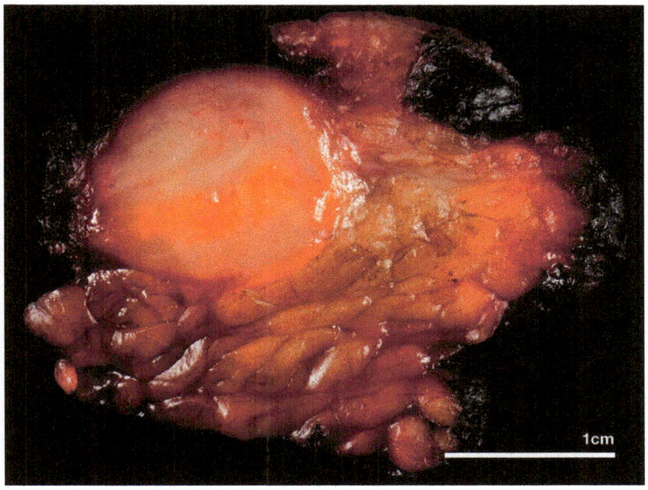

Fig. 4.10 (Gross examination) Circumscribed, metastatic lung adenocarcinoma

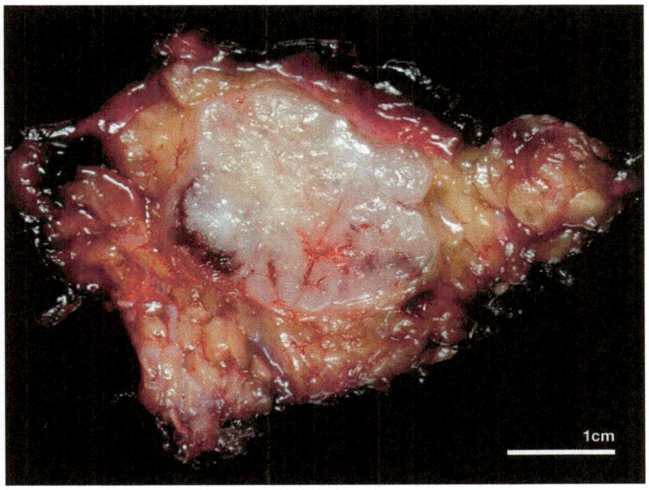

Fig. 4.11 (Gross examination) Nodular, pleomorphic adenoma

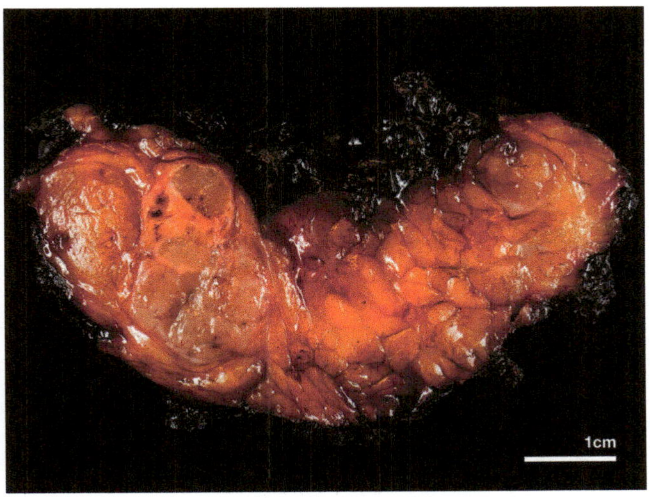

Fig. 4.12 (Gross examination) Nodular, basal cell adenoma

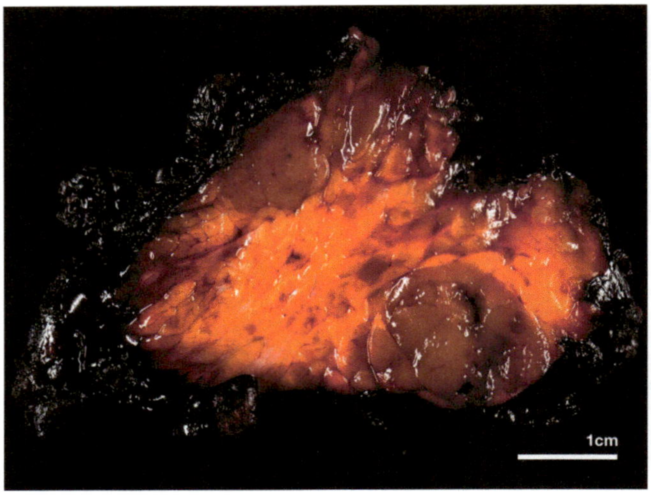

Fig. 4.13 (Gross examination) Nodular, oncocytoma

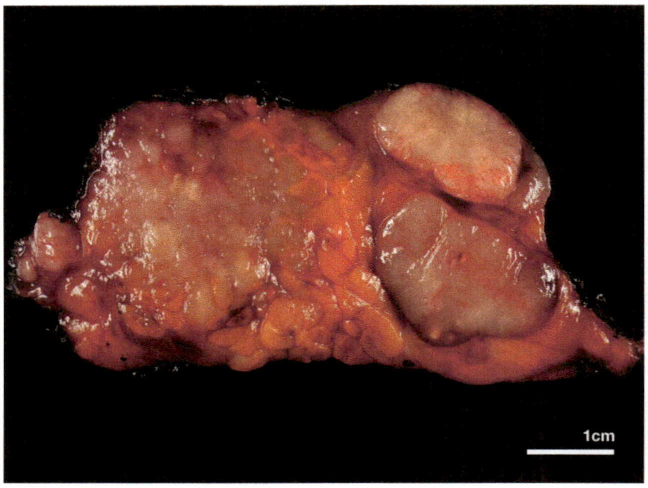

Fig. 4.14 (Gross examination) Nodular, salivary duct carcinoma

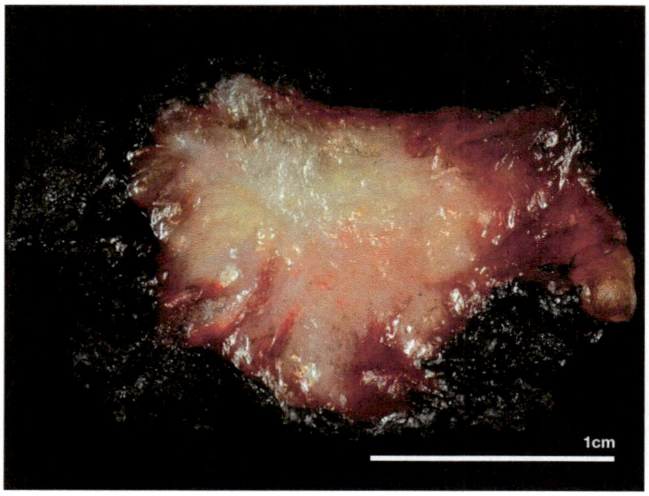

Fig. 4.15 (Gross examination) Infiltrative, mucoepidermoid carcinoma

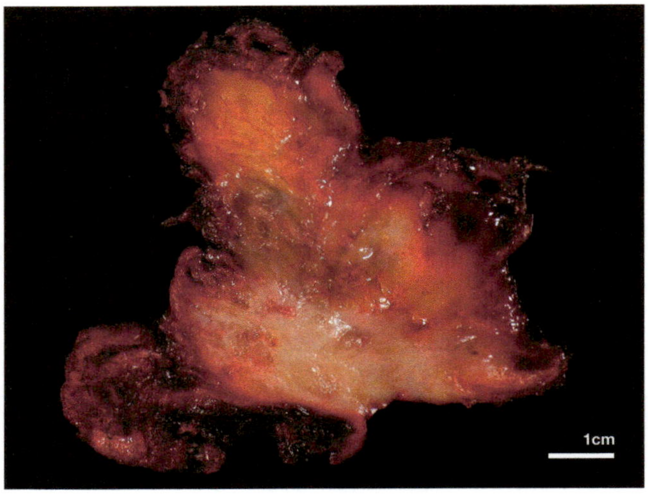

Fig. 4.16 (Gross examination) Infiltrative, adenoid cystic carcinoma

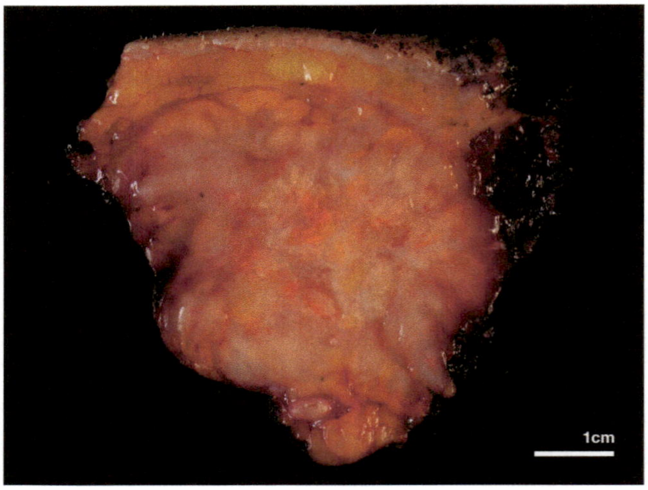

Fig. 4.17 (Gross examination) Infiltrative, carcinoma ex pleomorphic adenoma

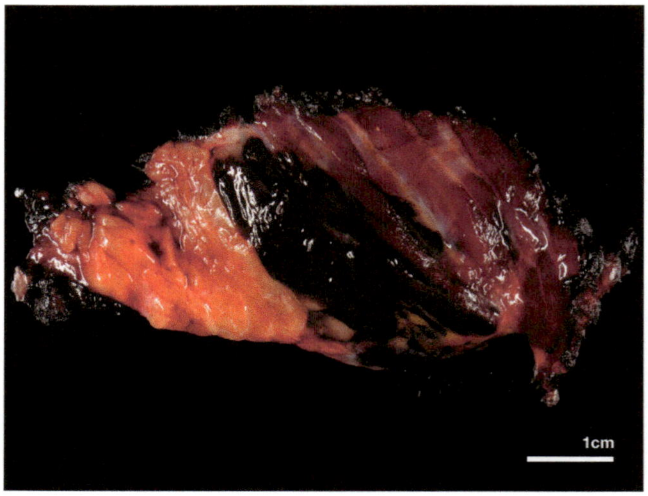

Fig. 4.18 (Gross examination) Infiltrative, metastatic melanoma

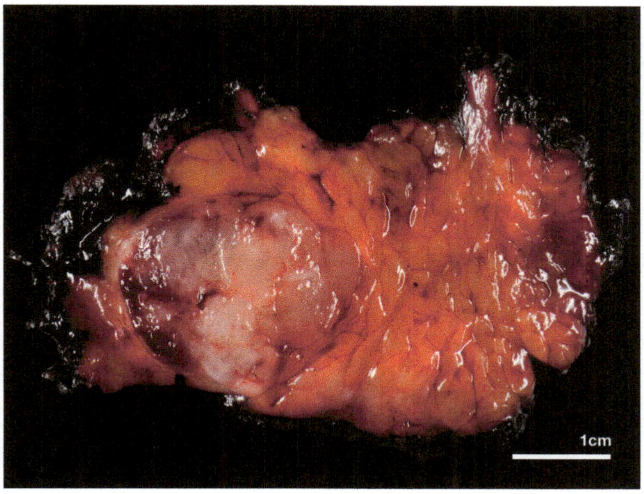

Fig. 4.19 (Gross examination) Chondroid, pleomorphic adenoma

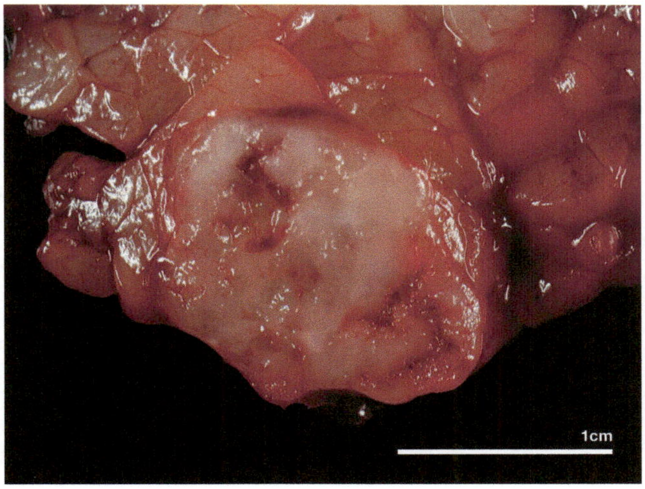

Fig. 4.20 (Gross examination) Chondroid, pleomorphic adenoma

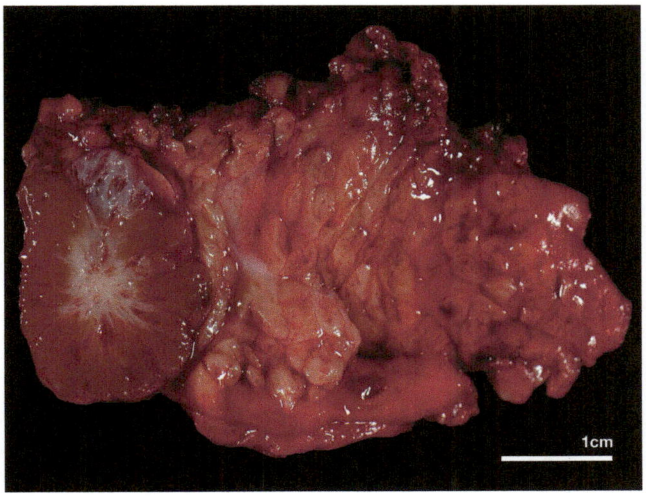

Fig. 4.21 (Gross examination) Oncocytic, oncocytoma

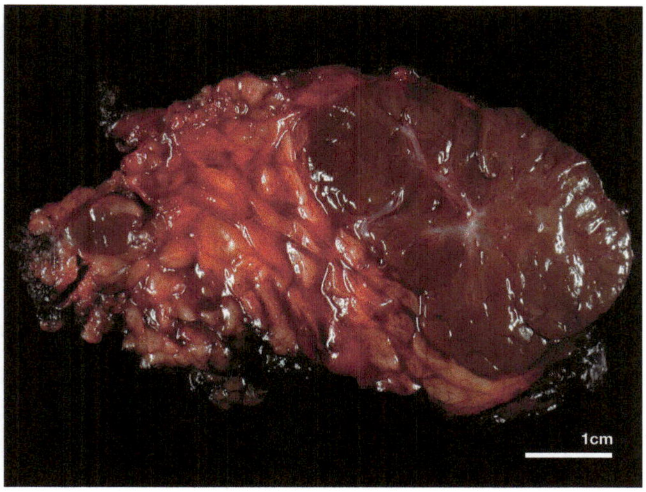

Fig. 4.22 (Gross examination) Oncocytic, oncocytoma

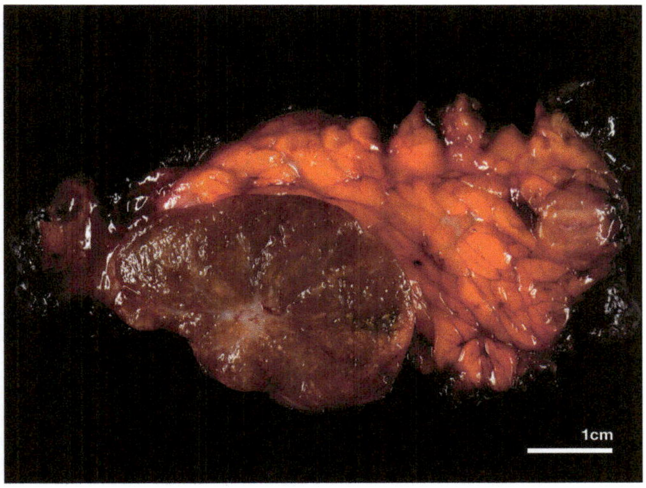

Fig. 4.23 (Gross examination) Oncocytic, Warthin's tumor

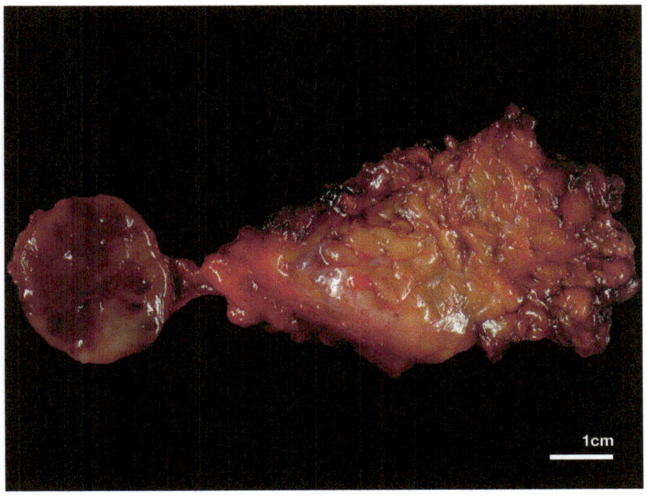

Fig. 4.24 (Gross examination) Oncocytic, basal cell adenoma

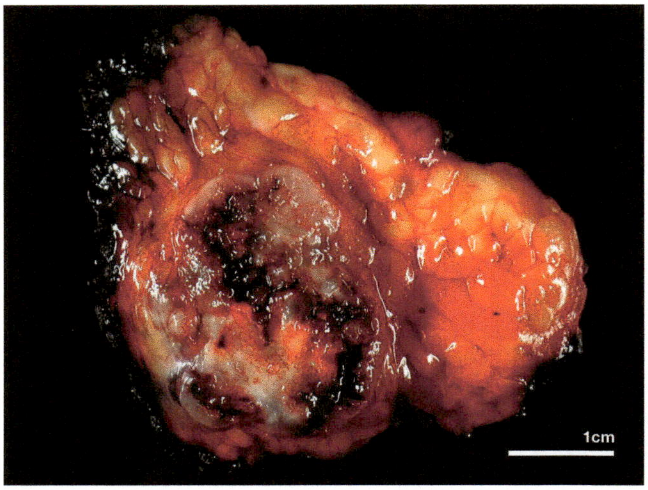

Fig. 4.25 (Gross examination) Hemorrhagic, pleomorphic adenoma

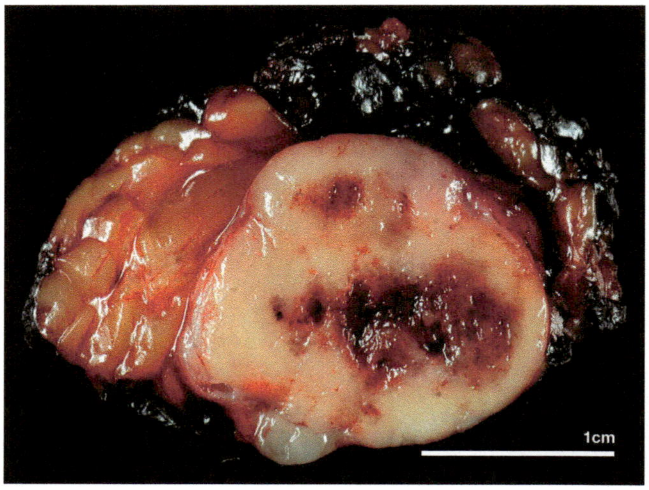

Fig. 4.26 (Gross examination) Hemorrhagic, basal cell adenoma

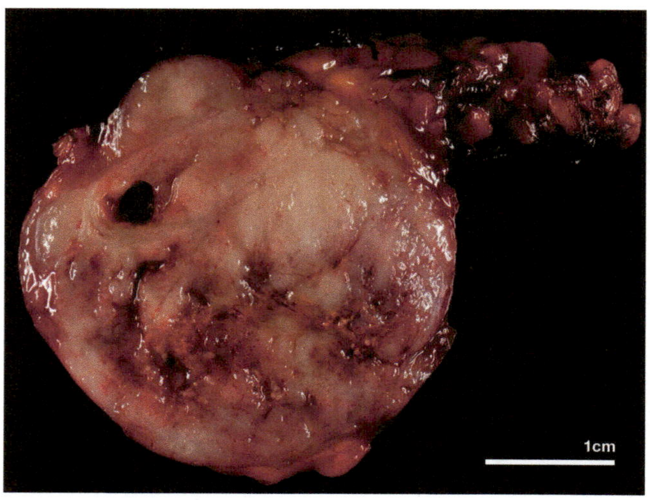

Fig. 4.27 (Gross examination) Hemorrhagic, acinic cell carcinoma

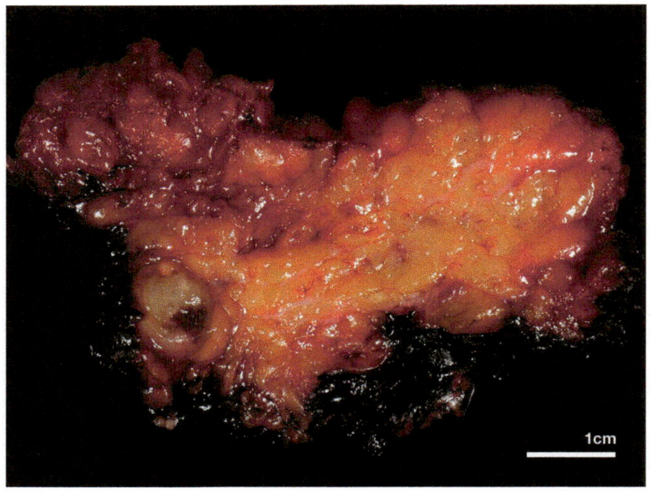

Fig. 4.28 (Gross examination) Hemorrhagic, epithelial-myoepithelial carcinoma

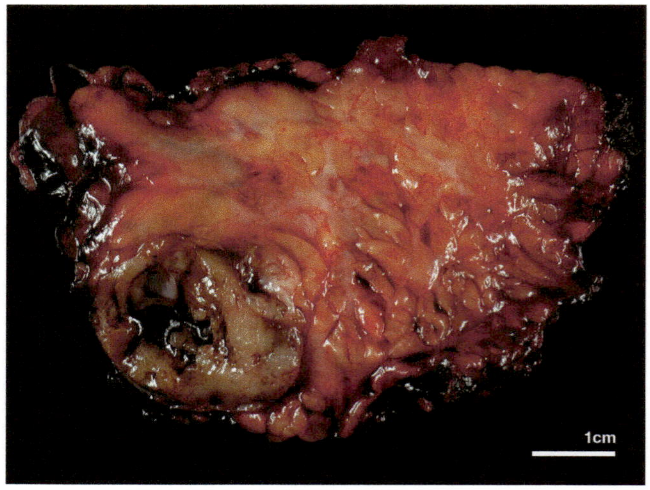

Fig. 4.29 (Gross examination) Cystic, basal cell adenoma

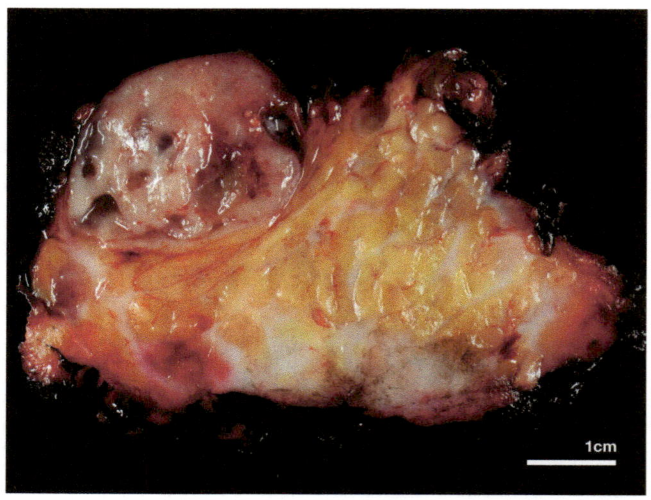

Fig. 4.30 (Gross examination) Cystic, lymphadenoma

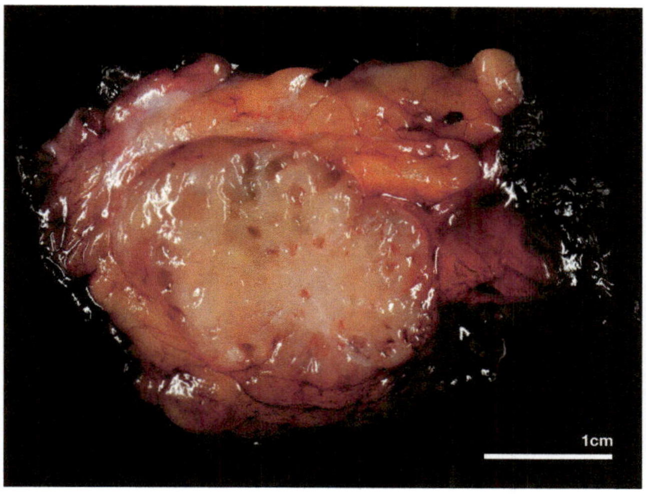

Fig. 4.31 (Gross examination) Cystic, mucoepidermoid carcinoma

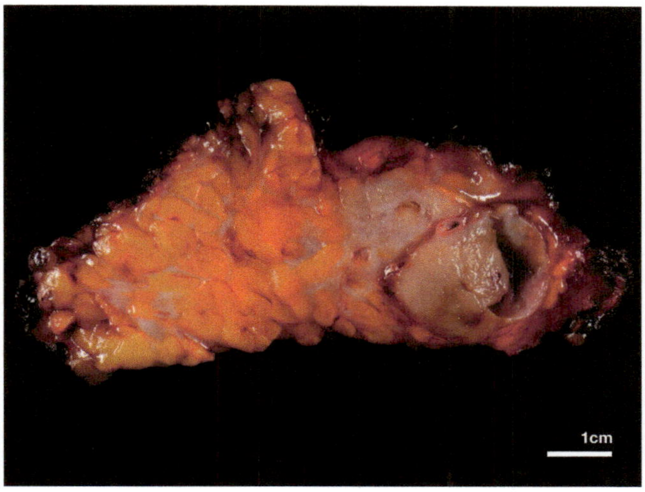

Fig. 4.32 (Gross examination) Cystic, acinic cell carcinoma

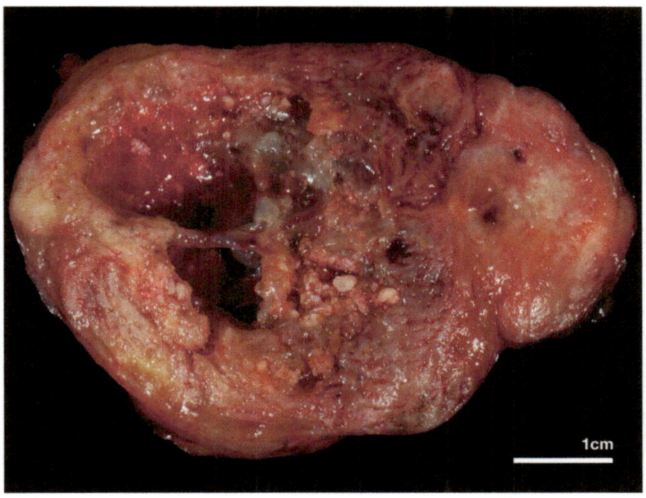

Fig. 4.33 (Gross examination) Necrotic, myoepithelioma

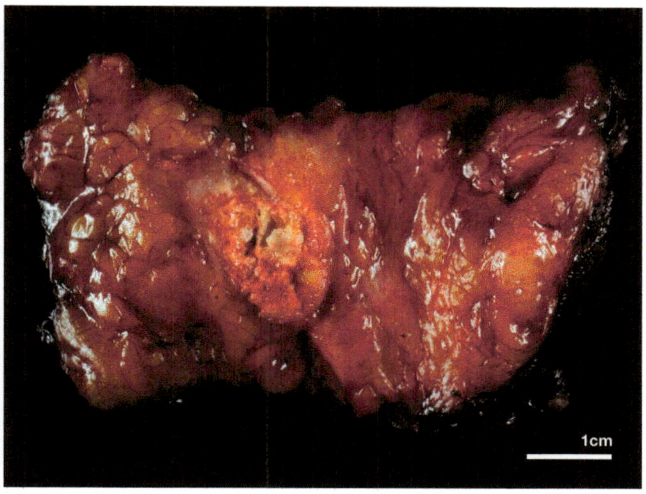

Fig. 4.34 (Gross examination) Necrotic, mucoepidermoid carcinoma

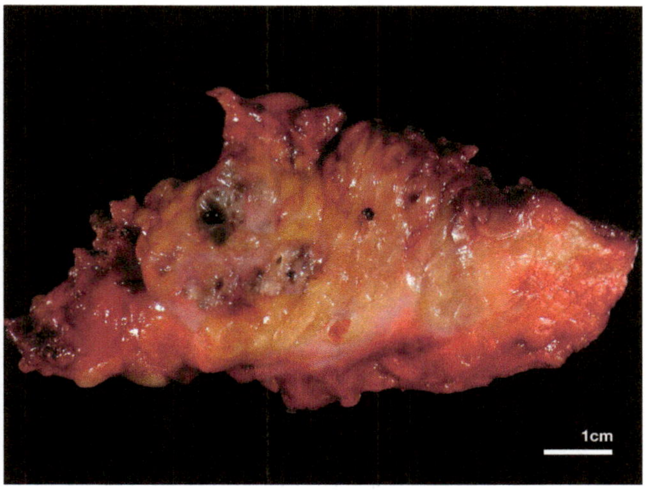

Fig. 4.35 (Gross examination) Necrotic, salivary duct carcinoma

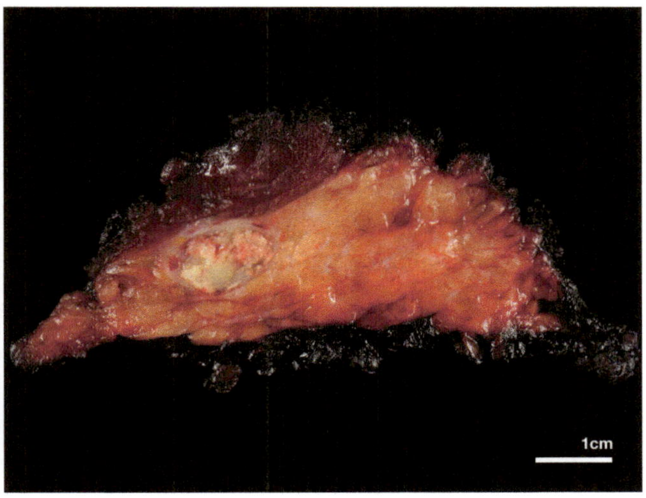

Fig. 4.36 (Gross examination) Necrotic, metastatic cutaneous squamous cell carcinoma

5 Microscopic Examination

The diagnostic complexity of salivary gland neoplasms is not to be underestimated. Although many cases are resolved at first microscopic glance, others require systematic evaluation to avoid diagnostic pitfalls. *Salivary Gland Pathology A, B, C, and D* represents the author's systematic approach to classifying neoplasms. The accuracy of this approach has limitations—a common theme in surgical pathology—and a subset of cases is best handled by consultation or committee (Figs. 5.1–5.35).

- *Architecture*—interface between neoplasm and adjacent parenchyma (e.g., circumscribed, infiltrative) often delineates benignity from malignancy
- *Biphasic*—number of cell phases/types (e.g., monophasic, biphasic, triphasic or more) often determines differential diagnostic considerations
- *Cytology*—cytology of cells (e.g., clear, oncocytic) often determines differential diagnostic considerations
- *Differential*—accurate classification often requires re-consideration of differential diagnostic considerations

J. J. García, *Atlas of Salivary Gland Pathology*, https://doi.org/10.1007/978-3-319-09021-4_5

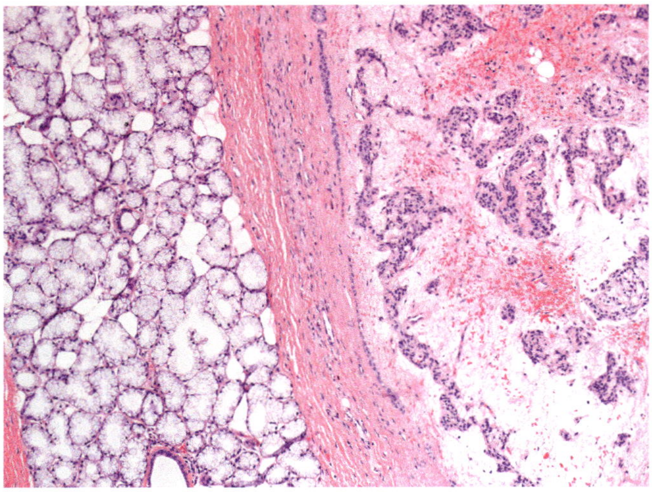

Fig. 5.1 (H&E, 100×) Encapsulated, pleomorphic adenoma

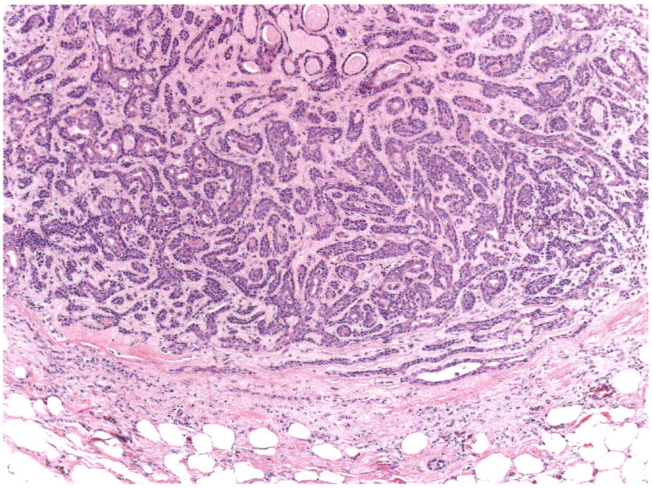

Fig. 5.2 (H&E, 100×) Circumscribed, basal cell adenoma

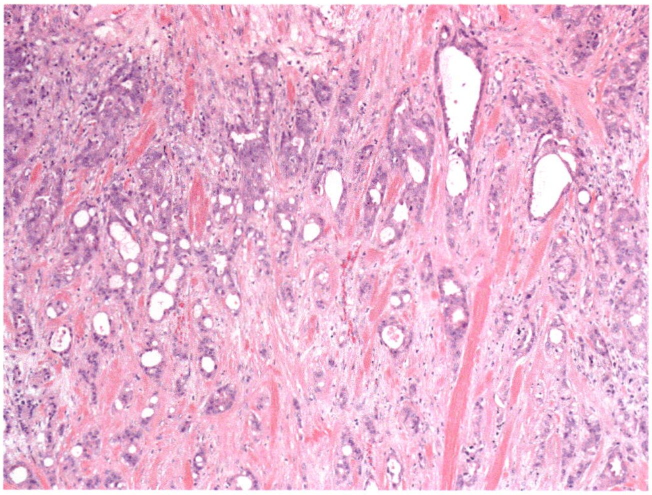

Fig. 5.3 (H&E, 100×) Infiltrative, salivary duct carcinoma

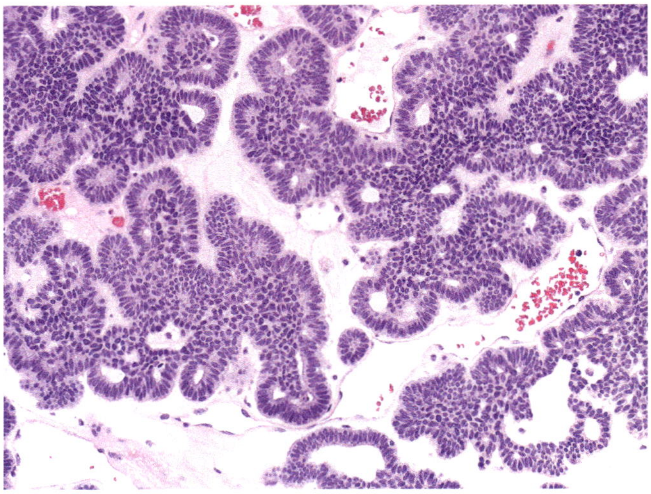

Fig. 5.4 (H&E, 200×) Monophasic, canalicular adenoma

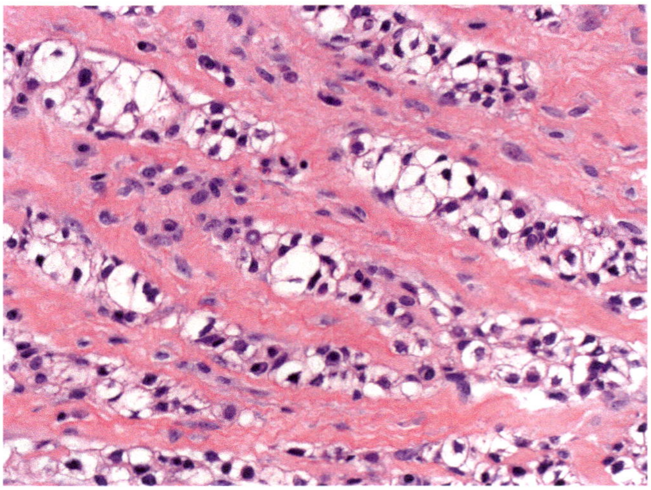

Fig. 5.5 (H&E, 400×) Monophasic, clear cell carcinoma

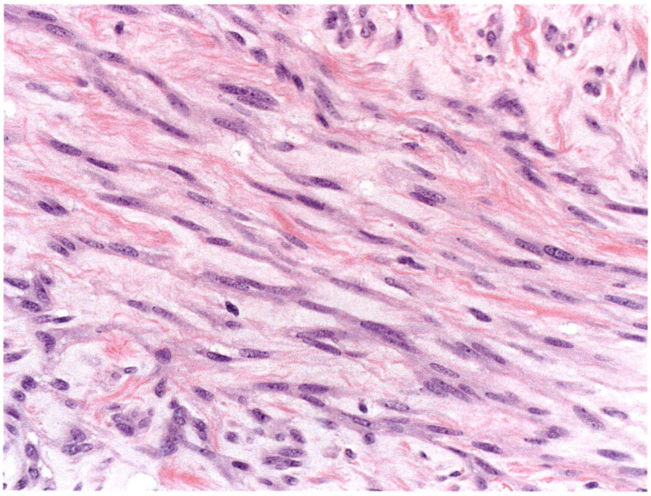

Fig. 5.6 (H&E, 400×) Monophasic, myoepithelioma

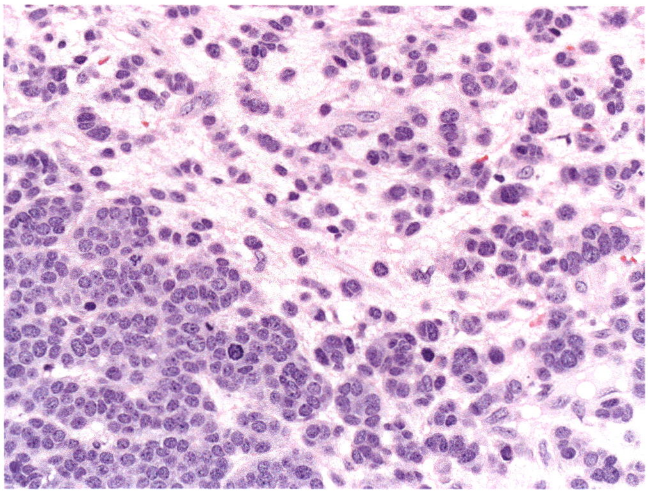

Fig. 5.7 (H&E, 400×) Monophasic, myoepithelial carcinoma

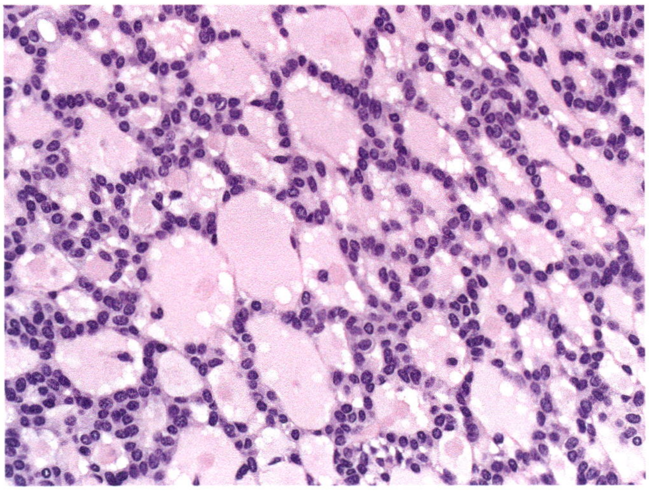

Fig. 5.8 (H&E, 400×) Monophasic, polymorphous adenocarcinoma

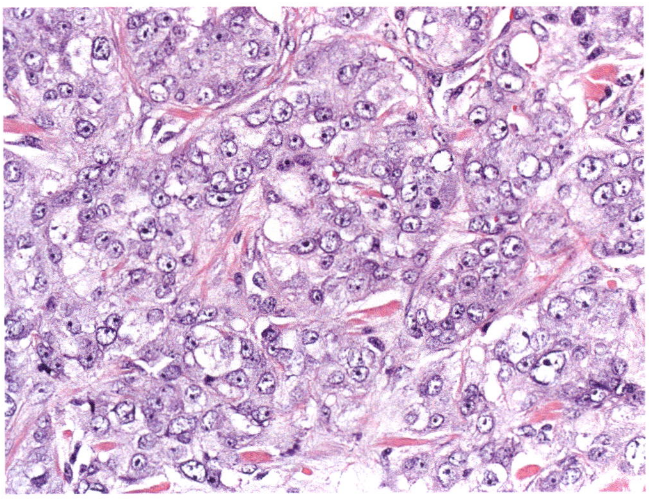

Fig. 5.9 (H&E, 400×) Monophasic, salivary duct carcinoma

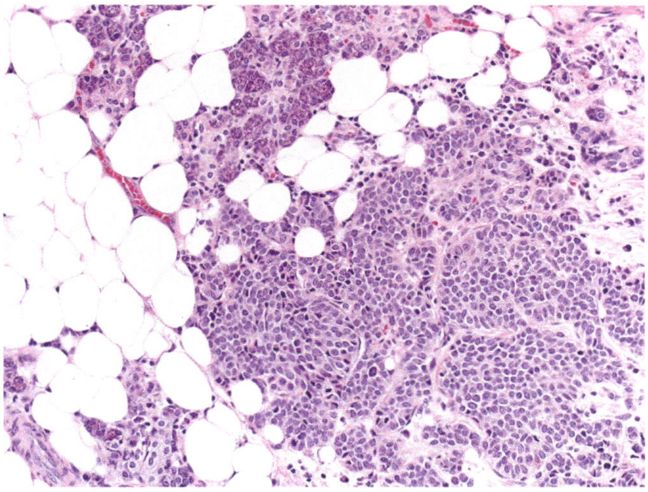

Fig. 5.10 (H&E, 200×) Monophasic, small cell neuroendocrine carcinoma

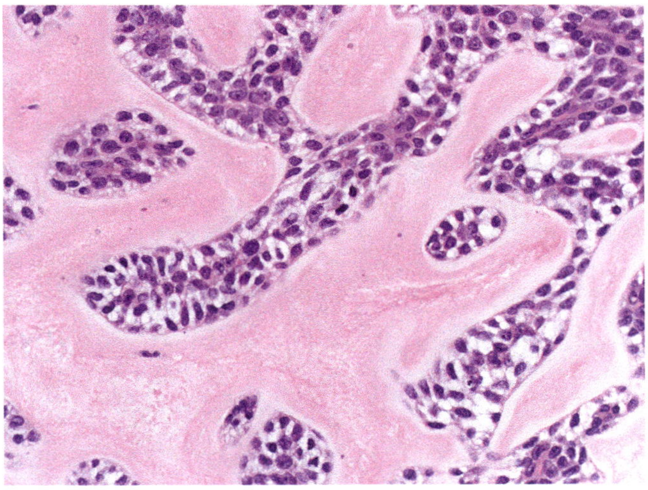

Fig. 5.11 (H&E, 400×) Biphasic, adenoid cystic carcinoma

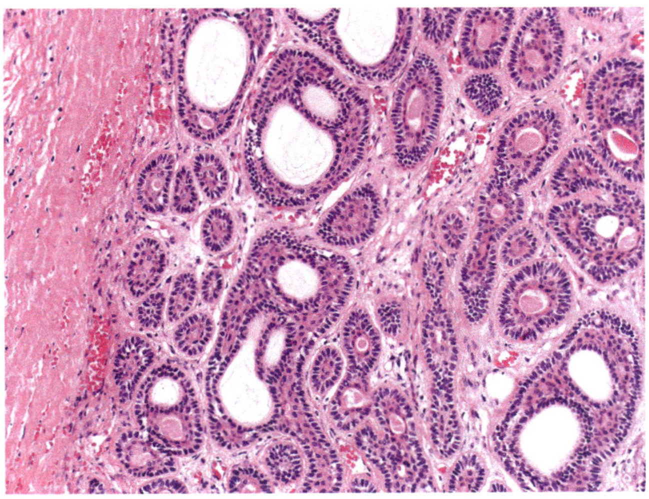

Fig. 5.12 (H&E, 200×) Biphasic, basal cell adenoma

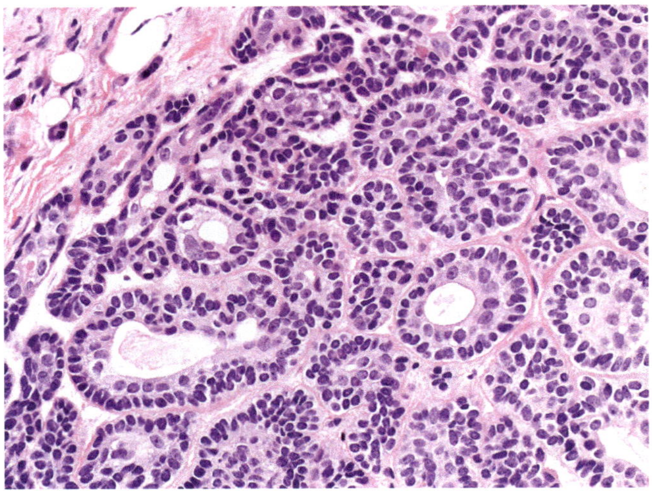

Fig. 5.13 (H&E, 400×) Biphasic, basal cell adenocarcinoma

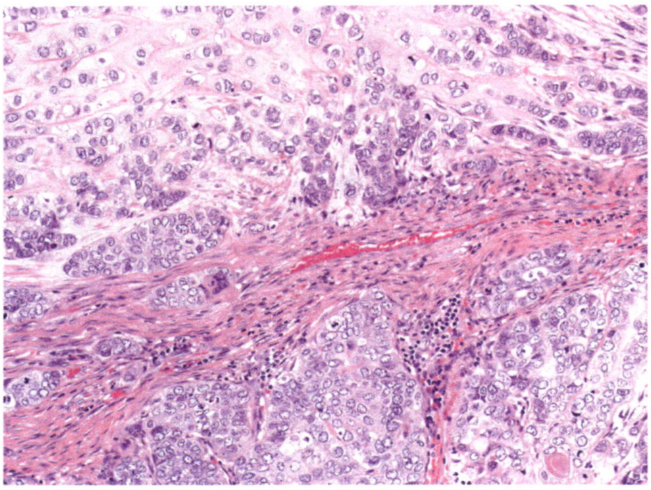

Fig. 5.14 (H&E, 200×) Biphasic, carcinosarcoma

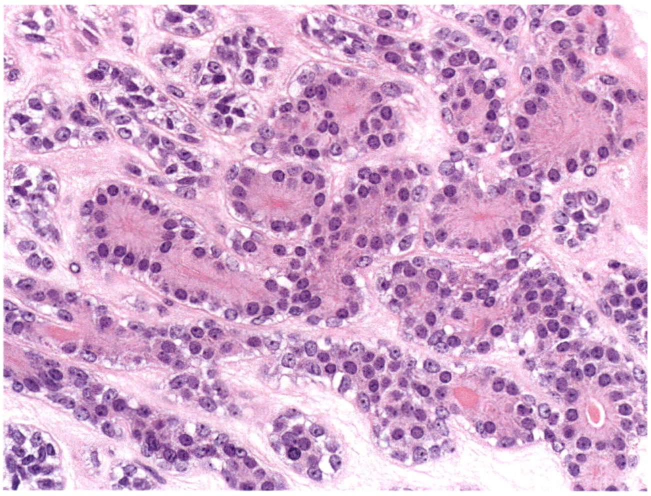

Fig. 5.15 (H&E, 400×) Biphasic, epithelial-myoepithelial carcinoma

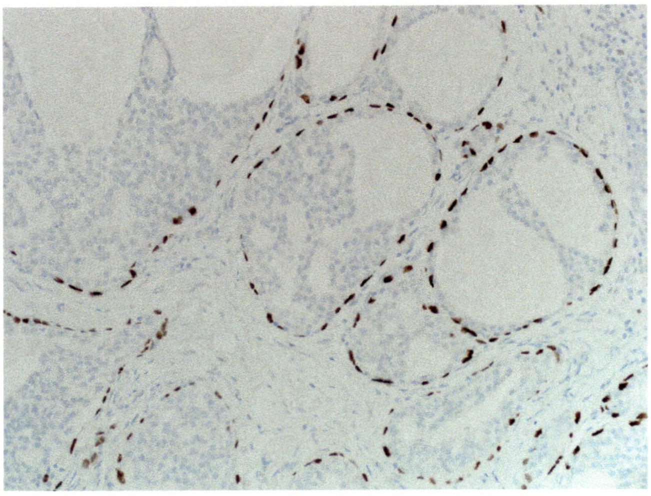

Fig. 5.16 (p63, 200×) Biphasic, intraductal carcinoma

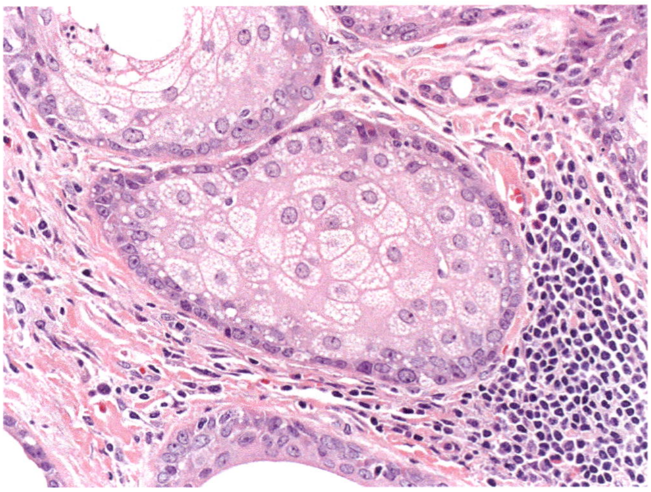

Fig. 5.17 (H&E, 400×) Biphasic, lymphadenoma

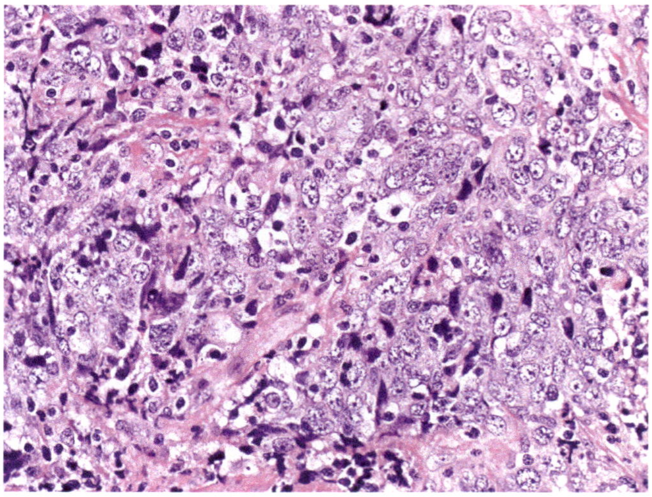

Fig. 5.18 (H&E, 400×) Biphasic, lymphoepithelial carcinoma

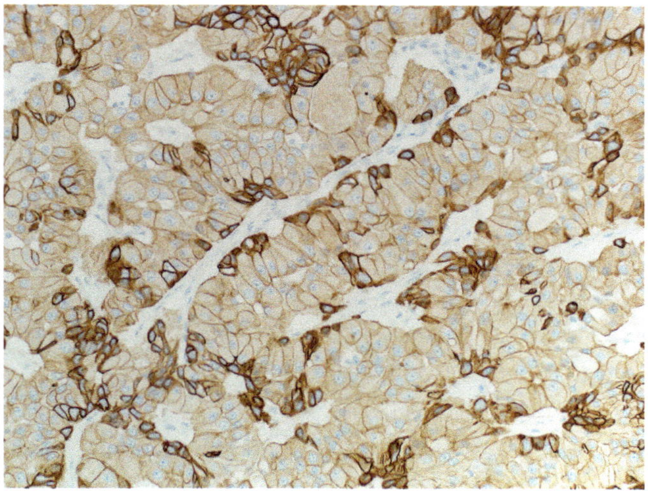

Fig. 5.19 (AE1/AE3, 200×) Biphasic, oncocytoma

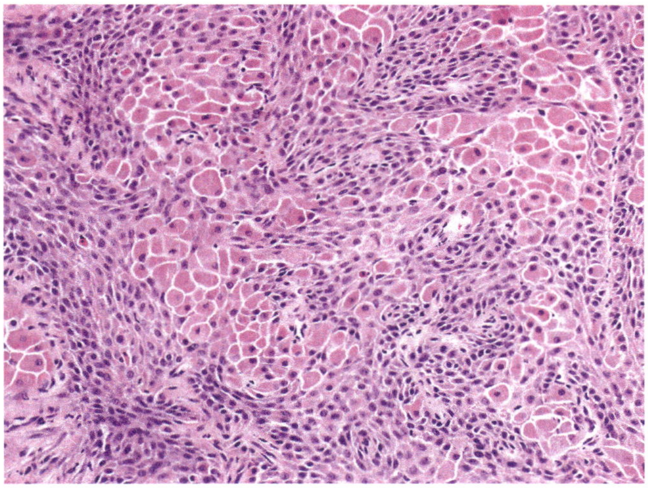

Fig. 5.20 (H&E, 200×) Biphasic, oncocytic carcinoma

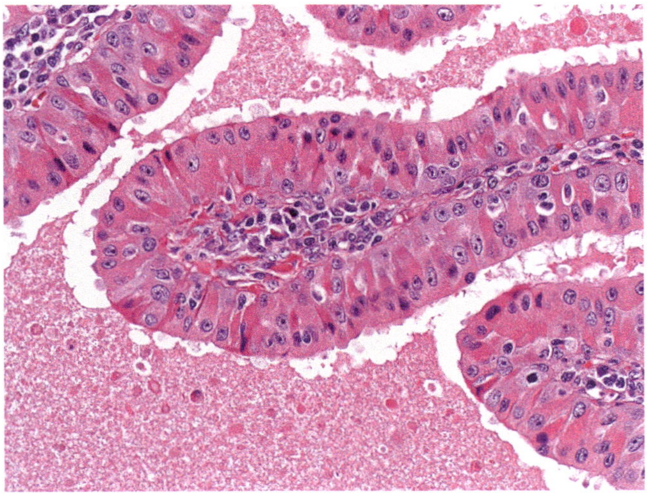

Fig. 5.21 (H&E, 400×) Biphasic, Warthin's tumor

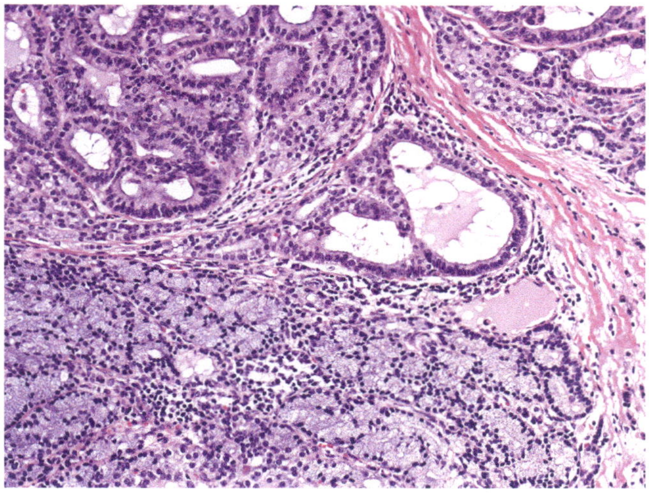

Fig. 5.22 (H&E, 200×) Triphasic or more, acinic cell carcinoma

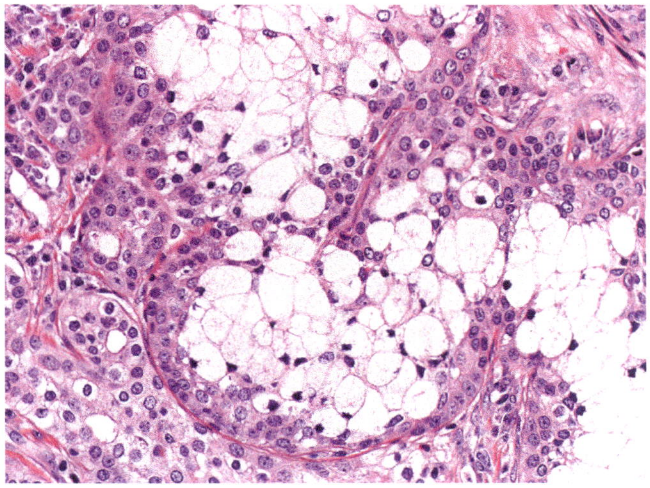

Fig. 5.23 (H&E, 400×) Triphasic or more, mucoepidermoid carcinoma

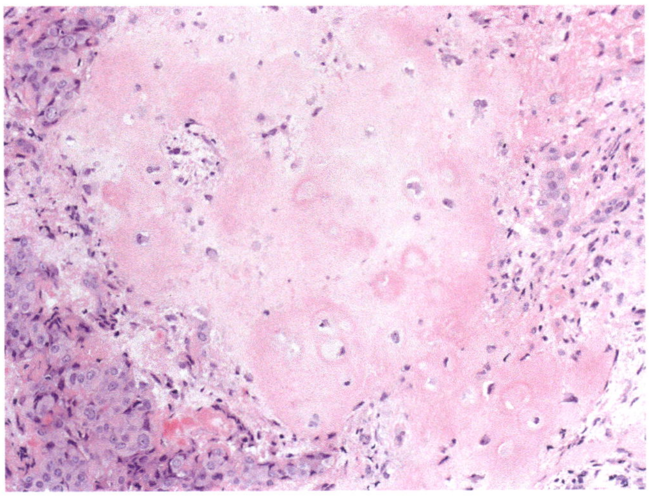

Fig. 5.24 (H&E, 200×) Triphasic or more, pleomorphic adenoma

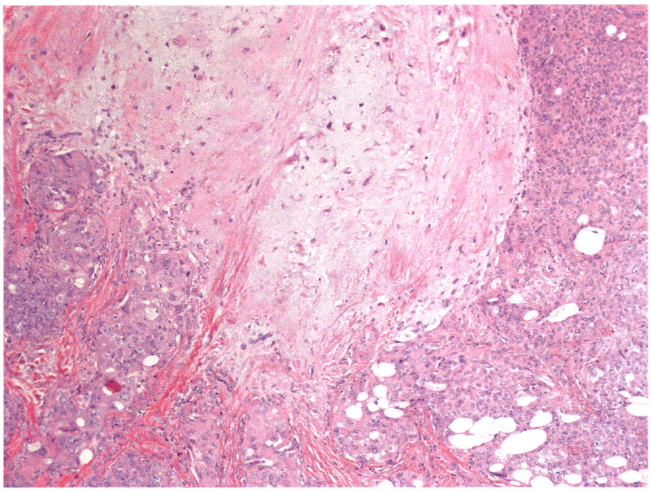

Fig. 5.25 (H&E, 100×) Triphasic or more, carcinoma ex pleomorphic adenoma

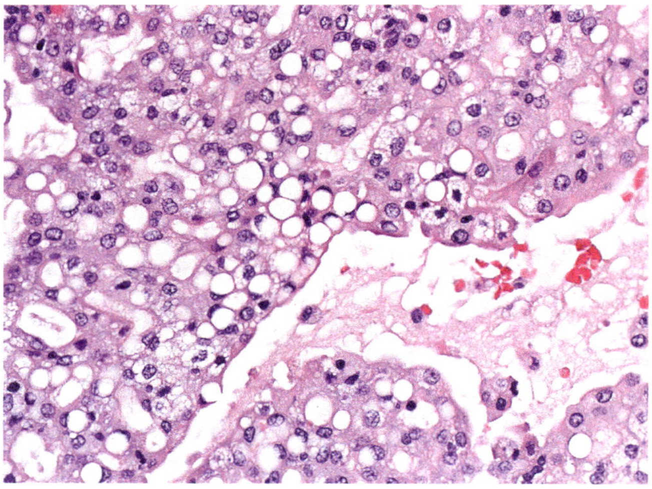

Fig. 5.26 (H&E, 400×) Triphasic or more, secretory carcinoma

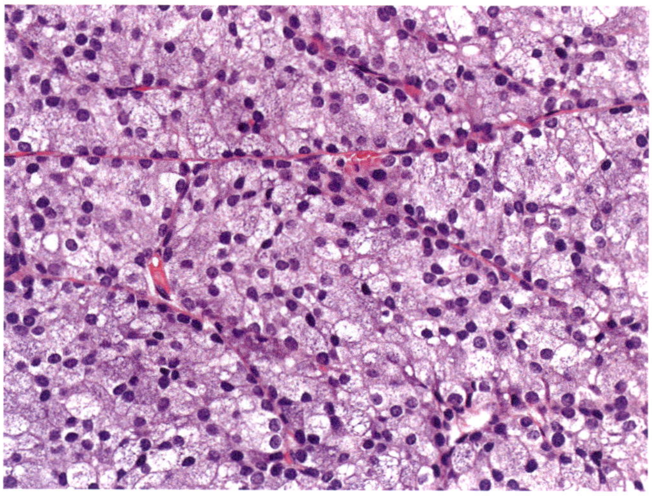

Fig. 5.27 (H&E, 400×) Acinar cells (serous), acinic cell carcinoma

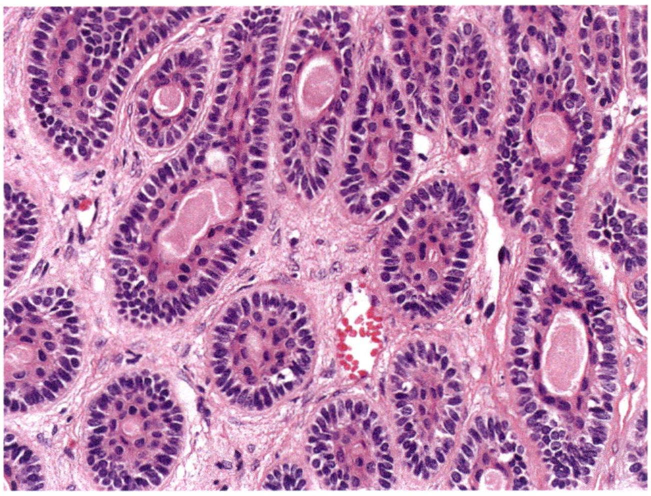

Fig. 5.28 (H&E, 400×) Basal cells, basal cell adenoma

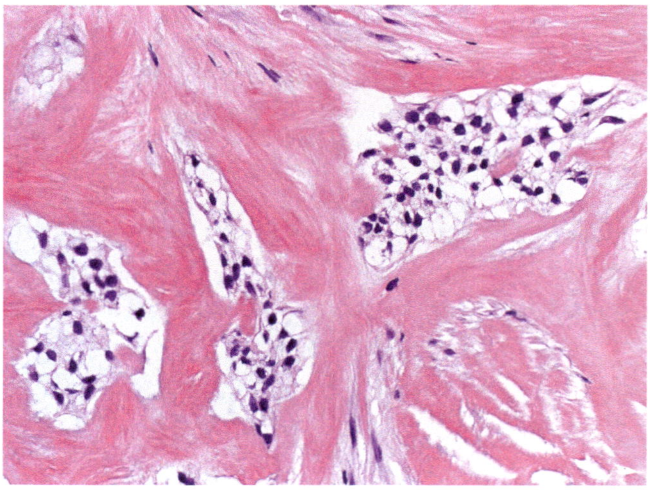

Fig. 5.29 (H&E, 400×) Clear cells, clear cell carcinoma

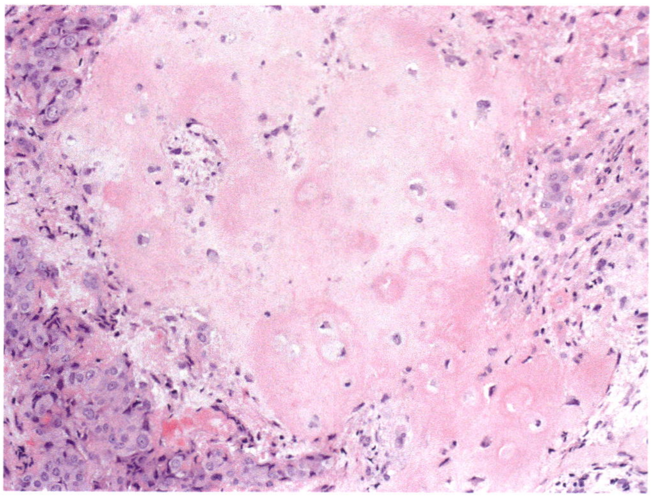

Fig. 5.30 (H&E, 200×) Chondrocytes, pleomorphic adenoma

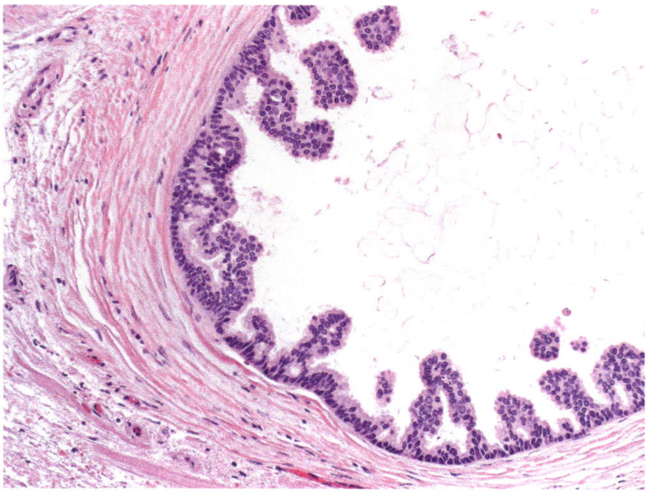

Fig. 5.31 (H&E, 200×) Ductal cells, intraductal carcinoma

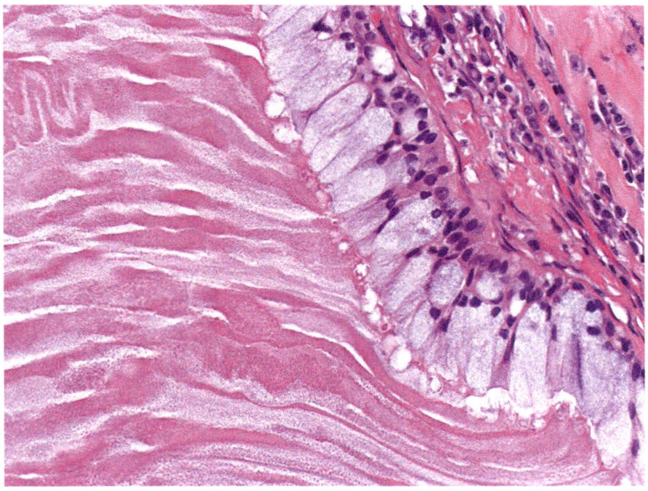

Fig. 5.32 (H&E, 400×) Mucous cells, mucoepidermoid carcinoma

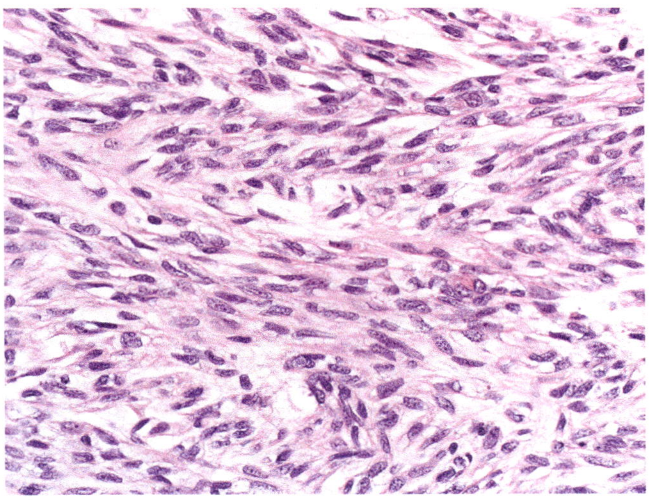

Fig. 5.33 (H&E, 400×) Myoepithelial cells, myoepithelioma

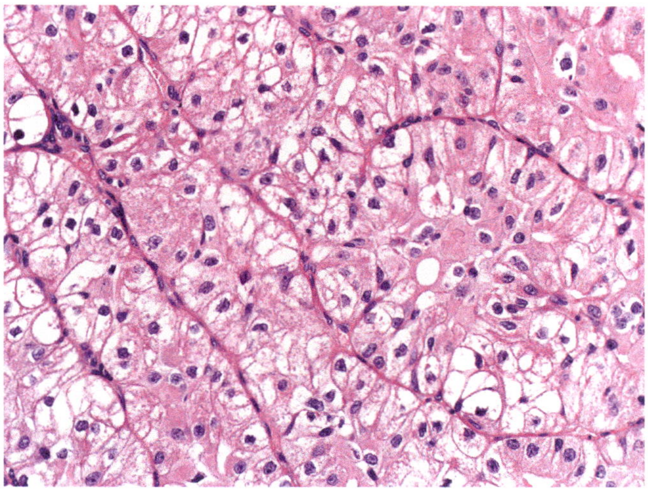

Fig. 5.34 (H&E, 400×) Oncocytes, oncytoma

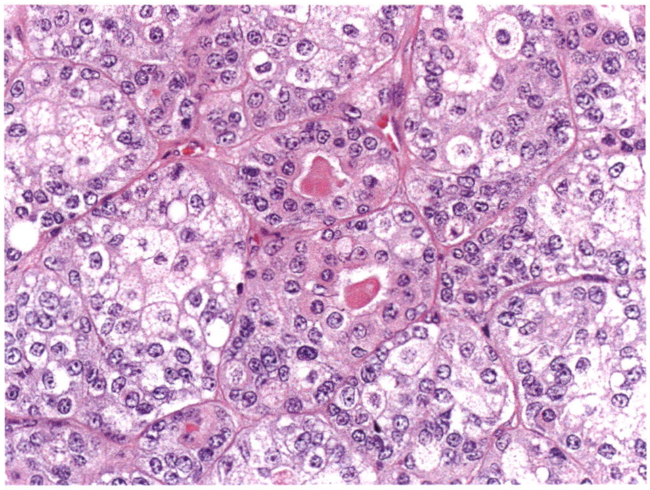

Fig. 5.35 (H&E, 400×) Sebaceous cells, epithelial-myoepithelial carcinoma

6 Acinic Cell Carcinoma

Acinic cell carcinoma affects children and adults and presents at a mean age of approximately 50 years. Women are involved slightly more than men. The majority of cases involve the parotid gland, presenting as single or multiple masses. Most cases of acinic cell carcinoma behave as low to intermediate-grade malignancies; however, a subset of cases with high-grade transformation (necrosis, elevated mitotic activity, and cytomorphologic atypia) are predisposed to recurrence, lymph node involvement, and distant metastasis. Acinic cell carcinoma may be circumscribed or infiltrative, comprised of multiple cell types (acinar, intercalated ductal, vacuolated, clear, and non-specific glandular), and exhibit a variety of architectural patterns (solid, follicular, papillary, and cystic) (Figs. 6.1–6.43).

J. J. García, *Atlas of Salivary Gland Pathology*, https://doi.org/10.1007/978-3-319-09021-4_6

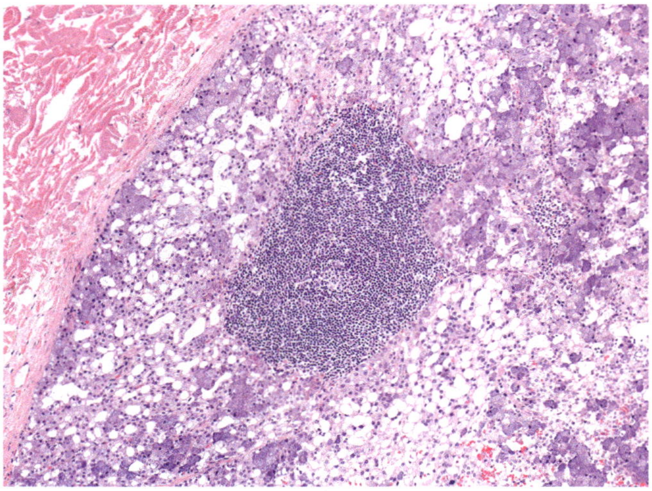

Fig. 6.1 (H&E, 100×) Acinic cell carcinoma, circumscribed

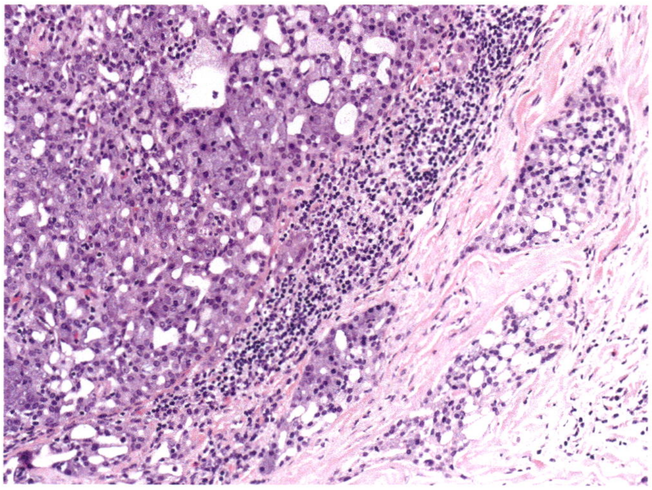

Fig. 6.2 (H&E, 200×) Acinic cell carcinoma, infiltrative

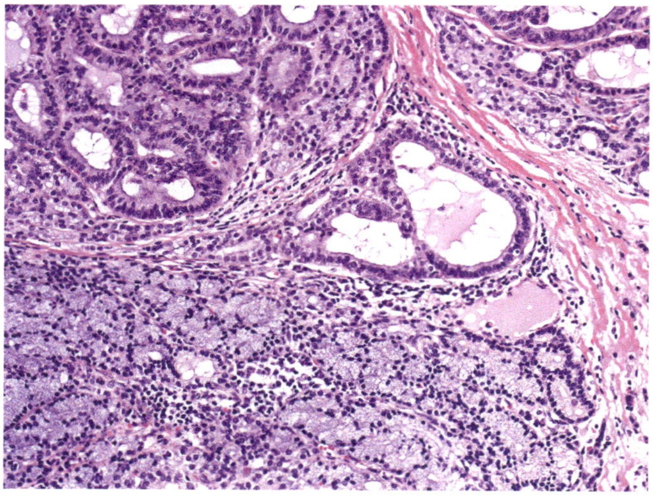

Fig. 6.3 (H&E, 200×) Acinic cell carcinoma, triphasic or more

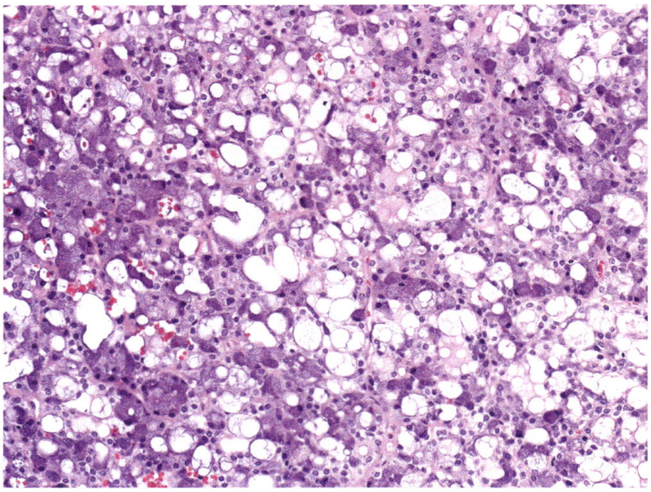

Fig. 6.4 (H&E, 200×) Acinic cell carcinoma, microcystic

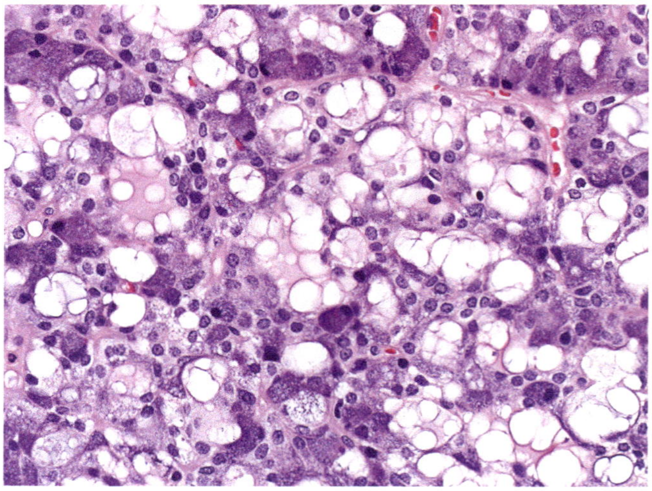

Fig. 6.5 (H&E, 400×) Acinic cell carcinoma, microcystic

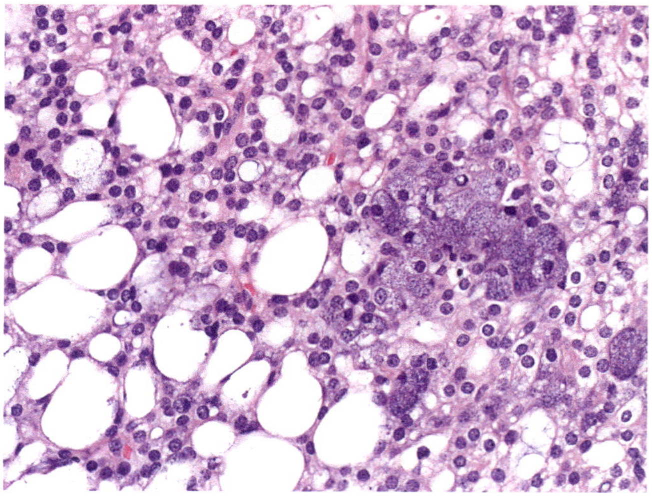

Fig. 6.6 (H&E, 400×) Acinic cell carcinoma, microcystic

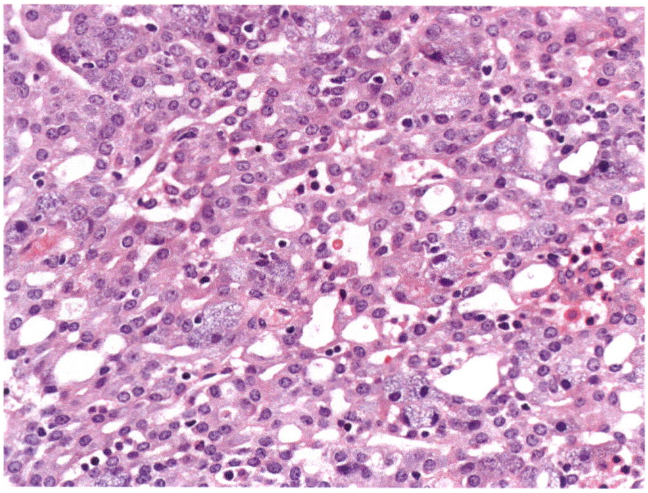

Fig. 6.7 (H&E, 400×) Acinic cell carcinoma, microcystic

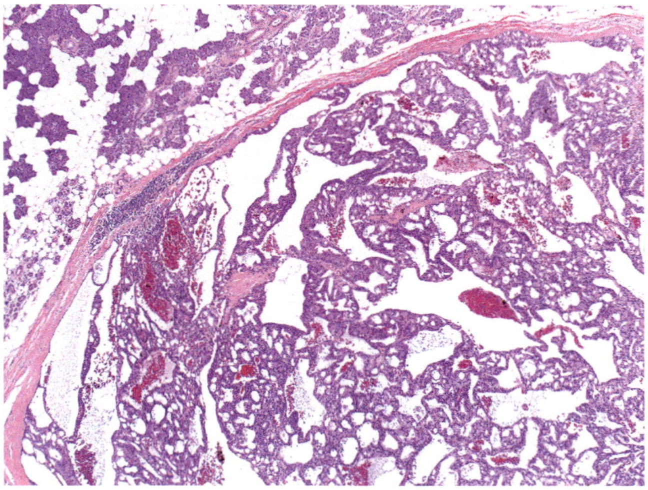

Fig. 6.8 (H&E, 40×) Acinic cell carcinoma, papillary-cystic

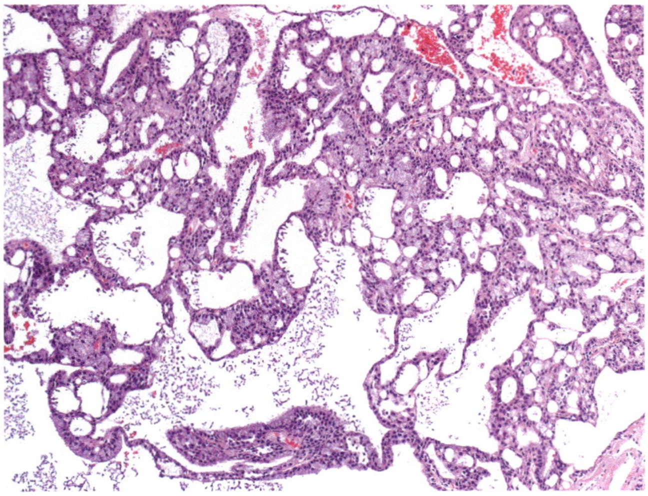

Fig. 6.9 (H&E, 100×) Acinic cell carcinoma, papillary-cystic

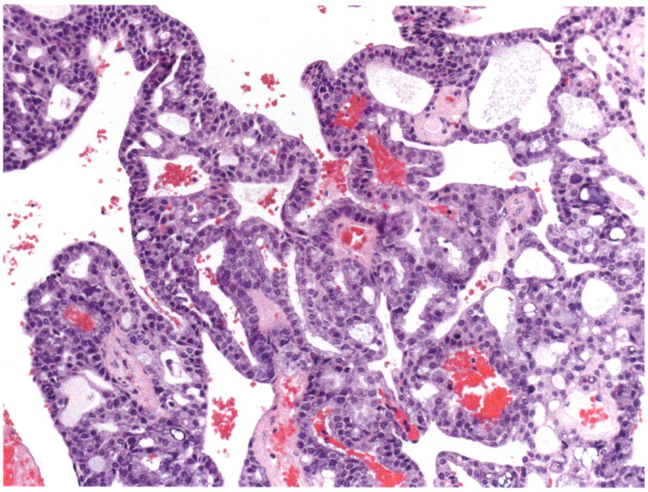

Fig. 6.10 (H&E, 200×) Acinic cell carcinoma, papillary-cystic

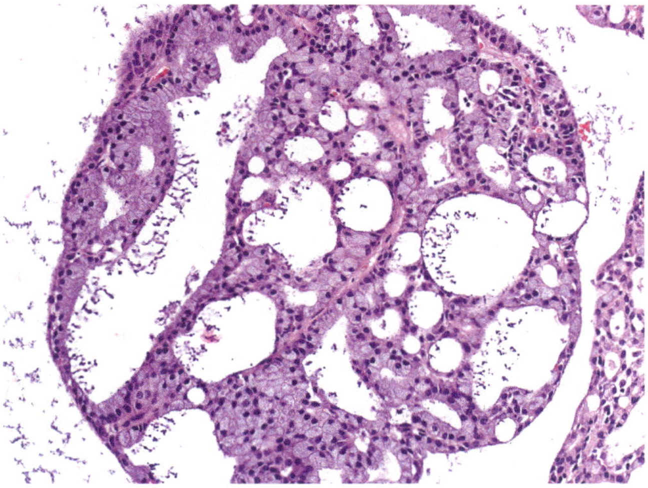

Fig. 6.11 (H&E, 200×) Acinic cell carcinoma, papillary-cystic

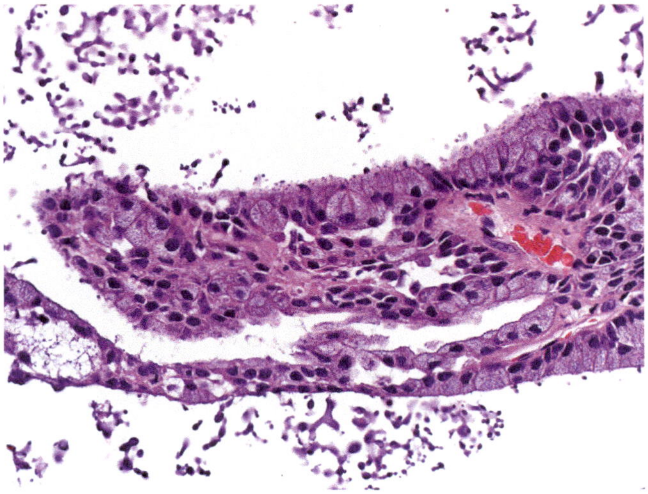

Fig. 6.12 (H&E, 400×) Acinic cell carcinoma, papillary-cystic

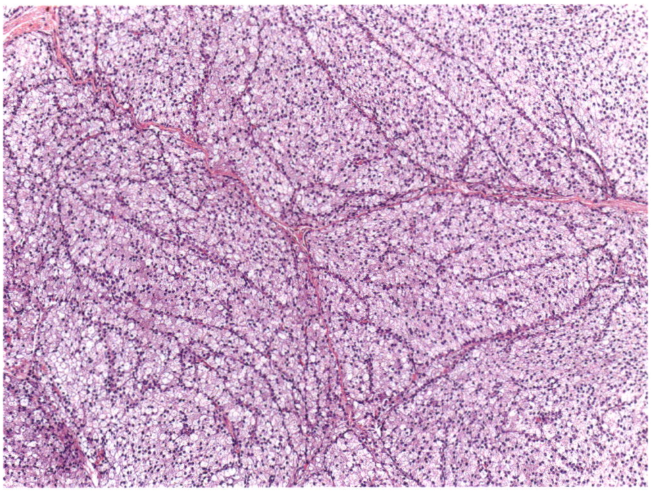

Fig. 6.13 (H&E, 100×) Acinic cell carcinoma, solid

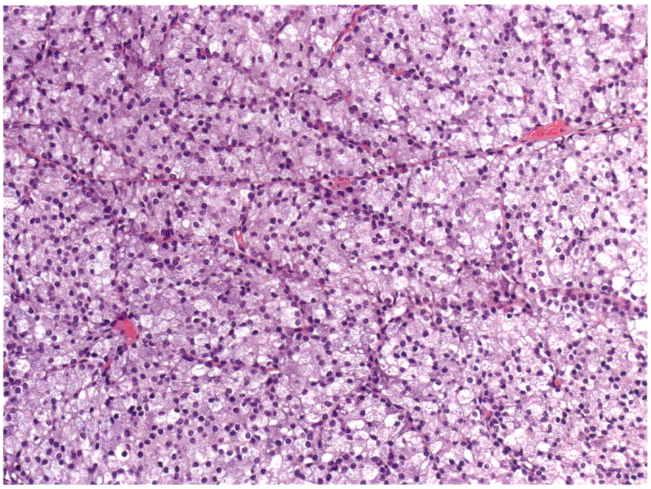

Fig. 6.14 (H&E, 200×) Acinic cell carcinoma, solid

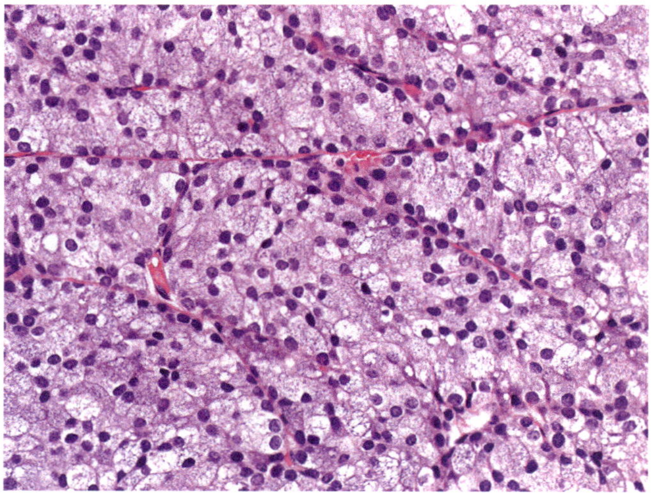

Fig. 6.15 (H&E, 400×) Acinic cell carcinoma, solid

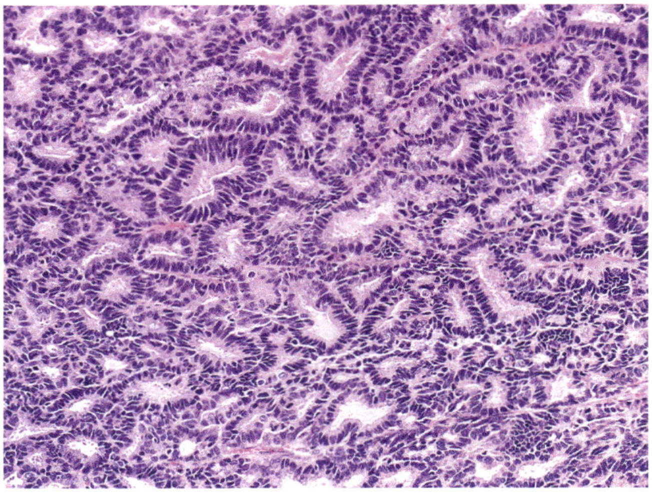

Fig. 6.16 (H&E, 200×) Acinic cell carcinoma, follicular

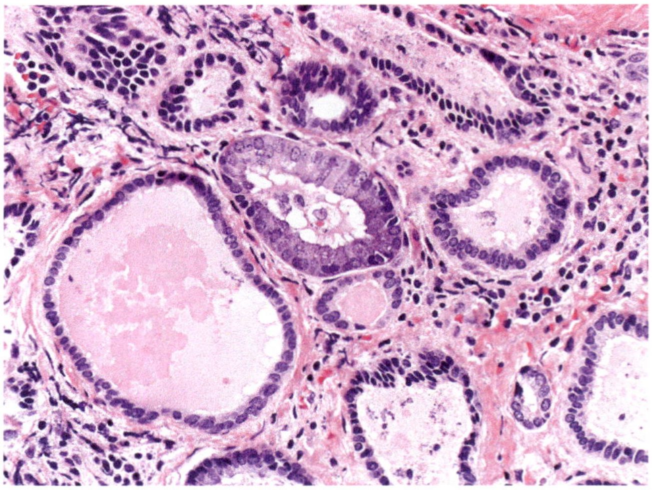

Fig. 6.17 (H&E, 400×) Acinic cell carcinoma, follicular

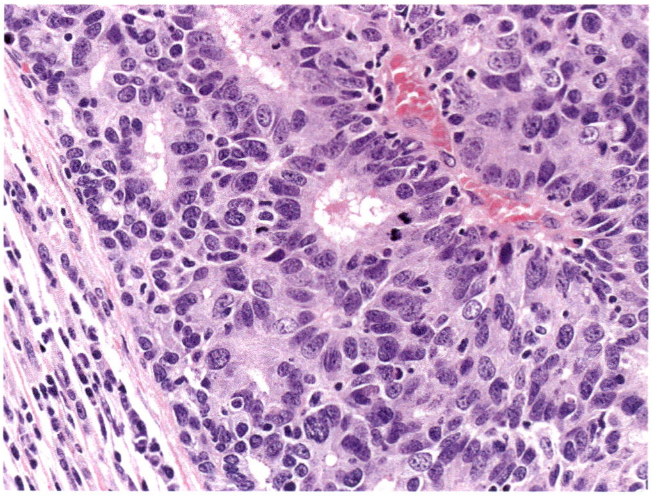

Fig. 6.18 (H&E, 400×) Acinic cell carcinoma, follicular

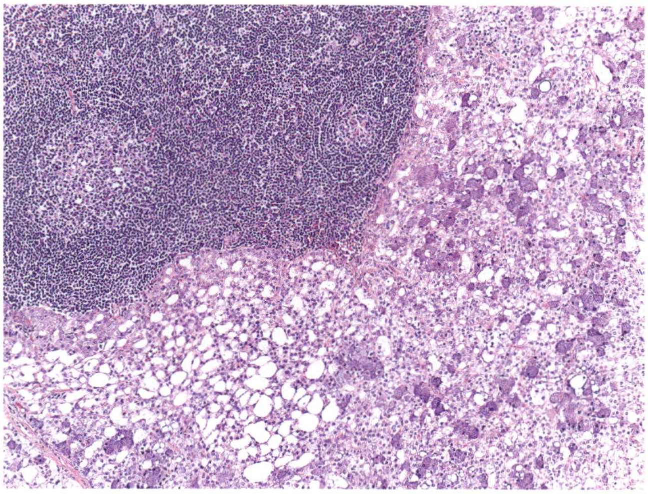

Fig. 6.19 (H&E, 100×) Acinic cell carcinoma, tumor-associated lymphoid proliferation

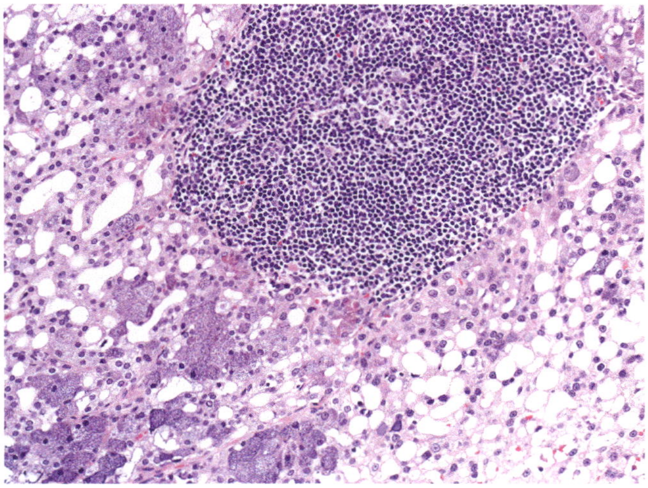

Fig. 6.20 (H&E, 200×) Acinic cell carcinoma, tumor-associated lymphoid proliferation

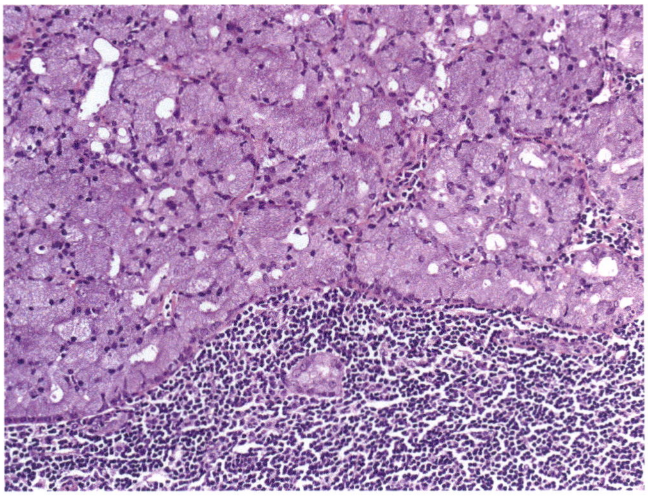

Fig. 6.21 (H&E, 200×) Acinic cell carcinoma, tumor-associated lymphoid proliferation

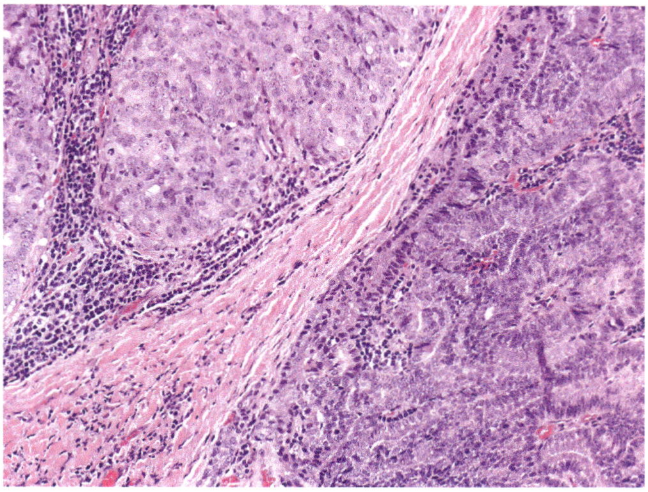

Fig. 6.22 (H&E, 200×) Acinic cell carcinoma, high-grade transformation, cytomorphologic atypia

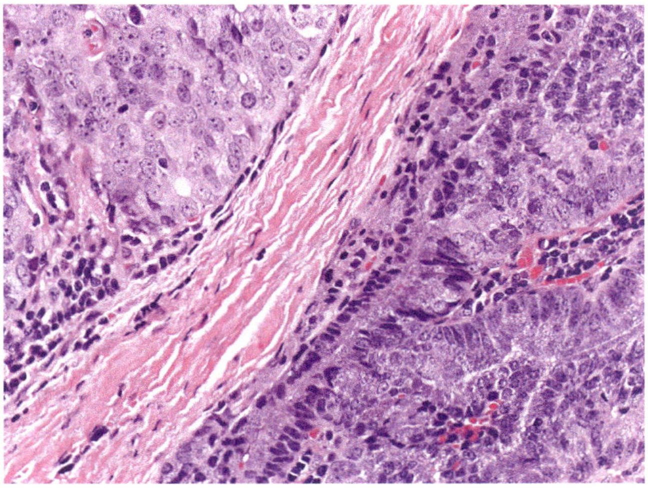

Fig. 6.23 (H&E, 400×) Acinic cell carcinoma, high-grade transformation, cytomorphologic atypia

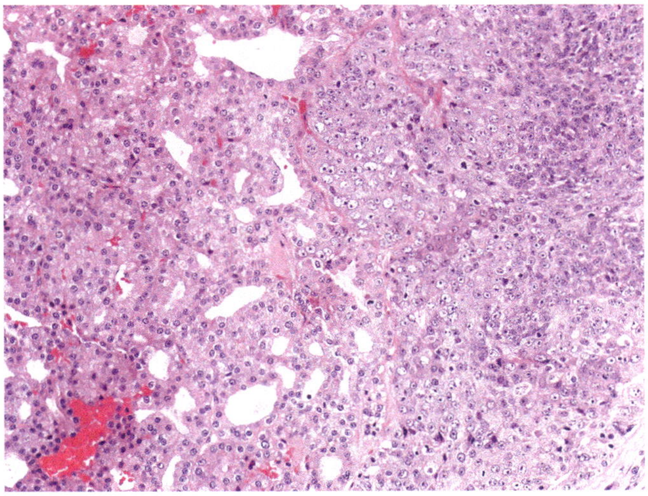

Fig. 6.24 (H&E, 200×) Acinic cell carcinoma, high-grade transformation, mitotic activity

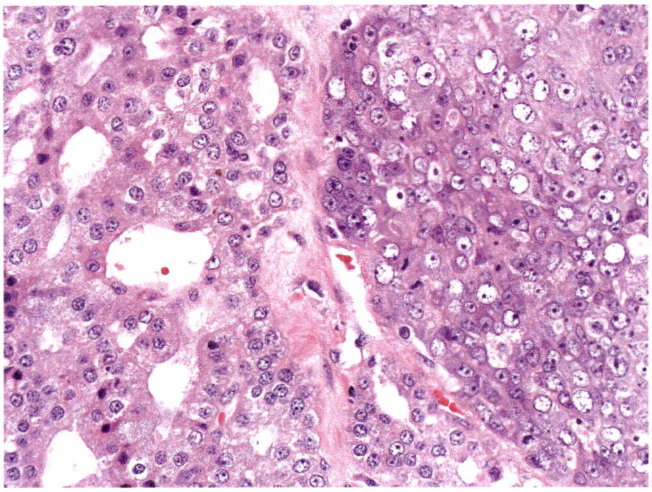

Fig. 6.25 (H&E, 400×) Acinic cell carcinoma, high-grade transformation, mitotic activity

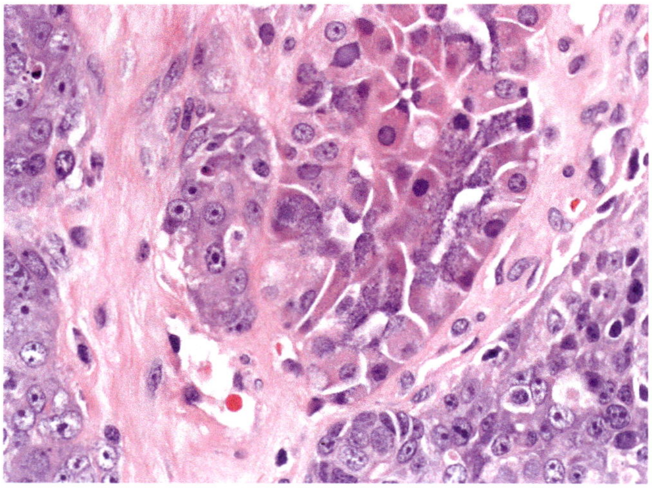

Fig. 6.26 (H&E, 600×) Acinic cell carcinoma, high-grade transformation, zymogen-like granules

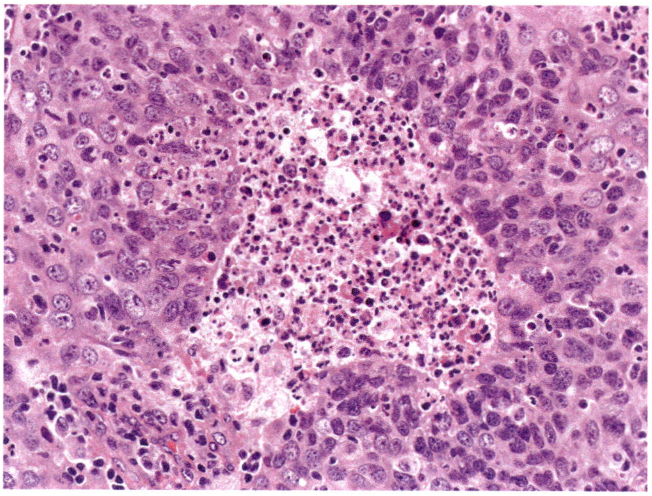

Fig. 6.27 (H&E, 400×) Acinic cell carcinoma, high-grade transformation, necrosis

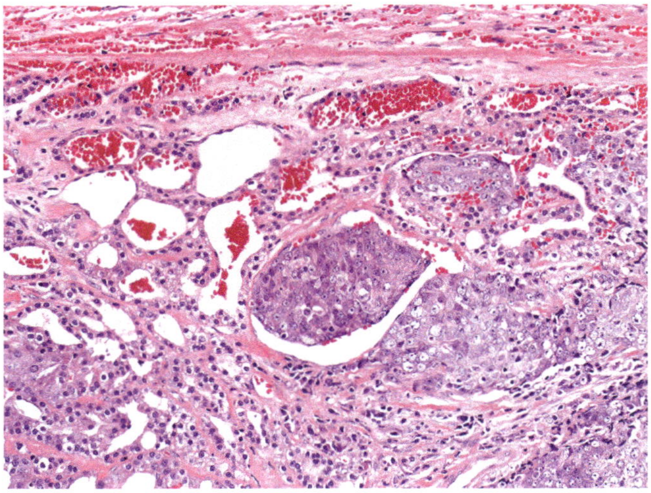

Fig. 6.28 (H&E, 200×) Acinic cell carcinoma, high-grade transformation, angiolymphatic invasion

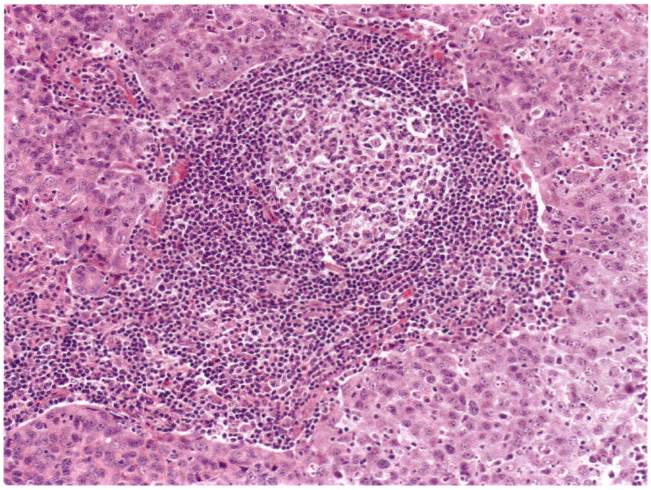

Fig. 6.29 (H&E, 200×) Acinic cell carcinoma, high-grade transformation, tumor-associated lymphoid proliferation

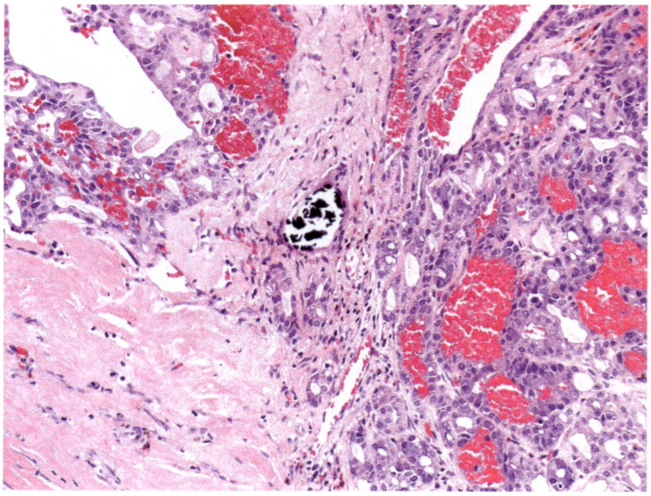

Fig. 6.30 (H&E, 200×) Acinic cell carcinoma, microcalcifications

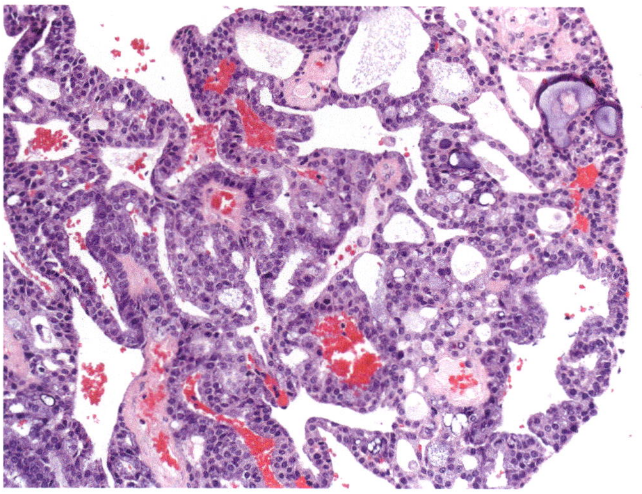

Fig. 6.31 (H&E, 200×) Acinic cell carcinoma, microcalcifications

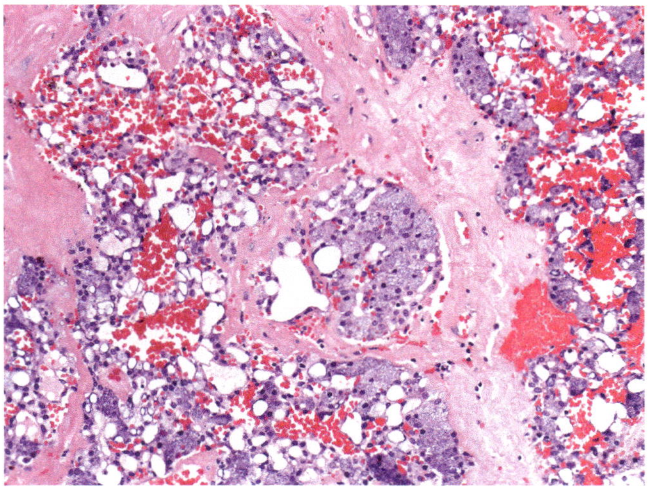

Fig. 6.32 (H&E, 200×) Acinic cell carcinoma, hemorrhagic

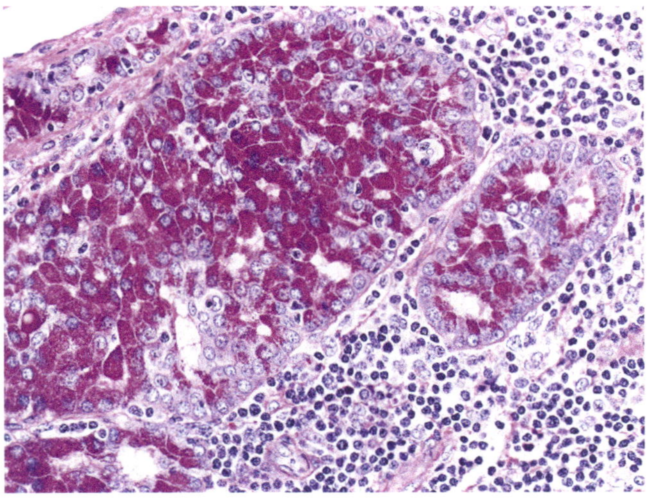

Fig. 6.33 (PAS-D, 400×) Acinic cell carcinoma, zymogen-like granules

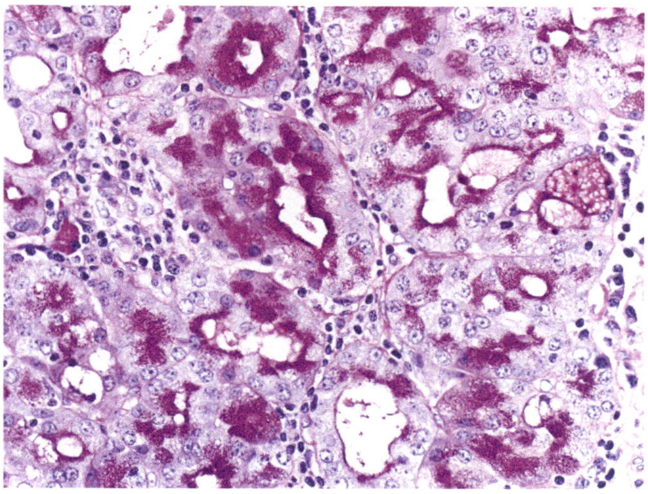

Fig. 6.34 (PAS-D, 400×) Acinic cell carcinoma, zymogen-like granules

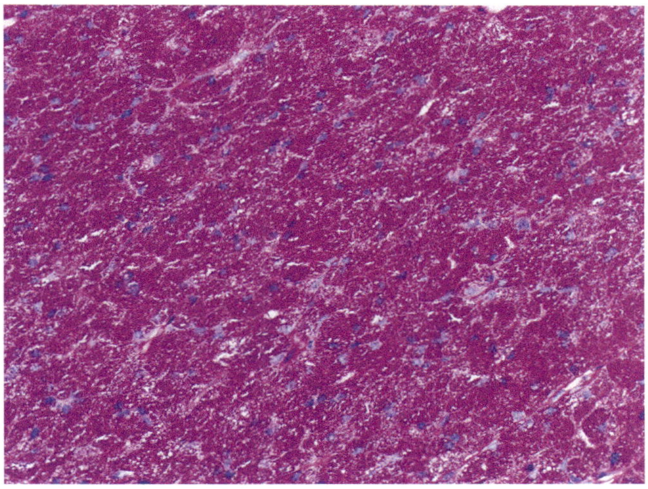

Fig. 6.35 (PAS-D, 400×) Acinic cell carcinoma, zymogen-like granules

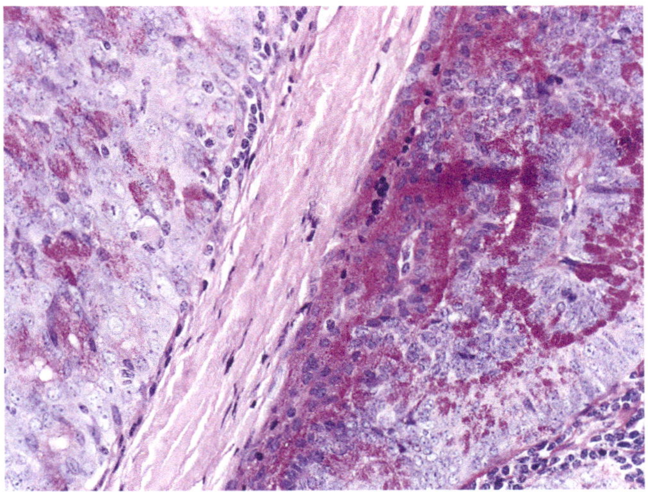

Fig. 6.36 (PAS-D, 400×) Acinic cell carcinoma, high-grade transformation, zymogen-like granules

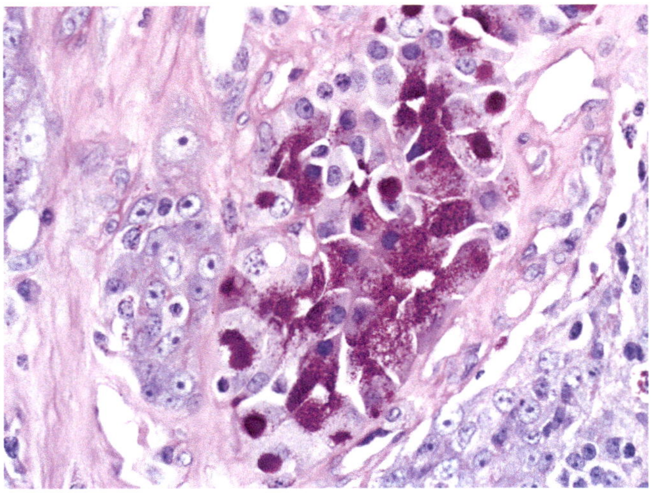

Fig. 6.37 (PAS-D, 600×) Acinic cell carcinoma, high-grade transformation, zymogen-like granules

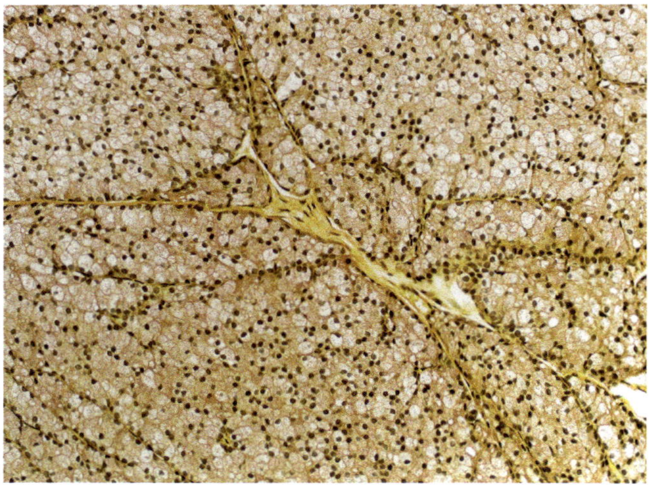

Fig. 6.38 (Mucicarmine, 200×) Acinic cell carcinoma, negative reactivity

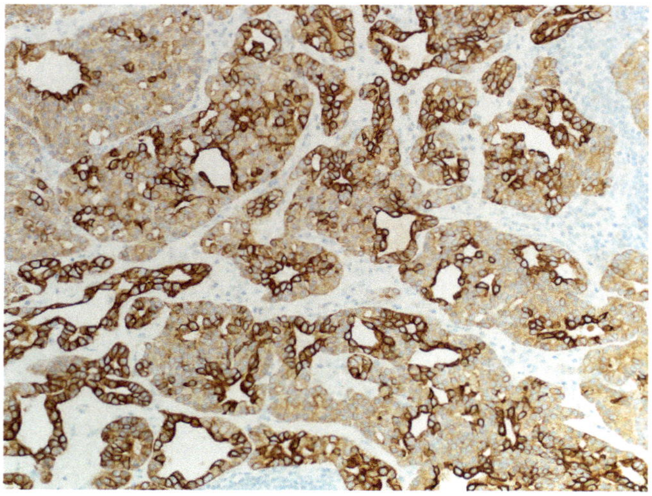

Fig. 6.39 (AE1/AE3, 200×) Acinic cell carcinoma, diffuse immunoreactivity

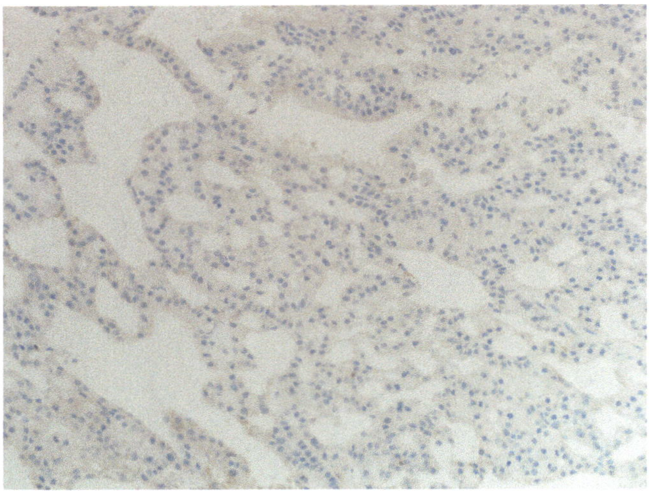

Fig. 6.40 (S-100, 200×) Acinic cell carcinoma, negative immunoreactivity

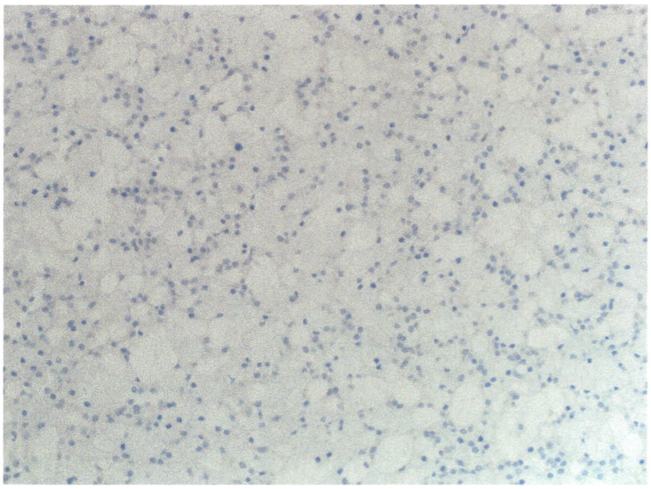

Fig. 6.41 (p63, 200×) Acinic cell carcinoma, negative immunoreactivity

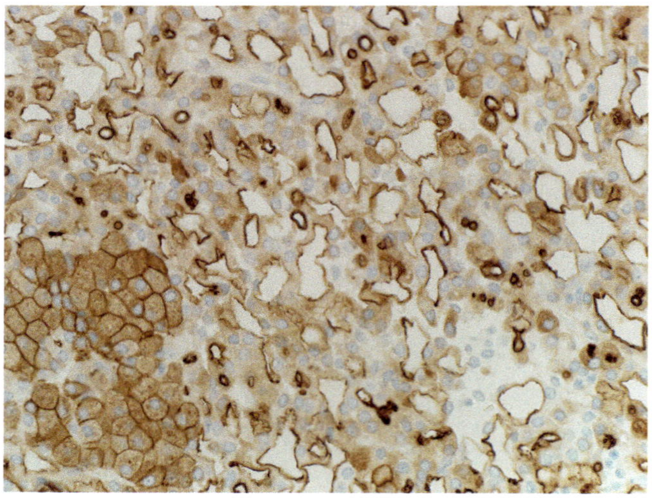

Fig. 6.42 (DOG1, 400×) Acinic cell carcinoma, diffuse immunoreactivity

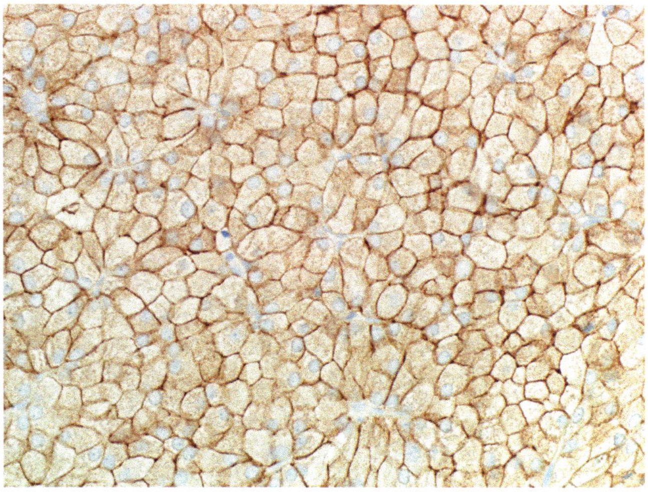

Fig. 6.43 (DOG1, 400×) Acinic cell carcinoma, diffuse immunoreactivity

Suggested Reading

Ali SZ. Acinic-cell carcinoma, papillary-cystic variant: a diagnostic dilemma in salivary gland aspiration. Diagn Cytopathol. 2002;27(4):244–50.

Bishop JA, Yonescu R, Batista D, Eisele DW, Westra WH. Most nonparotid "acinic cell carcinomas" represent mammary analog secretory carcinomas. Am J Surg Pathol. 2013;37(7):1053–7.

Chiosea SI, Griffith C, Assaad A, Seethala RR. The profile of acinic cell carcinoma after recognition of mammary analog secretory carcinoma. Am J Surg Pathol. 2012;36(3):343–50.

Gomez DR, Katabi N, Zhung J, Wolden SL, Zelefsky MJ, Kraus DH, et al. Clinical and pathologic prognostic features in acinic cell carcinoma of the parotid gland. Cancer. 2009;115(10):2128–37.

Ihrler S, Blasenbreu-Vogt S, Sendelhofert A, Lang S, Zietz C, Lohrs U. Differential diagnosis of salivary acinic cell carcinoma and adenocarcinoma (NOS). A comparison of (immuno-) histochemical markers. Pathol Res Pract. 2002;198(12):777–83.

Lei Y, Chiosea SI. Re-evaluating historic cohort of salivary acinic cell carcinoma with new diagnostic tools. Head Neck Pathol. 2012;6(2):166–70.

Lin WN, Huang HC, Wu CC, Liao CT, Chen IH, Kan CJ, et al. Analysis of acinic cell carcinoma of the parotid gland: 15 years experience. Acta Otolaryngol. 2010;130(12):1406–10.

Piana S, Cavazza A, Pedroni C, Scotti R, Serra L, Gardini G. Dedifferentiated acinic cell carcinoma of the parotid gland with myoepithelial features. Arch Pathol Lab Med. 2002;126(9):1104–5.

Roy S, Dhingra KK, Gupta P, Khurana N, Gupta B, Meher R. Acinic cell carcinoma with extensive neuroendocrine differentiation: a diagnostic challenge. Head Neck Pathol. 2009;3(2):163–8.

Skalova A, Sima R, Vanecek T, Muller S, Korabecna M, Nemcova J, et al. Acinic cell carcinoma with high-grade transformation: a report of 9 cases with immunohistochemical study and analysis of TP53 and HER-2/neu genes. Am J Surg Pathol. 2009;33(8):1137–45.

7 Adenoid Cystic Carcinoma

Adenoid cystic carcinoma affects children and adults and presents at a mean age of approximately 60 years. Women are involved slightly more than men. Major or minor salivary glands may be involved, presenting as single or multiple masses. Most cases of adenoid cystic carcinoma behave as low to intermediate-grade malignancies; however, a subset of cases with high-grade transformation (necrosis, elevated mitotic activity, and cytomorphologic atypia) are predisposed to recurrence, lymph node involvement, and distant metastasis. Adenoid cystic carcinoma may be circumscribed or infiltrative, comprised of multiple cell types (ductal and myoepithelial), and may exhibit a variety of architectural patterns (solid, cribriform, and tubular) (Figs. 7.1–7.37).

J. J. García, *Atlas of Salivary Gland Pathology*, https://doi.org/10.1007/978-3-319-09021-4_7

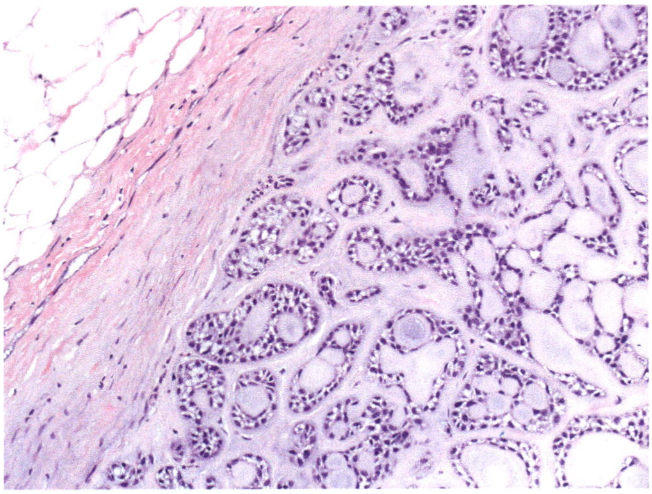

Fig. 7.1 (H&E, 200×) Adenoid cystic carcinoma, circumscribed

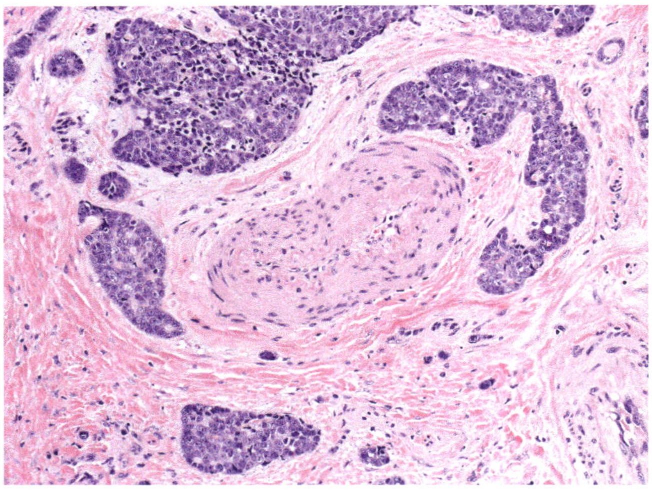

Fig. 7.2 (H&E, 200×) Adenoid cystic carcinoma, infiltrative

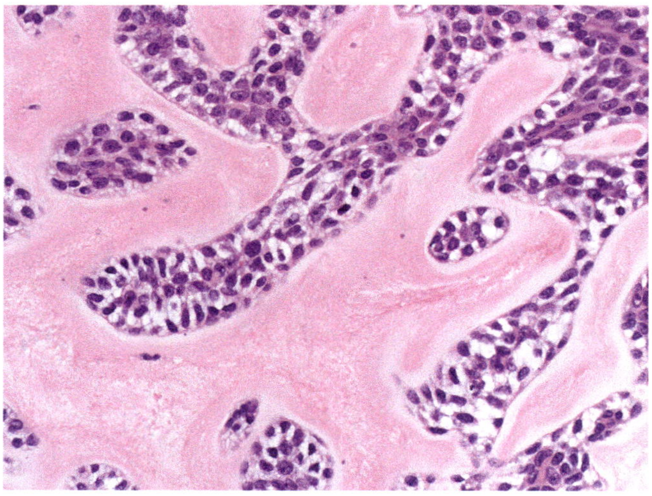

Fig. 7.3 (H&E, 400×) Adenoid cystic carcinoma, biphasic

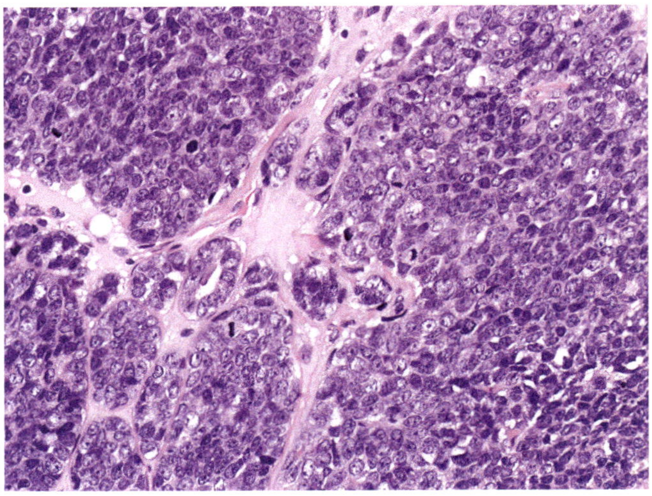

Fig. 7.4 (H&E, 400×) Adenoid cystic carcinoma, solid

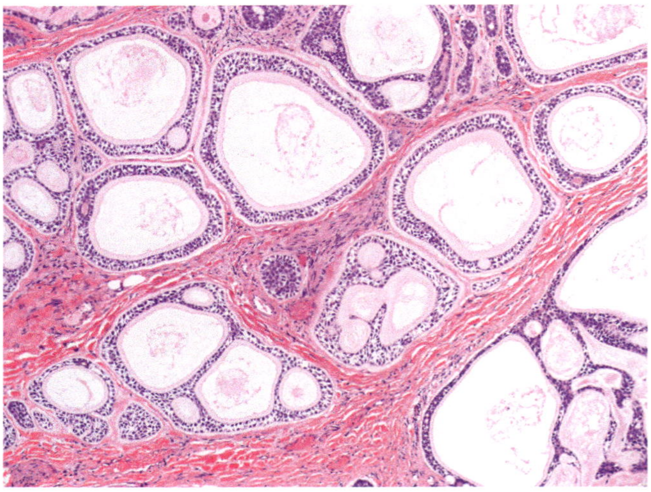

Fig. 7.5 (H&E, 100×) Adenoid cystic carcinoma, tubular

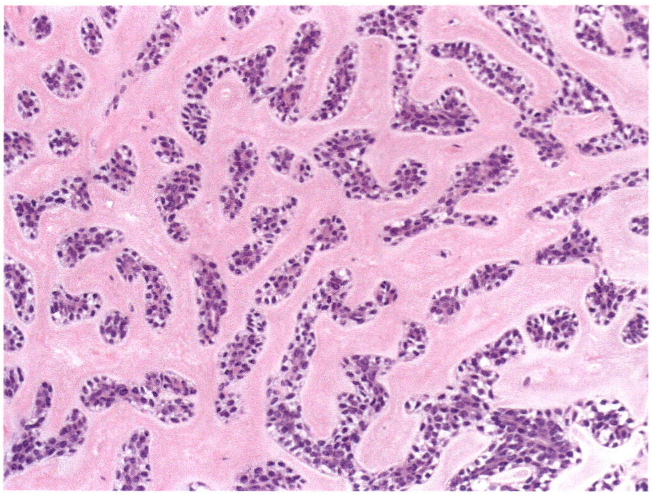

Fig. 7.6 (H&E, 200×) Adenoid cystic carcinoma, tubular

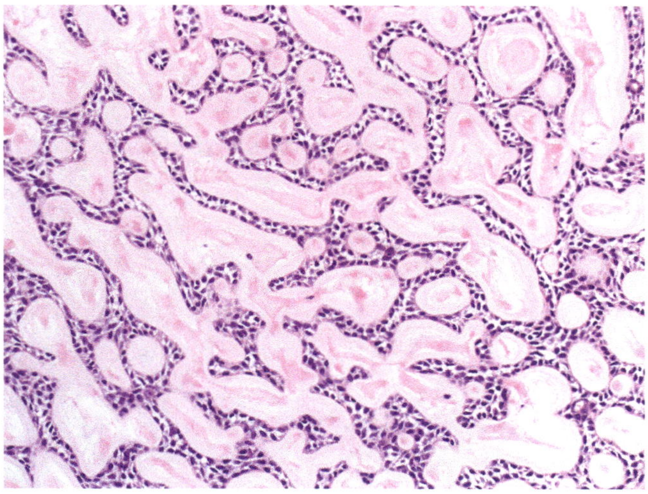

Fig. 7.7 (H&E, 200×) Adenoid cystic carcinoma, tubular

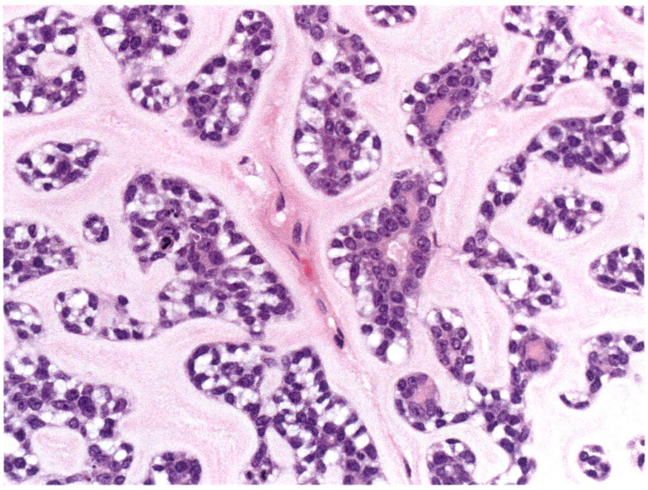

Fig. 7.8 (H&E, 400×) Adenoid cystic carcinoma, tubular

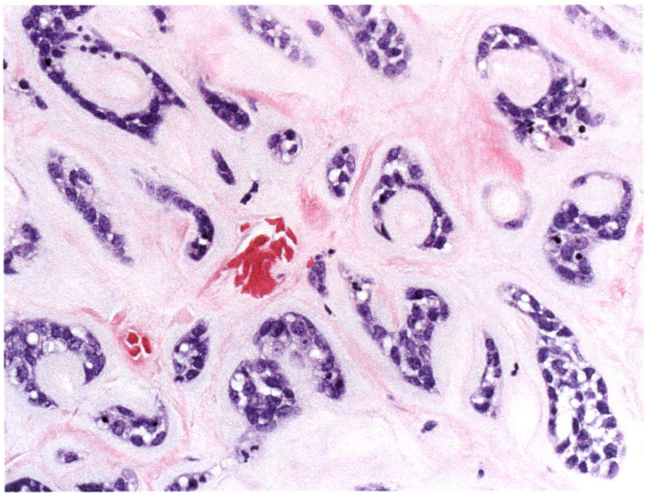

Fig. 7.9 (H&E, 400×) Adenoid cystic carcinoma, tubular

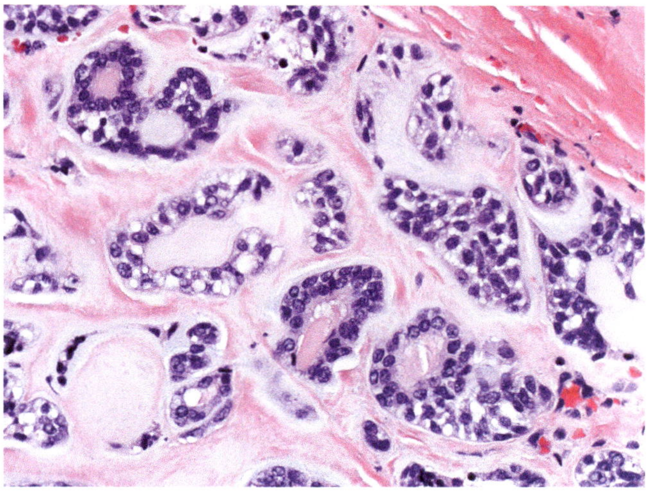

Fig. 7.10 (H&E, 400×) Adenoid cystic carcinoma, tubular

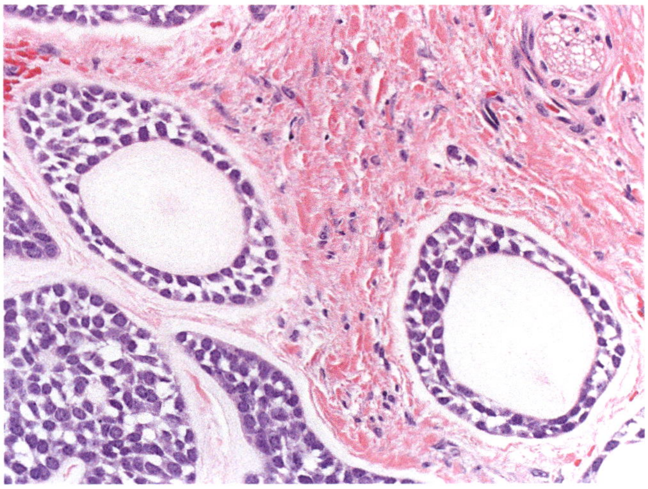

Fig. 7.11 (H&E, 400×) Adenoid cystic carcinoma, tubular

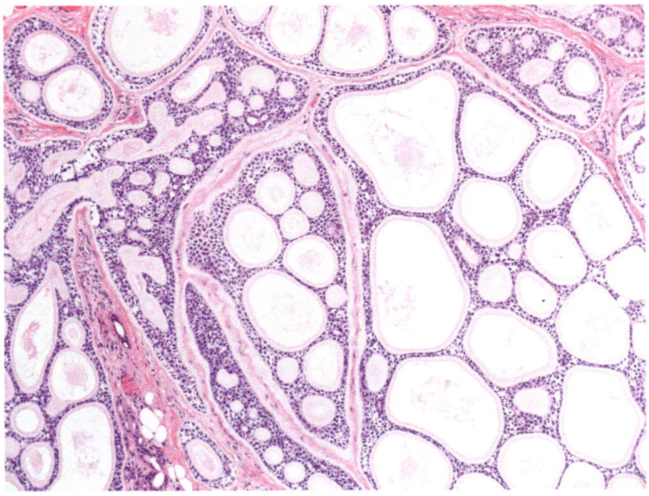

Fig. 7.12 (H&E, 100×) Adenoid cystic carcinoma, cribriform

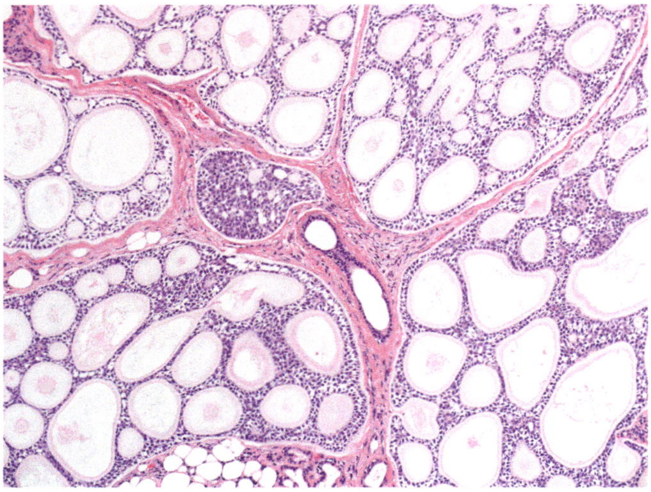

Fig. 7.13 (H&E, 100×) Adenoid cystic carcinoma, cribriform

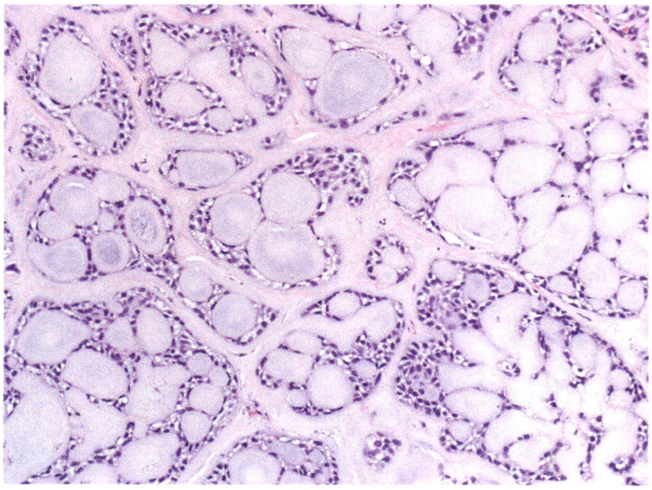

Fig. 7.14 (H&E, 200×) Adenoid cystic carcinoma, cribriform

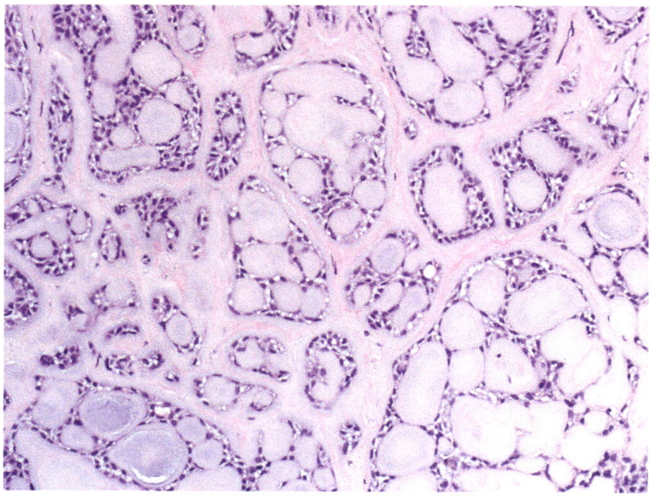

Fig. 7.15 (H&E, 200×) Adenoid cystic carcinoma, cribriform

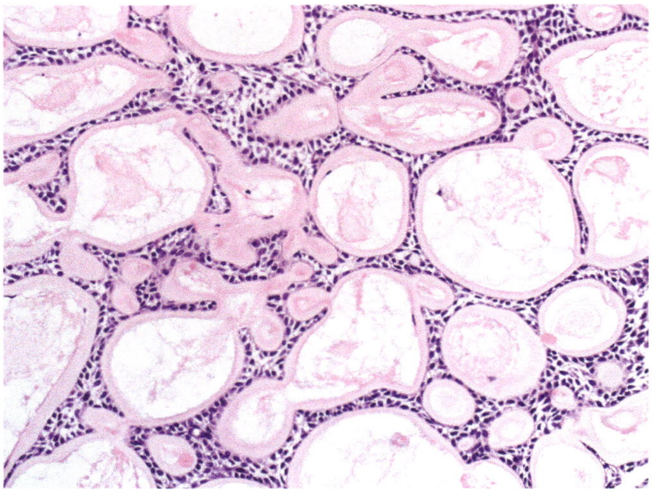

Fig. 7.16 (H&E, 200×) Adenoid cystic carcinoma, cribriform

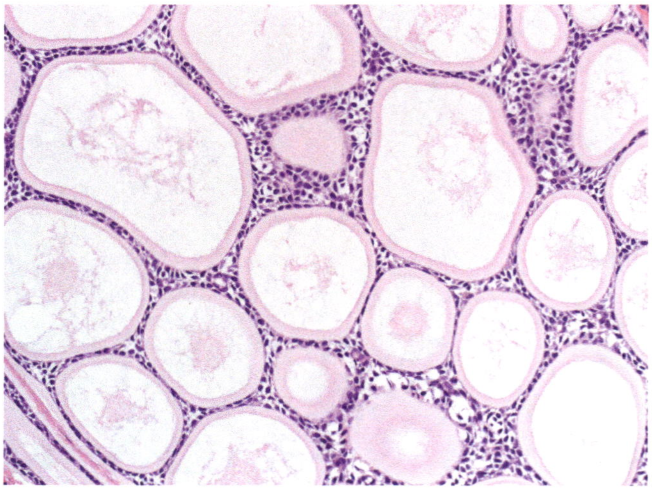

Fig. 7.17 (H&E, 200×) Adenoid cystic carcinoma, cribriform

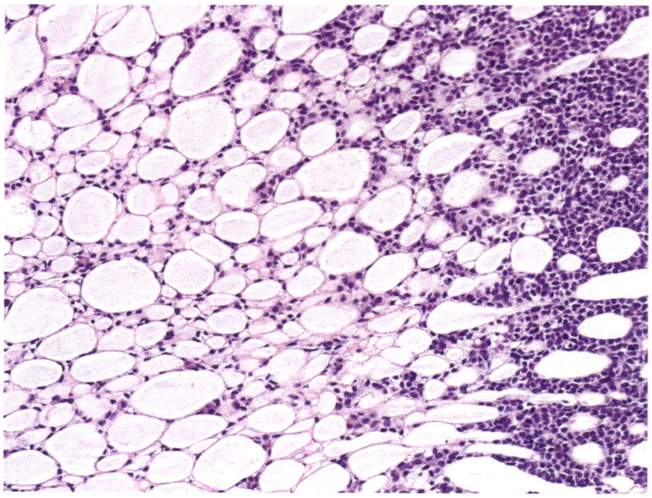

Fig. 7.18 (H&E, 200×) Adenoid cystic carcinoma, cribriform

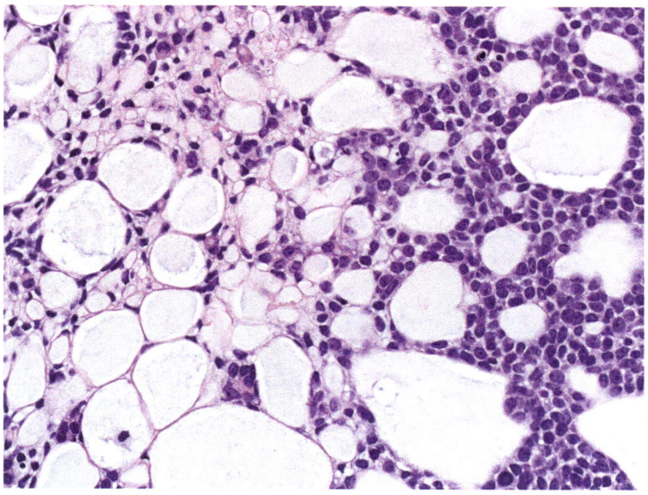

Fig. 7.19 (H&E, 400×) Adenoid cystic carcinoma, cribriform

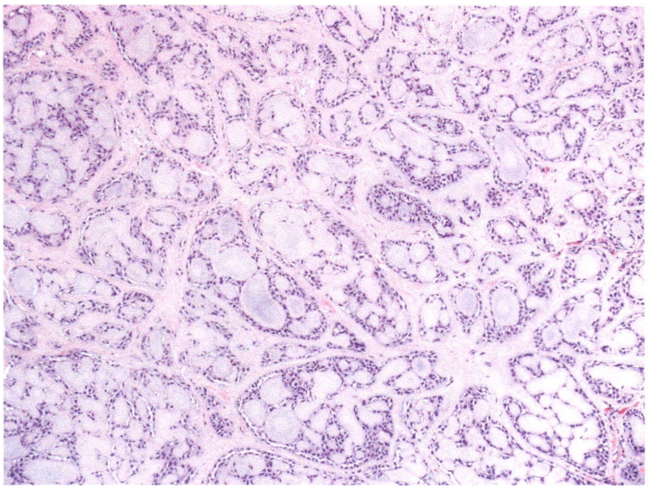

Fig. 7.20 (H&E, 100×) Adenoid cystic carcinoma, tubular and cribriform

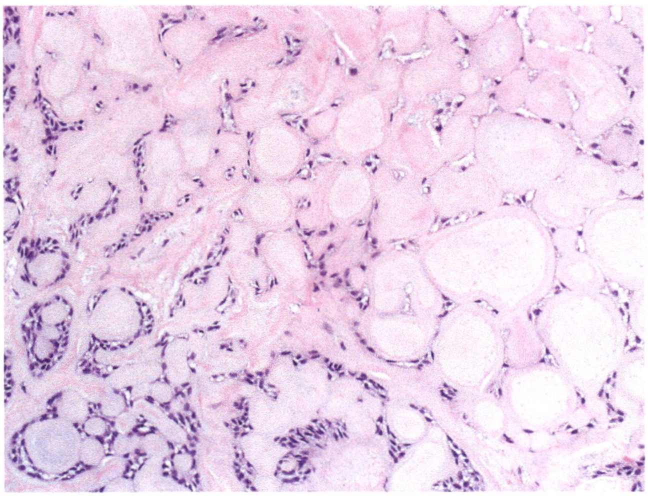

Fig. 7.21 (H&E, 200×) Adenoid cystic carcinoma, tubular and cribriform

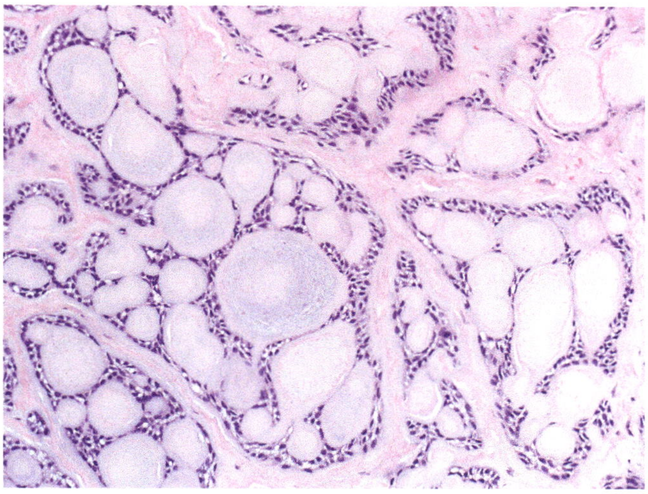

Fig. 7.22 (H&E, 200×) Adenoid cystic carcinoma, tubular and cribriform

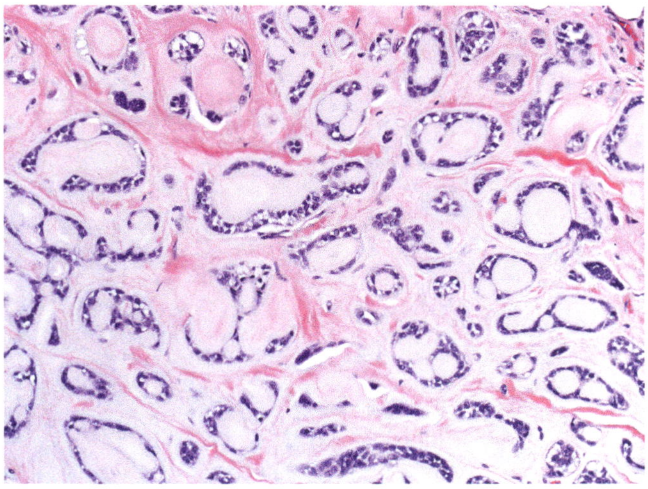

Fig. 7.23 (H&E, 200×) Adenoid cystic carcinoma, tubular and cribriform

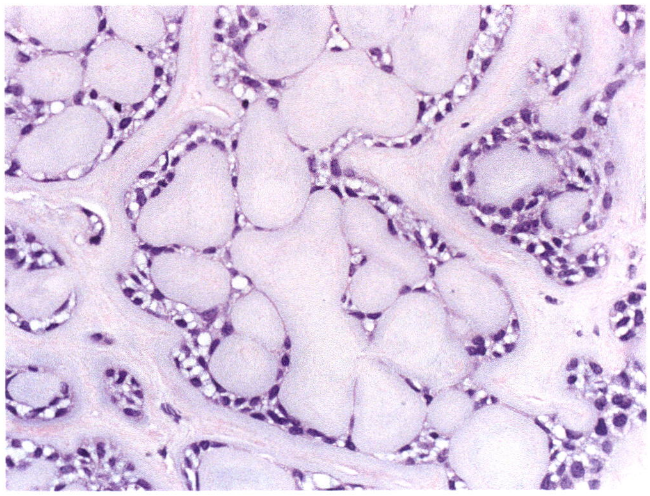

Fig. 7.24 (H&E, 400×) Adenoid cystic carcinoma, tubular and cribriform

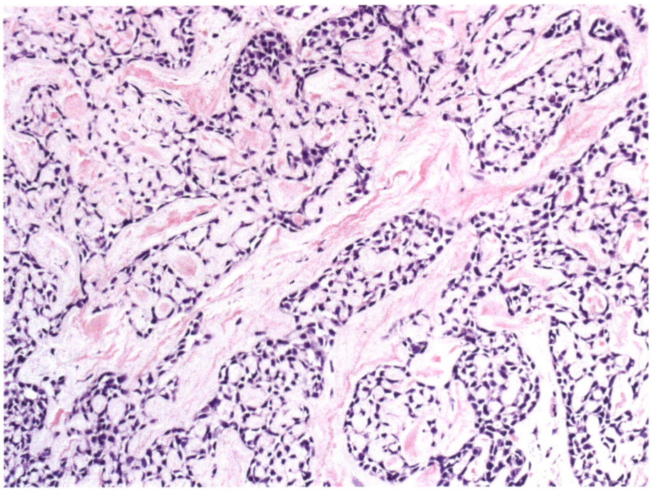

Fig. 7.25 (H&E, 200×) Adenoid cystic carcinoma, hyalinized

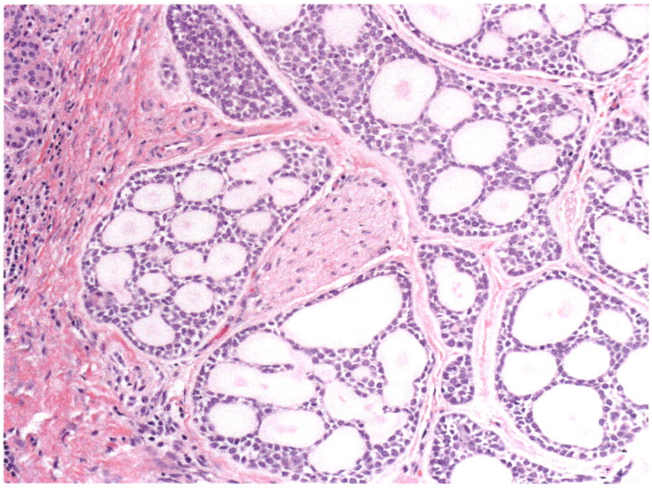

Fig. 7.26 (H&E, 200×) Adenoid cystic carcinoma, perineural invasion

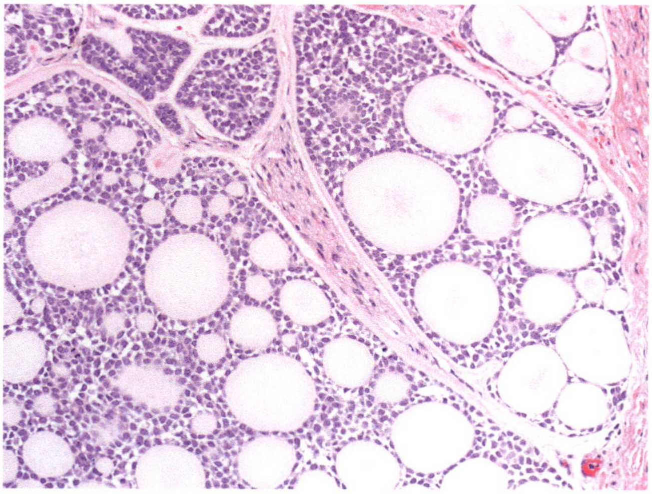

Fig. 7.27 (H&E, 200×) Adenoid cystic carcinoma, perineural invasion

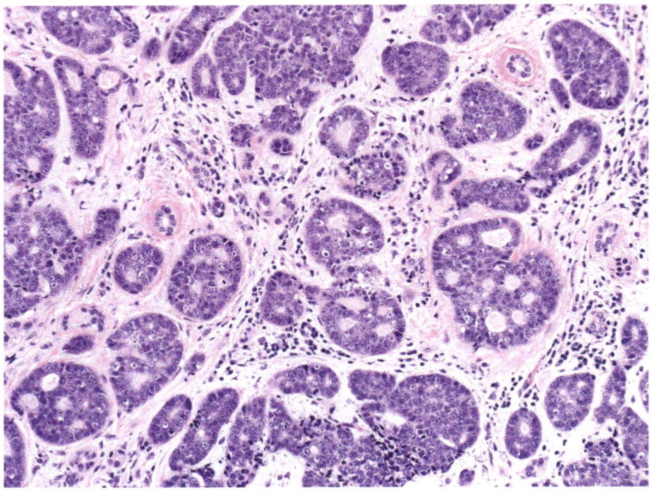

Fig. 7.28 (H&E, 200×) Adenoid cystic carcinoma, high-grade transformation, cytomorphologic atypia

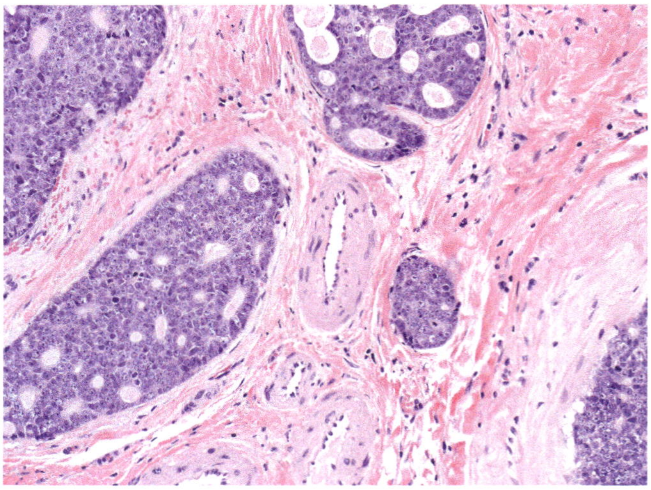

Fig. 7.29 (H&E, 200×) Adenoid cystic carcinoma, high-grade transformation, cytomorphologic atypia

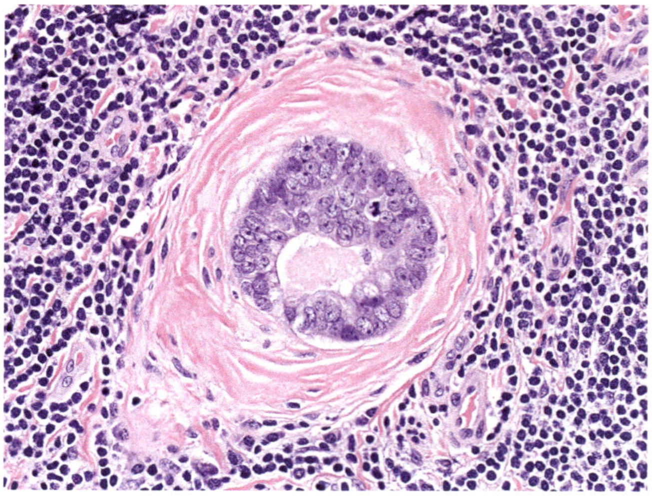

Fig. 7.30 (H&E, 400×) Adenoid cystic carcinoma, high-grade transformation, cytomorphologic atypia

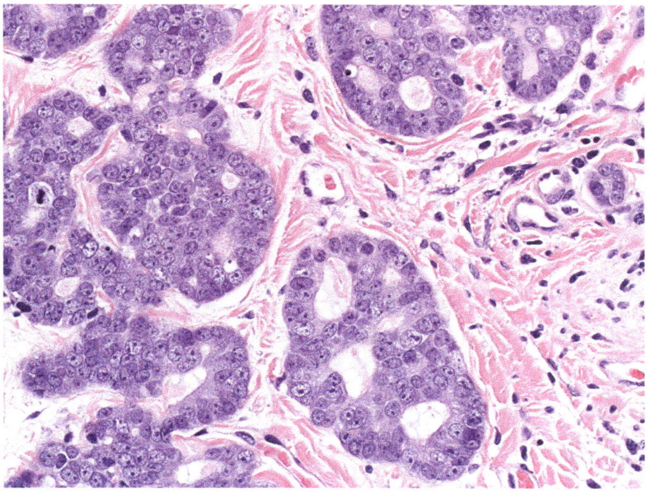

Fig. 7.31 (H&E, 400×) Adenoid cystic carcinoma, high-grade transformation, mitotic activity

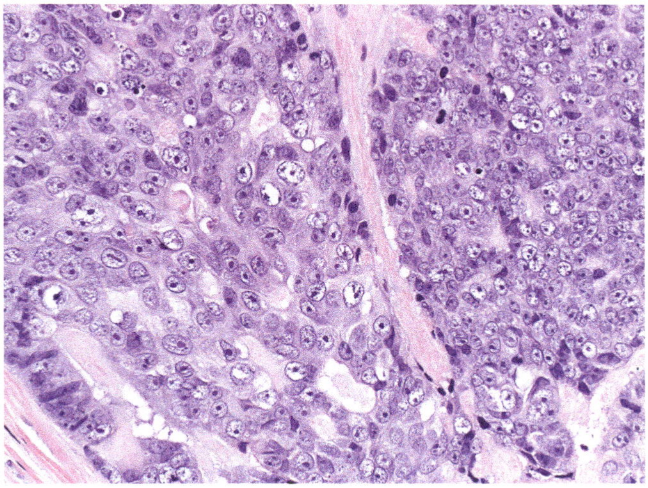

Fig. 7.32 (H&E, 400×) Adenoid cystic carcinoma, high-grade transformation, mitotic activity

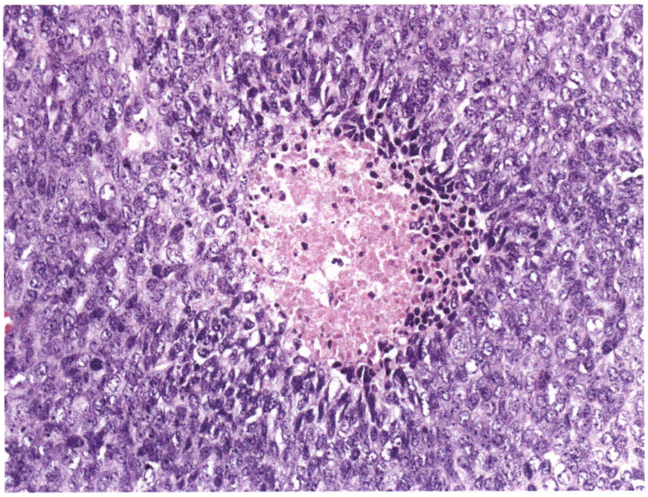

Fig. 7.33 (H&E, 400×) Adenoid cystic carcinoma, high-grade transformation, necrosis

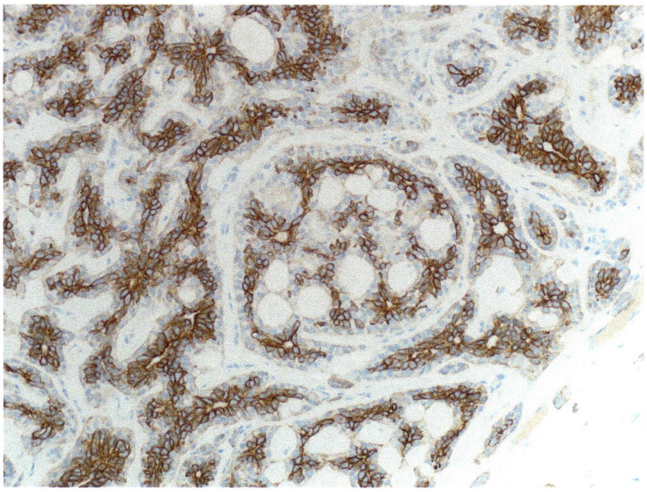

Fig. 7.34 (AE1/AE3, 200×) Adenoid cystic carcinoma, ductal immunoreactivity

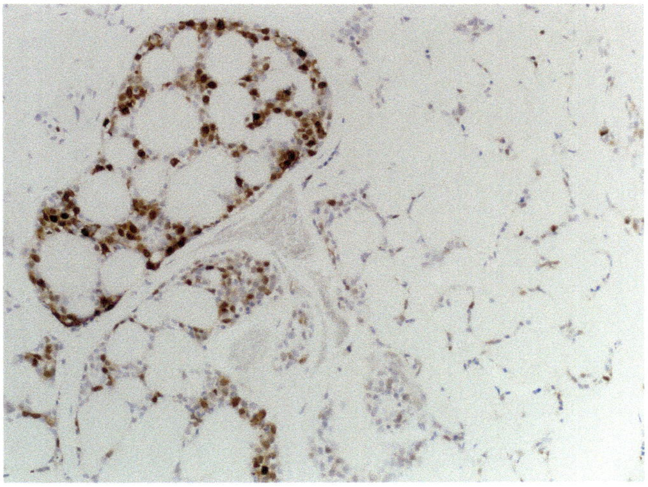

Fig. 7.35 (S-100, 200×) Adenoid cystic carcinoma, myoepithelial immunoreactivity

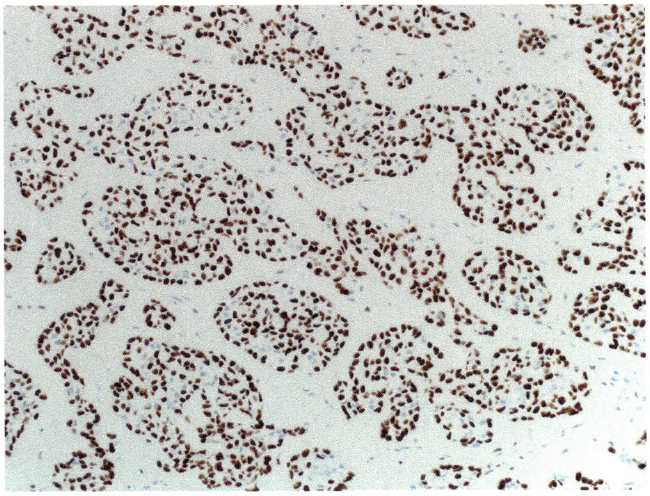

Fig. 7.36 (p63, 200×) Adenoid cystic carcinoma, myoepithelial immunoreactivity

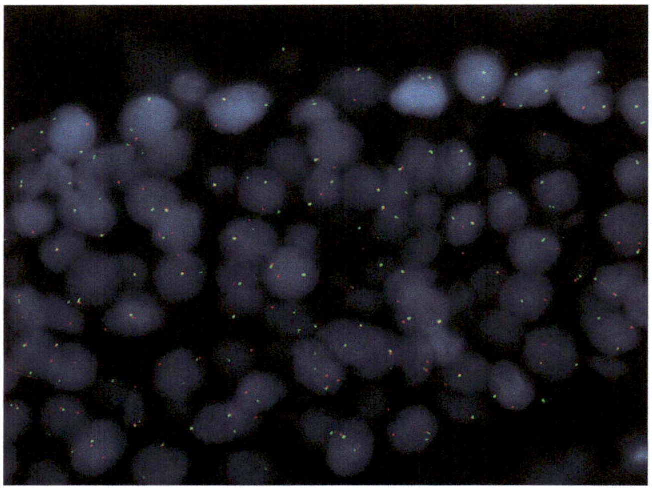

Fig. 7.37 (Fluorescent in situ hybridization, 600×) Adenoid cystic carcinoma, *MYB* rearrangement

Suggested Reading

Bhaijee F, Pepper DJ, Pitman KT, Bell D. New developments in the molecular pathogenesis of head and neck tumors: a review of tumor-specific fusion oncogenes in mucoepidermoid carcinoma, adenoid cystic carcinoma, and NUT midline carcinoma. Ann Diagn Pathol. 2011;15(1):69–77.

Brill LB 2nd, Kanner WA, Fehr A, Andrén Y, Moskaluk CA, Löning T, et al. Analysis of MYB expression and MYB-NFIB gene fusions in adenoid cystic carcinoma and other salivary neoplasms. Mod Pathol. 2011;24(9):1169–76.

Cohen AN, Damrose EJ, Huang RY, Nelson SD, Blackwell KE, Calcaterra TC. Adenoid cystic carcinoma of the submandibular gland: a 35-year review. Otolaryngol Head Neck Surg. 2004;131(6):994–1000.

da Cruz Perez DE, de Abreu AF, Nobuko Nishimoto I, de Almeida OP, Kowalski LP. Prognostic factors in head and neck adenoid cystic carcinoma. Oral Oncol. 2006;42(2):139–46.

Darling MR, Schneider JW, Phillips VM. Polymorphous low-grade adenocarcinoma and adenoid cystic carcinoma: a review and comparison of immunohistochemical markers. Oral Oncol. 2002;38(7):641–5.

Edwards PC, Bhuiya T, Kelsch RD. Assessment of p63 expression in the salivary gland neoplasms adenoid cystic carcinoma, polymorphous low-grade adenocarcinoma, and basal cell and canalicular adenomas. Oral Surg Oral Med Oral Pathol Oral Radiol Endod. 2004;97(5):613–9.

Friedrich RE, Bleckmann V. Adenoid cystic carcinoma of salivary and lacrimal gland origin: localization, classification, clinical pathological correlation, treatment results and long-term follow-up control in 84 patients. Anticancer Res. 2003;23(2A):931–40.

Ho AS, Kannan K, Roy DM, Morris LG, Ganly I, Katabi N, et al. The mutational landscape of adenoid cystic carcinoma. Nat Genet. 2013;45(7):791–8.

Kokemueller H, Eckardt A, Brachvogel P, Hausamen JE. Adenoid cystic carcinoma of the head and neck--a 20 years experience. Int J Oral Maxillofac Surg. 2004;33(1):25–31.

Lupinetti AD, Roberts DB, Williams MD, Kupferman ME, Rosenthal DI, Demonte F, et al. Sinonasal adenoid cystic carcinoma: the M. D Anderson Cancer center experience. Cancer. 2007;110(12):2726–31.

Mino M, Pilch BZ, Faquin WC. Expression of KIT (CD117) in neoplasms of the head and neck: an ancillary marker for adenoid cystic carcinoma. Mod Pathol. 2003;16(12):1224–31.

Mitani Y, Li J, Rao PH, Zhao YJ, Bell D, Lippman SM, et al. Comprehensive analysis of the MYB-NFIB gene fusion in salivary adenoid cystic carcinoma: incidence, variability, and clinicopathologic significance. Clin Cancer Res. 2010;16(19):4722–31.

Mitani Y, Rao PH, Futreal PA, Roberts DB, Stephens PJ, Zhao YJ, et al. Novel chromosomal rearrangements and break points at the t(6;9) in salivary adenoid cystic carcinoma: association with MYB-NFIB chimeric fusion, MYB expression, and clinical outcome. Clin Cancer Res. 2011;17(22):7003–14.

Penner CR, Folpe AL, Budnick SD. C-kit expression distinguishes salivary gland adenoid cystic carcinoma from polymorphous low-grade adenocarcinoma. Mod Pathol. 2002;15(7):687–91.

Persson M, Andrén Y, Moskaluk CA, Frierson HF Jr, Cooke SL, Futreal PA, et al. Clinically significant copy number alterations and complex rearrangements of MYB and NFIB in head and neck adenoid cystic carcinoma. Genes Chromosomes Cancer. 2012;51(8):805–17.

Rapidis AD, Givalos N, Gakiopoulou H, Faratzis G, Stavrianos SD, Vilos GA, et al. Adenoid cystic carcinoma of the head and neck. Clinicopathological analysis of 23 patients and review of the literature. Oral Oncol. 2005;41(3):328–35.

Seethala RR, Cieply K, Barnes EL, Dacic S. Progressive genetic alterations of adenoid cystic carcinoma with high-grade transformation. Arch Pathol Lab Med. 2011;135(1):123–30.

West RB, Kong C, Clarke N, Gilks T, Lipsick JS, Cao H, et al. MYB expression and translocation in adenoid cystic carcinomas and other salivary gland tumors with clinicopathologic correlation. Am J Surg Pathol. 2011;35(1):92–9.

Basal Cell Adenoma

8

Basal cell adenoma is the benign counterpart of basal cell adenocarcinoma. Basal cell adenoma affects primarily adults and presents at a mean age of approximately 65 years. Women are involved slightly more than men. The majority of cases involve the parotid gland, presenting as single or multiple masses. Basal cell adenoma may be encapsulated, circumscribed, or multi-nodular, comprised of multiple cell types (ductal, myoepithelial, and basal), and exhibit a variety of architectural patterns (solid, trabecular, tubular, and membranous) (Figs. 8.1–8.28).

J. J. García, *Atlas of Salivary Gland Pathology*, https://doi.org/10.1007/978-3-319-09021-4_8

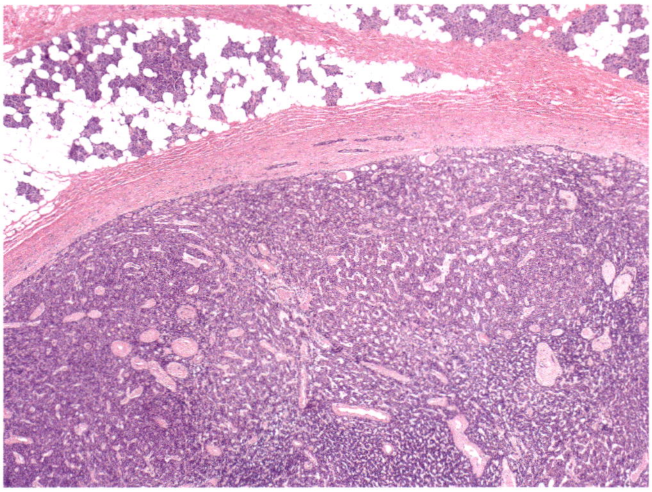

Fig. 8.1 (H&E, 40×) Basal cell adenoma, encapsulated

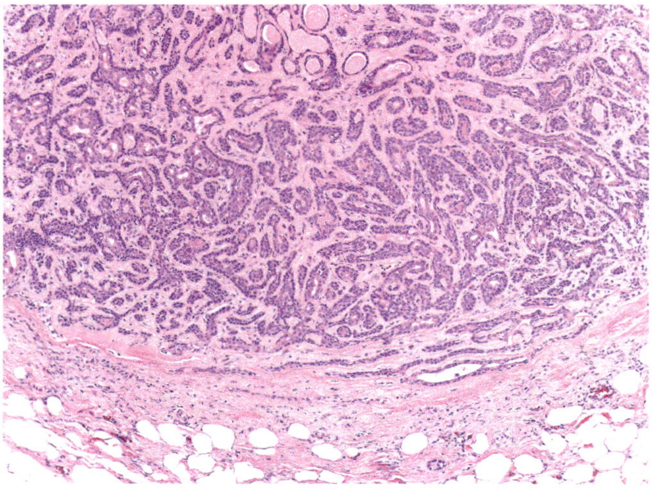

Fig. 8.2 (H&E, 100×) Basal cell adenoma, circumscribed

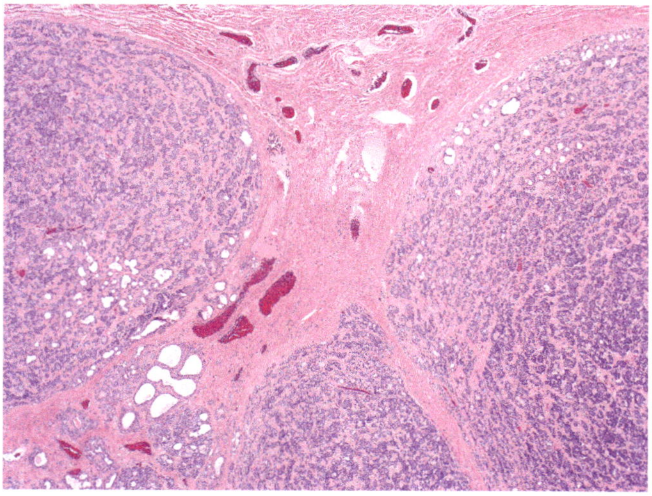

Fig. 8.3 (H&E, 40×) Basal cell adenoma, nodular

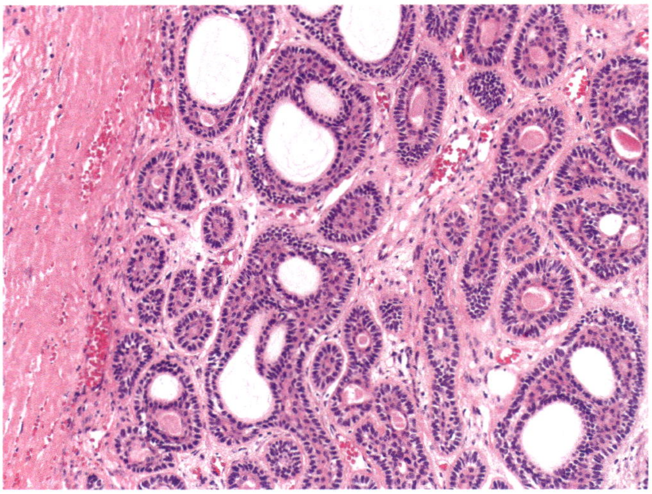

Fig. 8.4 (H&E, 200×) Basal cell adenoma, biphasic

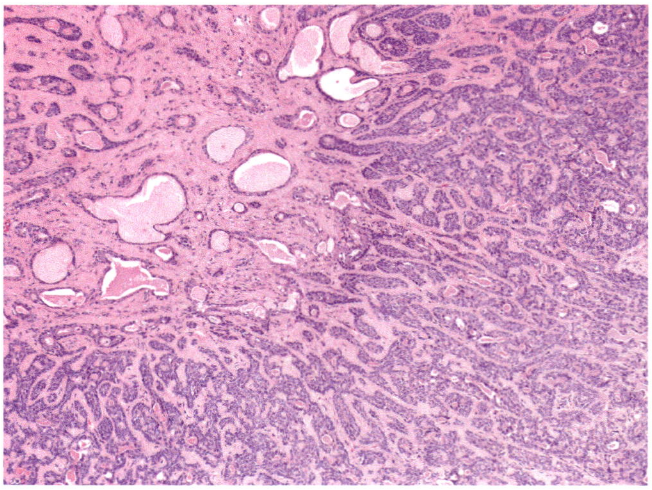

Fig. 8.5 (H&E, 100×) Basal cell adenoma, trabecular

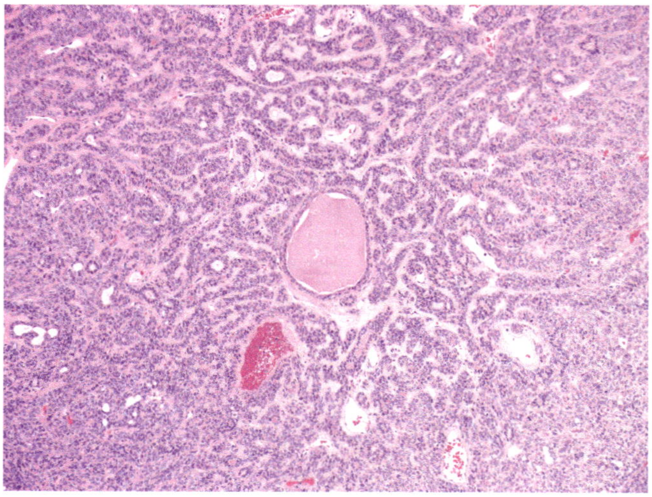

Fig. 8.6 (H&E, 100×) Basal cell adenoma, trabecular

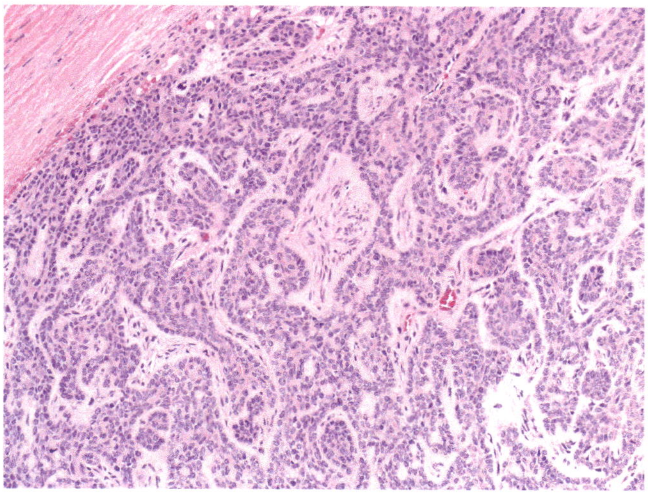

Fig. 8.7 (H&E, 200×) Basal cell adenoma, trabecular

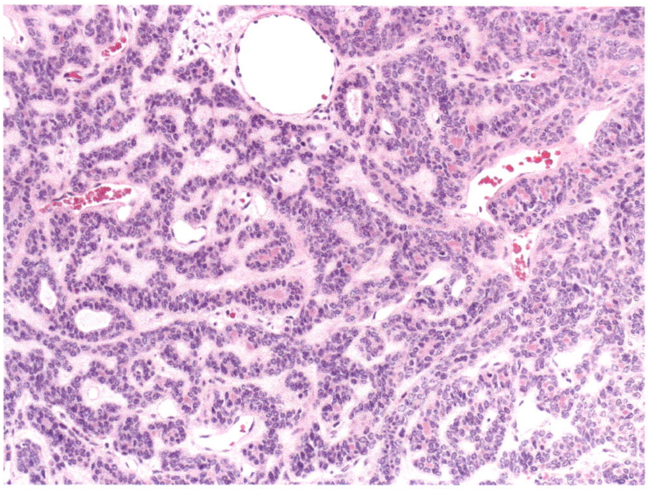

Fig. 8.8 (H&E, 200×) Basal cell adenoma, trabecular

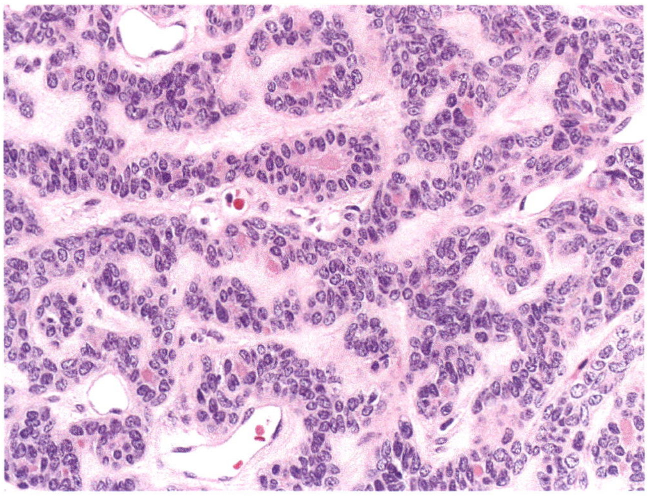

Fig. 8.9 (H&E, 400×) Basal cell adenoma, trabecular

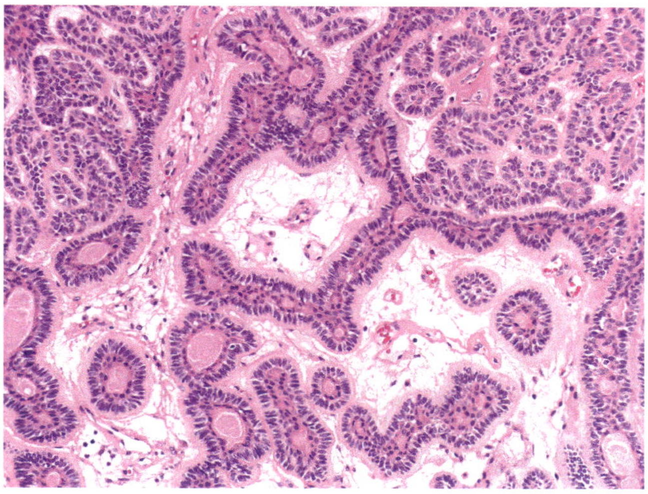

Fig. 8.10 (H&E, 200×) Basal cell adenoma, tubular

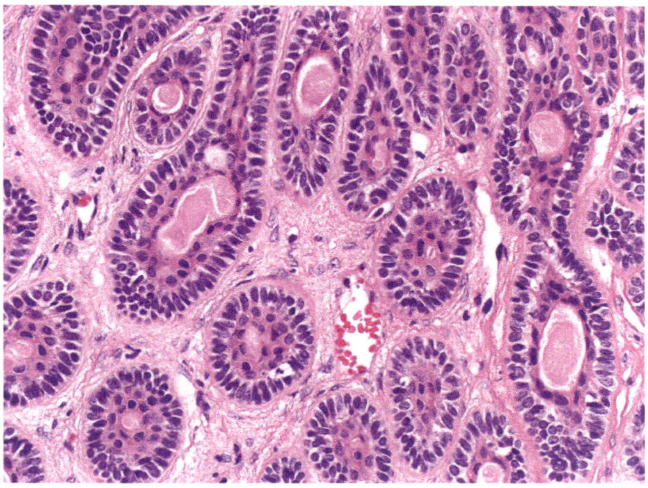

Fig. 8.11 (H&E, 400×) Basal cell adenoma, tubular

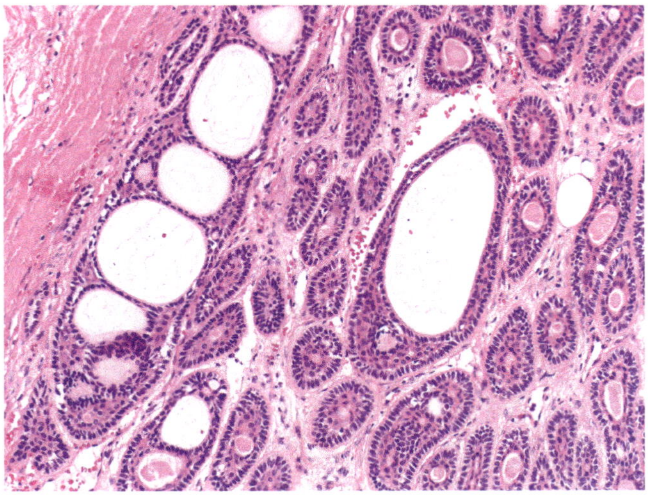

Fig. 8.12 (H&E, 200×) Basal cell adenoma, tubular and cribriform

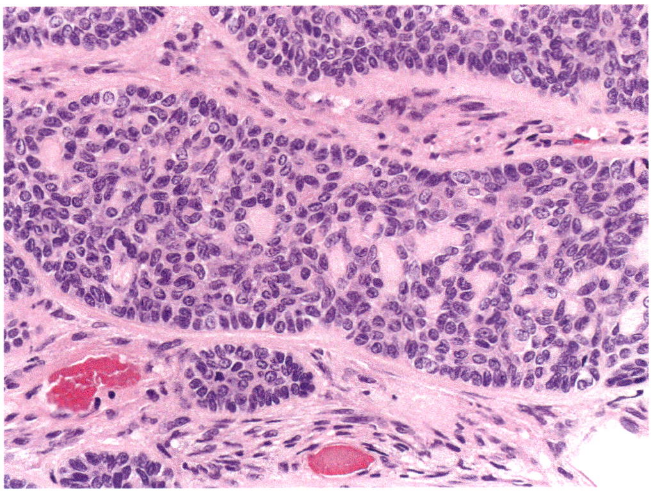

Fig. 8.13 (H&E, 400×) Basal cell adenoma, tubular and cribriform

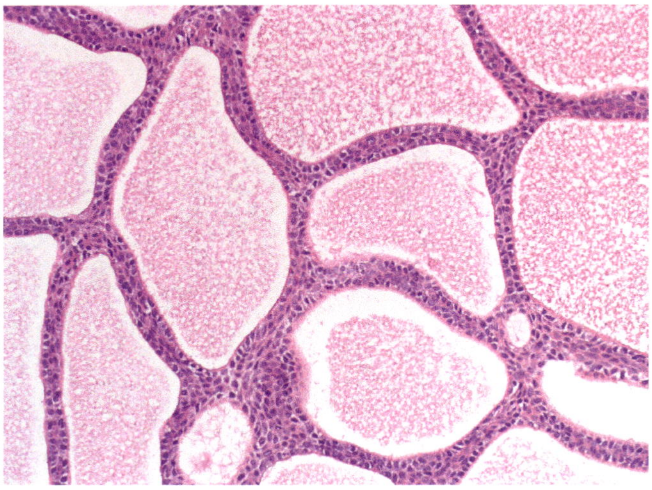

Fig. 8.14 (H&E, 200×) Basal cell adenoma, tubular and cystic

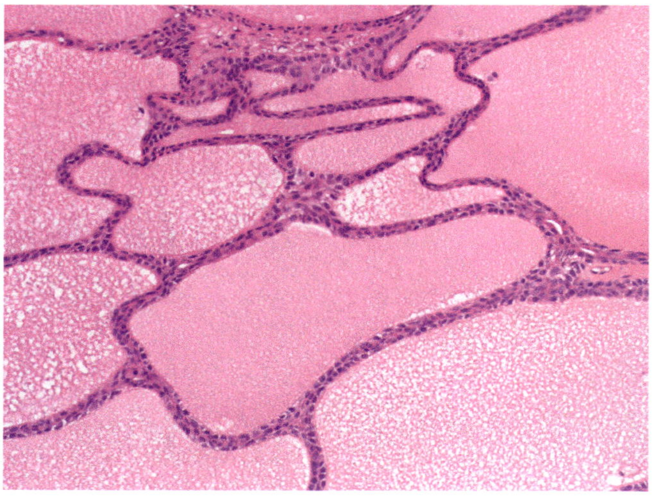

Fig. 8.15 (H&E, 200×) Basal cell adenoma, tubular and cystic

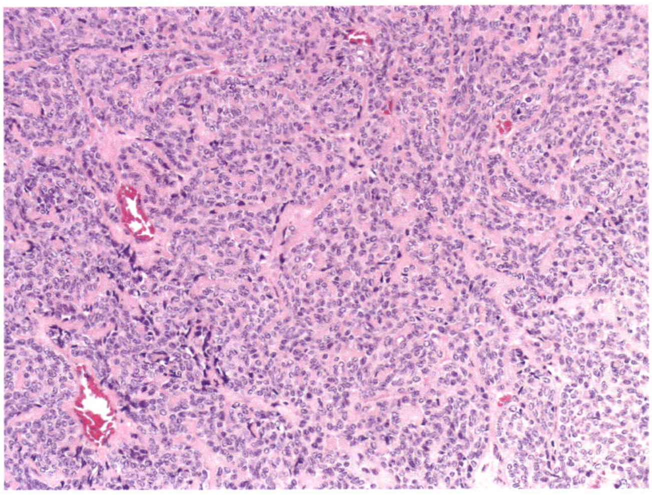

Fig. 8.16 (H&E, 200×) Basal cell adenoma, solid

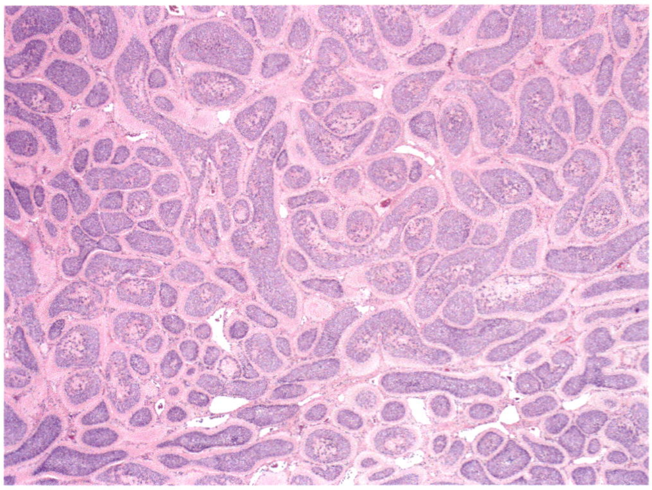

Fig. 8.17 (H&E, 40×) Basal cell adenoma, membranous

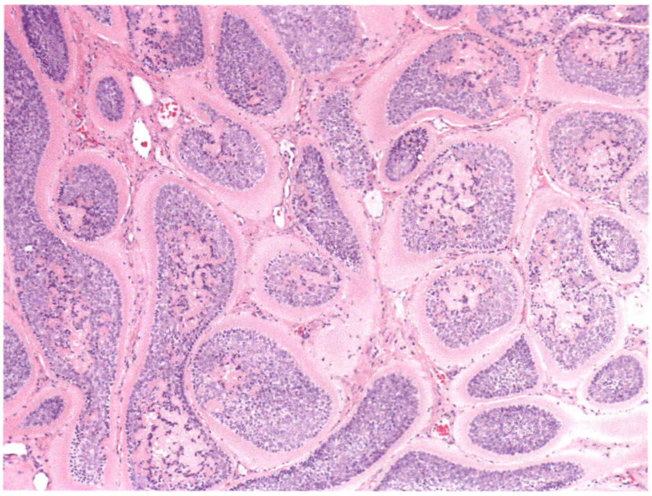

Fig. 8.18 (H&E, 100×) Basal cell adenoma, membranous

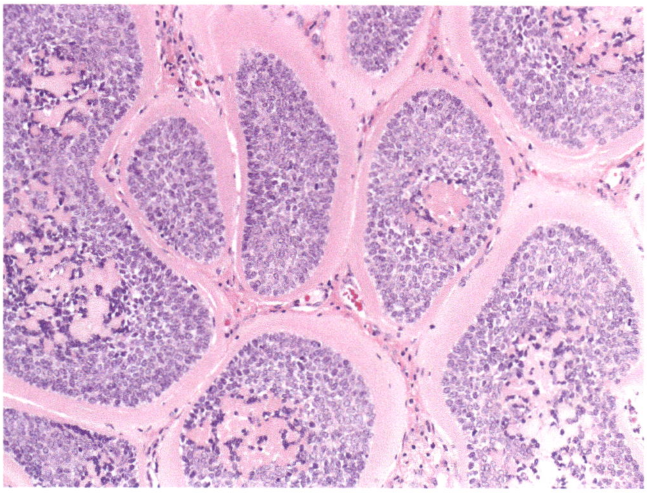

Fig. 8.19 (H&E, 200×) Basal cell adenoma, membranous

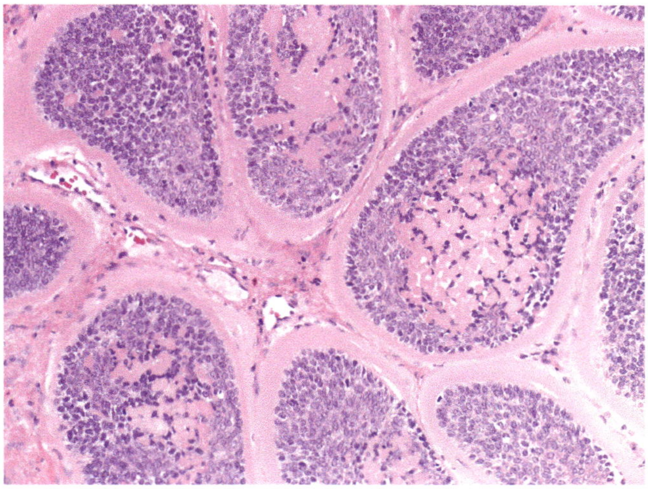

Fig. 8.20 (H&E, 200×) Basal cell adenoma, membranous

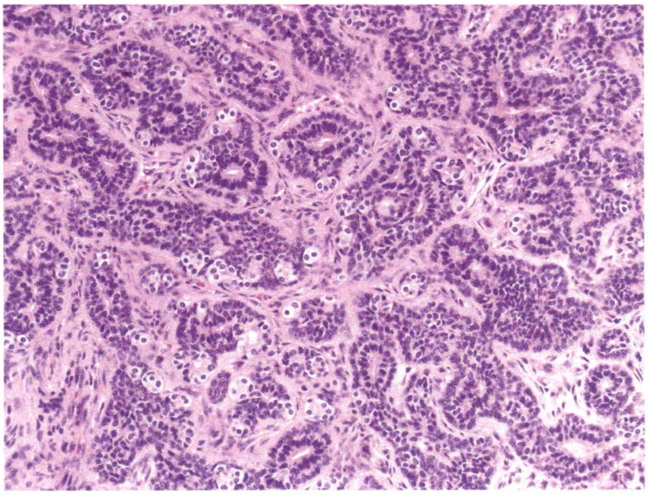

Fig. 8.21 (H&E, 200×) Basal cell adenoma, clear cells

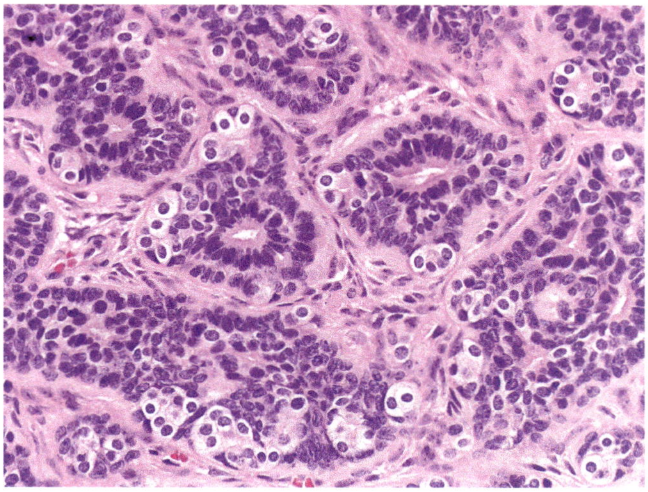

Fig. 8.22 (H&E, 400×) Basal cell adenoma, clear cells

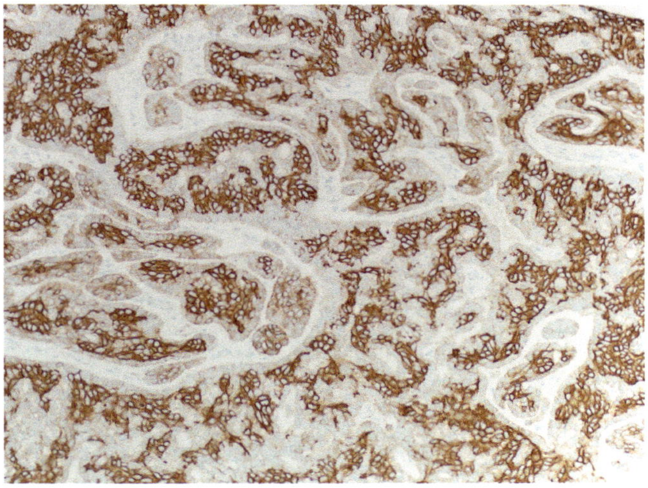

Fig. 8.23 (AE1/AE3, 200×) Basal cell adenoma, ductal immunoreactivity

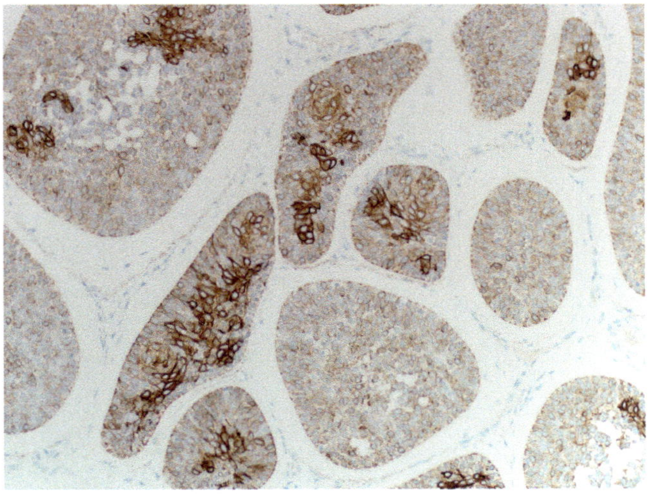

Fig. 8.24 (AE1/AE3, 200×) Basal cell adenoma, ductal immunoreactivity

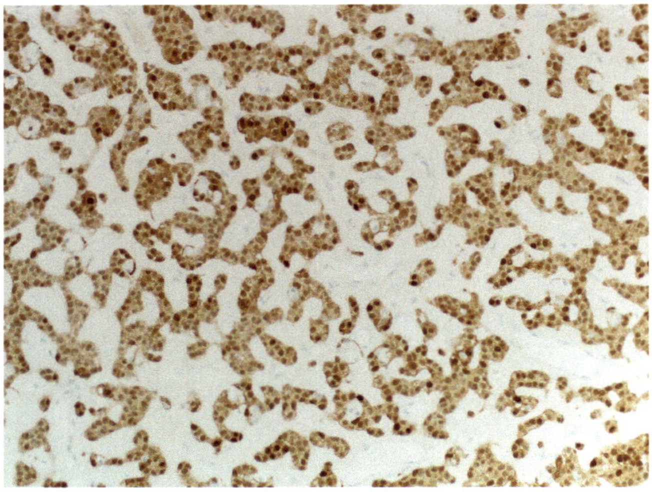

Fig. 8.25 (S-100, 200×) Basal cell adenoma, diffuse immunoreactivity

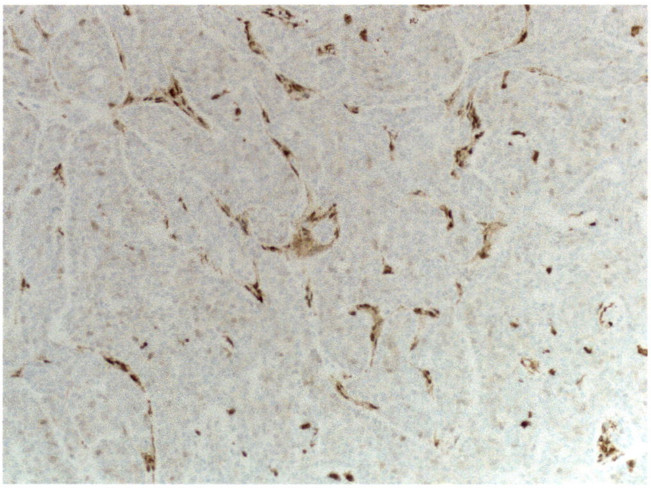

Fig. 8.26 (S-100, 200×) Basal cell adenoma, focal immunoreactivity

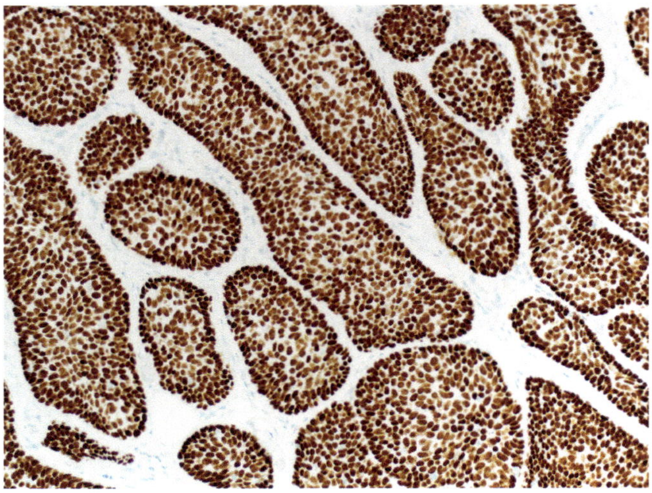

Fig. 8.27 (p63, 200×) Basal cell adenoma, diffuse immunoreactivity

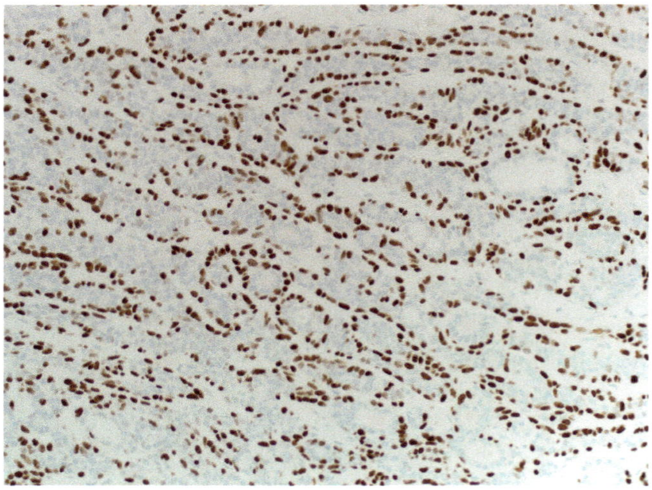

Fig. 8.28 (p63, 200×) Basal cell adenoma, basal immunoreactivity

Suggested Reading

Bastakis JG, Luna MA, el-Naggar AK. Basaloid monorphic adenomas. Ann Otol Rhinol Laryngol. 1991;100:687–90.

Chhieng DC, Paulino AF. Basaloid tumors of the salivary glands. Ann Diagn Pathol. 2002;6(6):364–72.

Edwards PC, Bhuiya T, Kelsch RD. Assessment of p63 expression in the salivary gland neoplasms adenoid cystic carcinoma, polymorphous low-grade adenocarcinoma, and basal cell and canalicular adenomas. Oral Surg Oral Med Oral Pathol Oral Radiol Endod. 2004;97(5):613–9.

Ethunandan M, Pratt CA, Macpherson DW. Changing frequency of parotid gland neoplasms—analysis of 560 tumors treated in a district general hospital. Ann R Coll Surg Engl. 2002;84:1–6.

Hyman BA, Scheithauer BW, Weiland LH, Irons GB. Membranous basal cell adenoma of the parotid gland. Malignant transformation in a patient with multiple dermal cylindromas. Arch Pathol Lab Med. 1988;112:209–11.

Klijanienko J, El-Naggar AK, Vielh P. Comparative cytologic and histologic study of fifteen salivary basal-cell tumors: differential diagnostic considerations. Diagn Cytopathol. 1999;21(1):30–4.

Machado de Sousa SO, Soares de Araújo N, Corrêa L, Pires Soubhia AM, Cavalcanti de Araújo V. Immunohistochemical aspects of basal cell adenoma and canalicular adenoma of salivary glands. Oral Oncol. 2001;37(4):365–8.

Nagao T, Sugano I, Ishida Y, Hasegawa M, Matsuzaki O, Konno A, et al. Basal cell adenocarcinoma of the salivary glands: comparison with basal cell adenoma through assessment of cell proliferation, apoptosis, and expression of p53 and bcl-2. Cancer. 1998;82(3):439–47.

Scott AR, Faquin WC, Deschler DG. Parotid mass in a woman with multiple cutaneous cylindromas. Head Neck. 2010;32:684–7.

Tian Z, Li L, Wang L, Hu Y, Li J. Salivary gland neoplasms in oral and maxillofacial regions: a 23-year retrospective study of 6982 case in an eastern Chinese population. Int J Oral Maxillofac Surg. 2010;39:235–42.

Wilson TC, Robinson RA. Basal cell adenocarcinoma and basal cell adenoma of the salivary glands: a clinicopathological review of seventy tumors with comparison of morphologic features and growth control indices. Head Neck Pathol. 2015;9:205–13.

Yu GY, Ubmüller J, Donath K. Membranous basal cell adenoma of the salivary gland: a clinicopathologic study of 12 cases. Acta Otolaryngol. 1998;118:588–93.

Zarbo RJ, Prasad AR, Regezi JA, Gown AM, Savera AT. Salivary gland basal cell and canalicular adenomas: immunohistochemical demonstration of myoepithelial cell participation and morphogenetic considerations. Arch Pathol Lab Med. 2000;124(3):401–5.

9 Basal Cell Adenocarcinoma

Basal cell adenocarcinoma is the malignant counterpart of basal cell adenoma. Basal cell adenocarcinoma affects primarily adults and presents at a mean age of approximately 65 years. Women and men are involved with similar frequency. The majority of cases involve the parotid gland, presenting as single or multiple masses. Basal cell adenocarcinoma may be circumscribed or infiltrative, comprised of multiple cell types (ductal, myoepithelial, and basal), and may exhibit a variety of architectural patterns (solid, trabecular, tubular, and membranous) (Figs. 9.1–9.28).

J. J. García, *Atlas of Salivary Gland Pathology*, https://doi.org/10.1007/978-3-319-09021-4_9

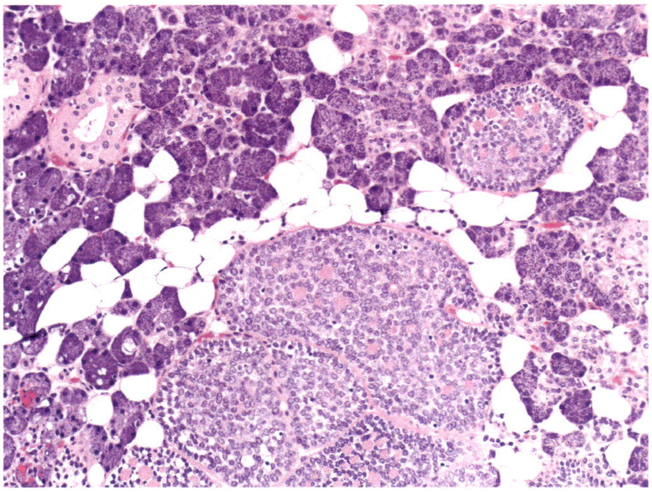

Fig. 9.1 (H&E, 200×) Basal cell adenocarcinoma, infiltrative

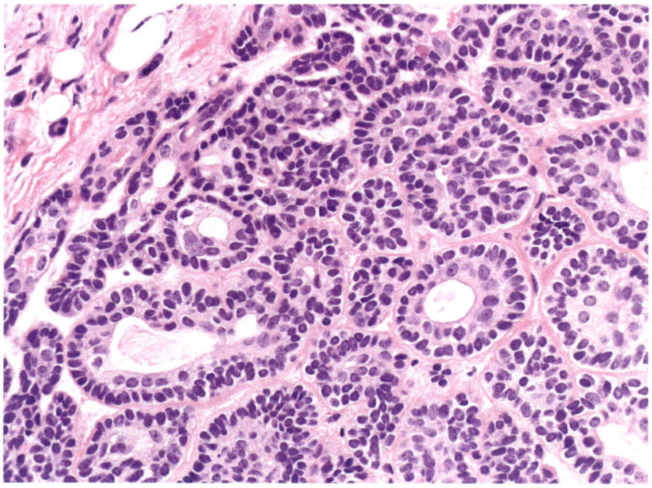

Fig. 9.2 (H&E, 400×) Basal cell adenocarcinoma, biphasic

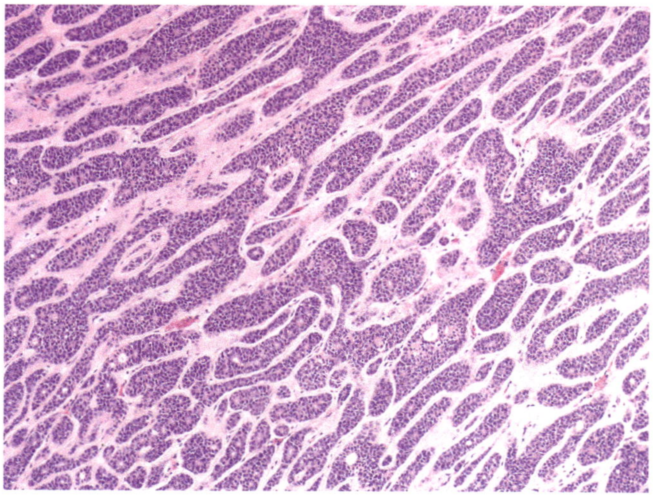

Fig. 9.3 (H&E, 100×) Basal cell adenocarcinoma, trabecular

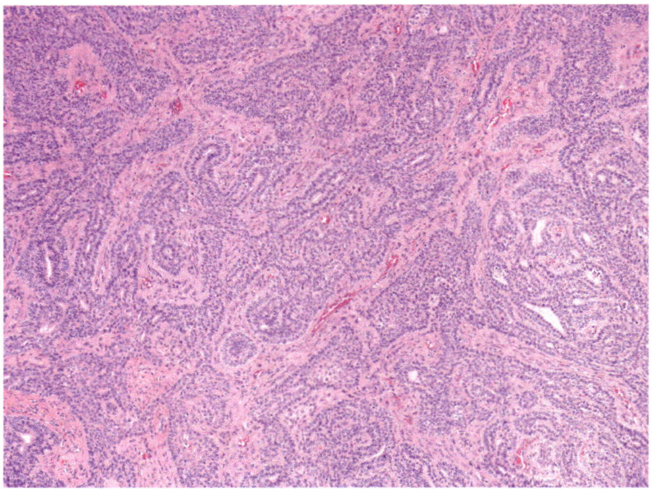

Fig. 9.4 (H&E, 100×) Basal cell adenocarcinoma, trabecular

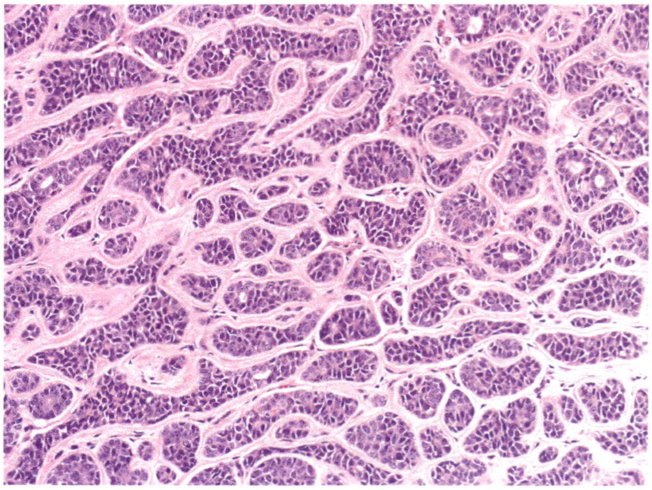

Fig. 9.5 (H&E, 200×) Basal cell adenocarcinoma, tubular

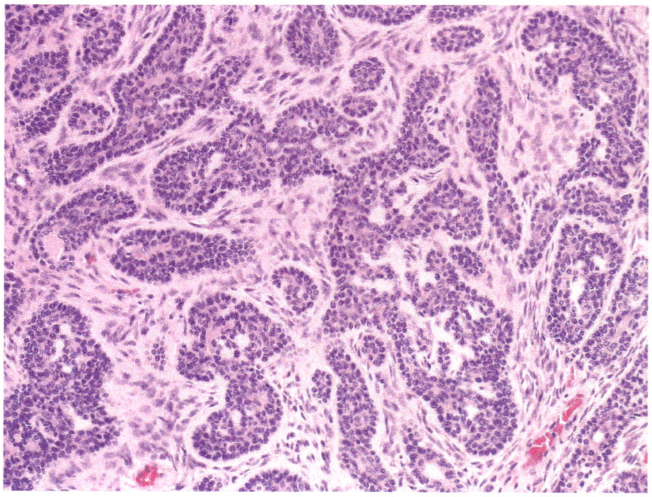

Fig. 9.6 (H&E, 200×) Basal cell adenocarcinoma, tubular

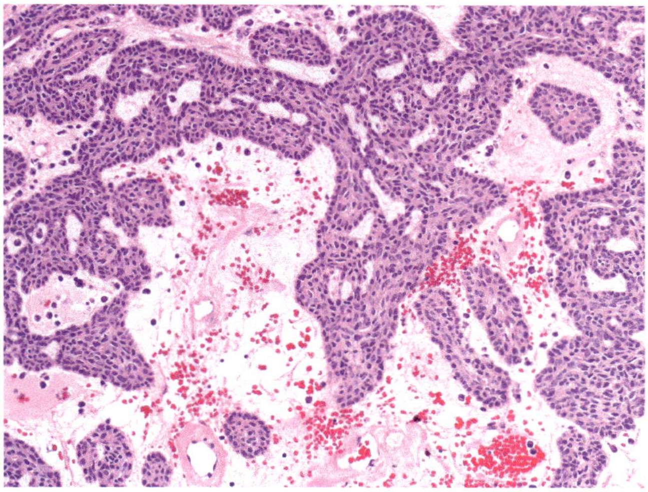

Fig. 9.7 (H&E, 200×) Basal cell adenocarcinoma, tubular

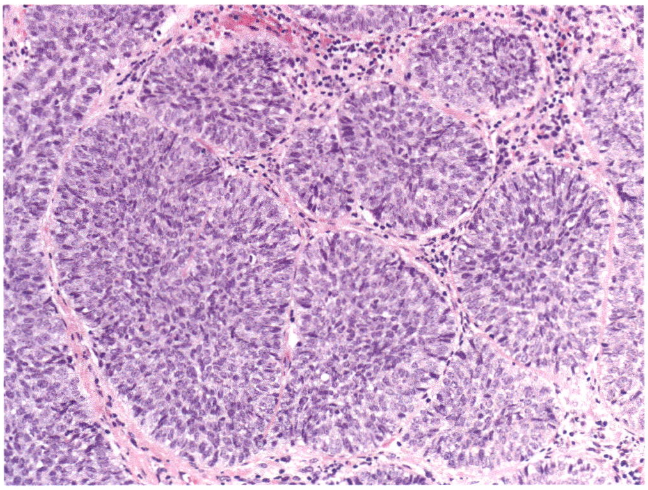

Fig. 9.8 (H&E, 200×) Basal cell adenocarcinoma, solid

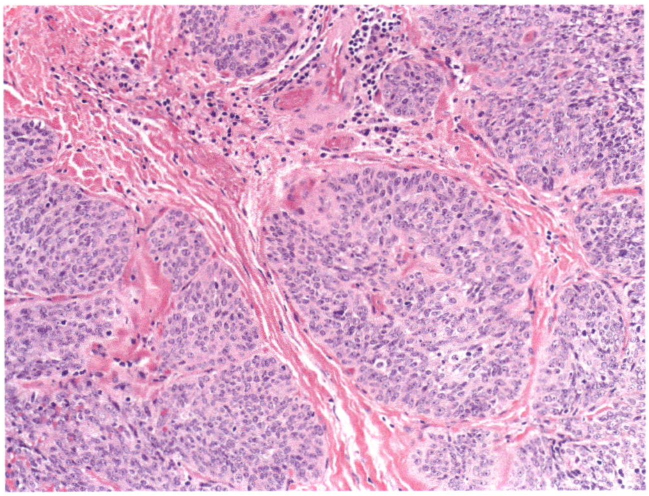

Fig. 9.9 (H&E, 200×) Basal cell adenocarcinoma, solid

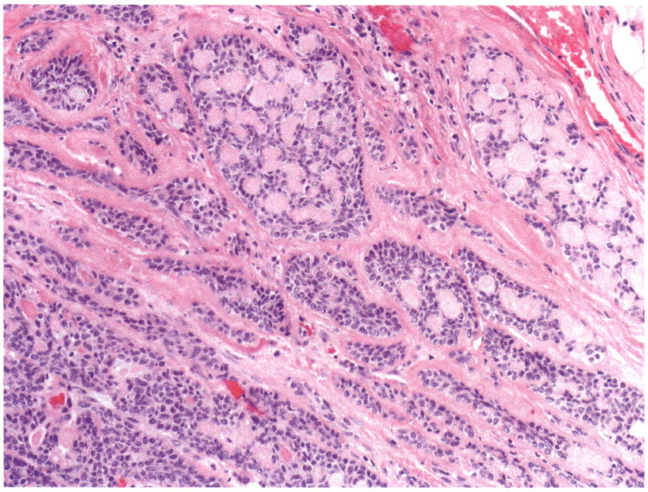

Fig. 9.10 (H&E, 200×) Basal cell adenocarcinoma, tubular and cribriform

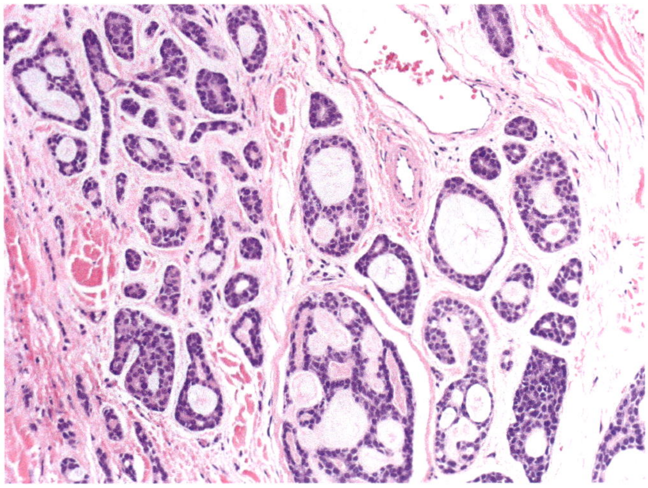

Fig. 9.11 (H&E, 200×) Basal cell adenocarcinoma, tubular and cribriform

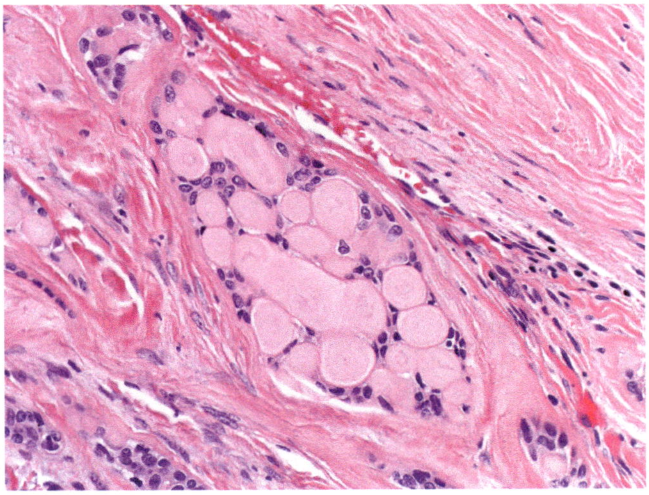

Fig. 9.12 (H&E, 400×) Basal cell adenocarcinoma, tubular and cribriform

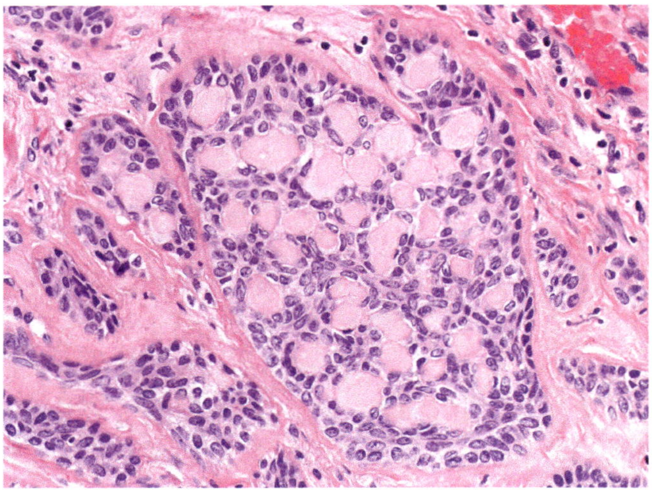

Fig. 9.13 (H&E, 400×) Basal cell adenocarcinoma, tubular and cribriform

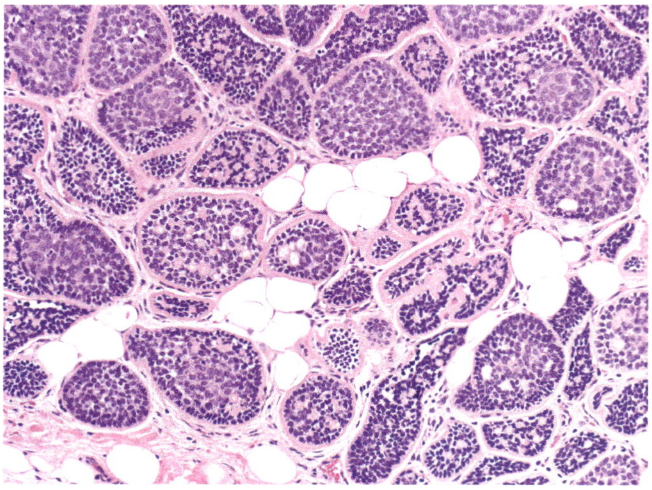

Fig. 9.14 (H&E, 200×) Basal cell adenocarcinoma, solid and cribriform

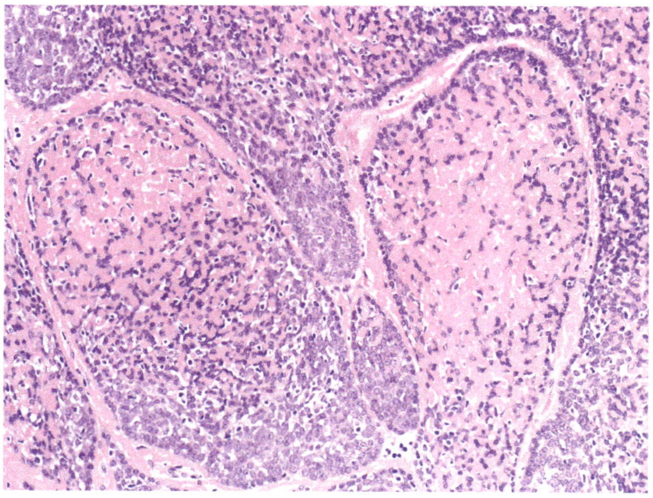

Fig. 9.15 (H&E, 200×) Basal cell adenocarcinoma, membranous

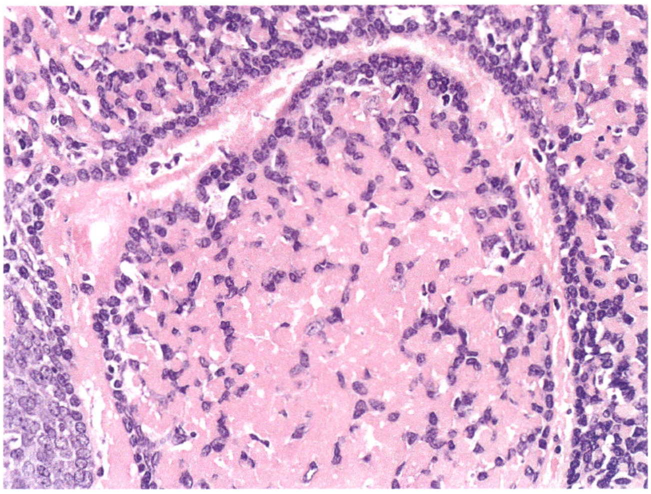

Fig. 9.16 (H&E, 400×) Basal cell adenocarcinoma, membranous

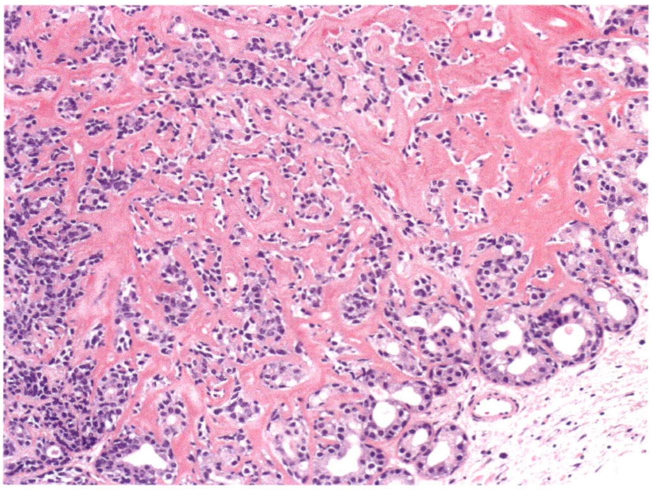

Fig. 9.17 (H&E, 200×) Basal cell adenocarcinoma, hyalinized

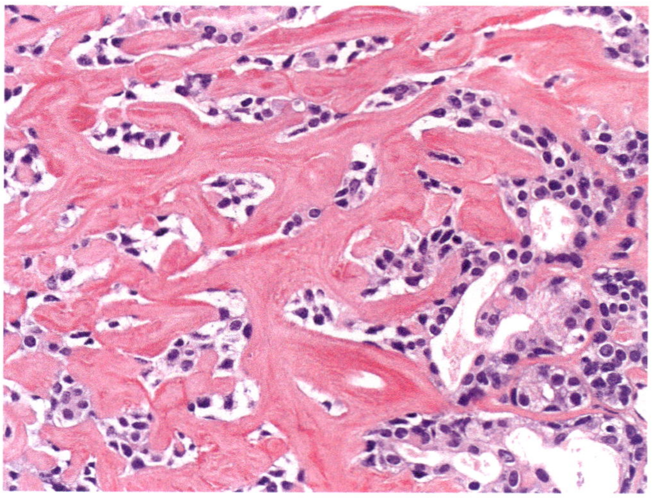

Fig. 9.18 (H&E, 400×) Basal cell adenocarcinoma, hyalinized

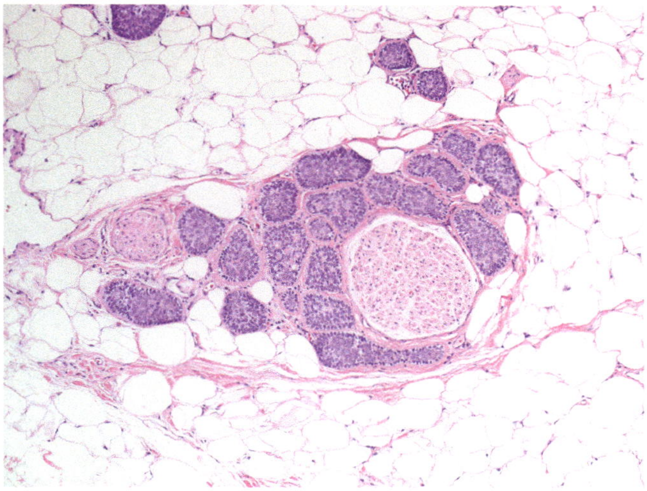

Fig. 9.19 (H&E, 100×) Basal cell adenocarcinoma, perineural invasion

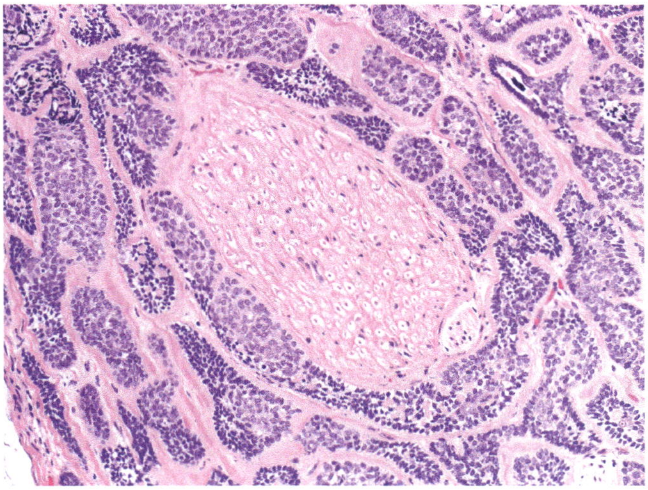

Fig. 9.20 (H&E, 200×) Basal cell adenocarcinoma, perineural invasion

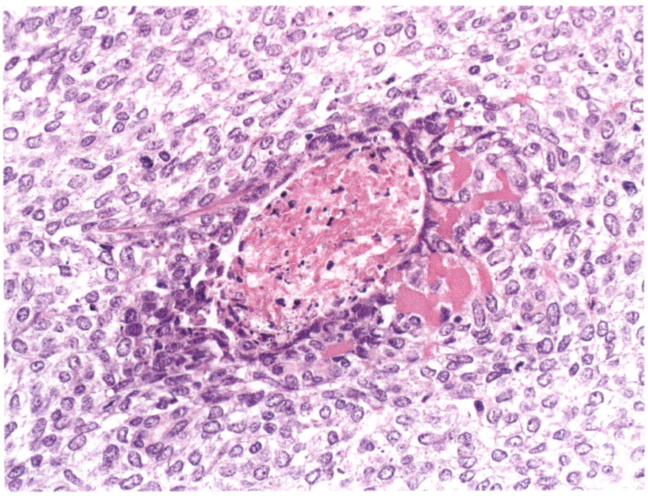

Fig. 9.21 (H&E, 400×) Basal cell adenocarcinoma, high-grade transformation, necrosis

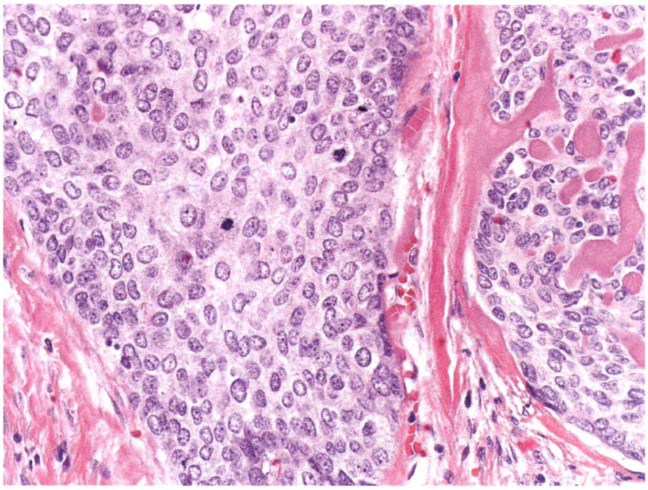

Fig. 9.22 (H&E, 400×) Basal cell adenocarcinoma, high-grade transformation, mitotic activity

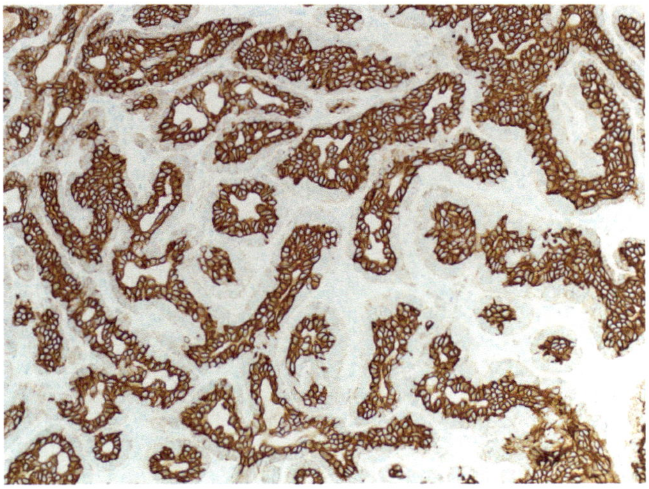

Fig. 9.23 (AE1/AE3, 200×) Basal cell adenocarcinoma, ductal immunoreactivity

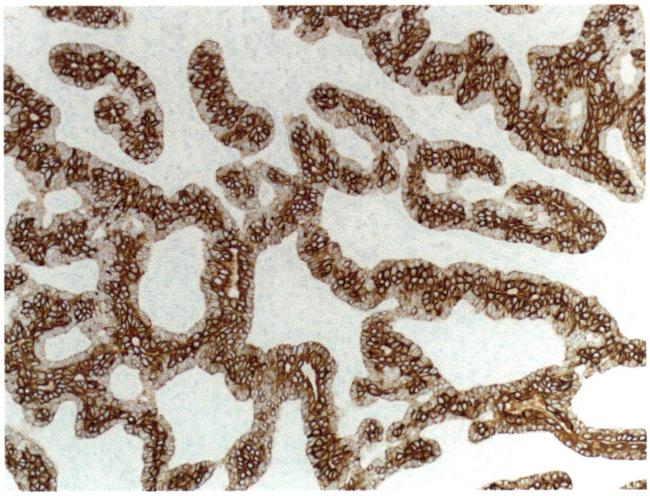

Fig. 9.24 (AE1/AE3, 200×) Basal cell adenocarcinoma, diffuse immunoreactivity

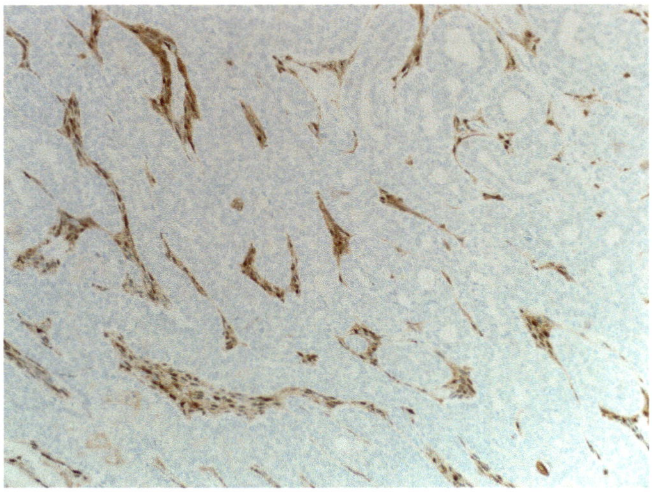

Fig. 9.25 (S-100, 200×) Basal cell adenocarcinoma, focal immunoreactivity

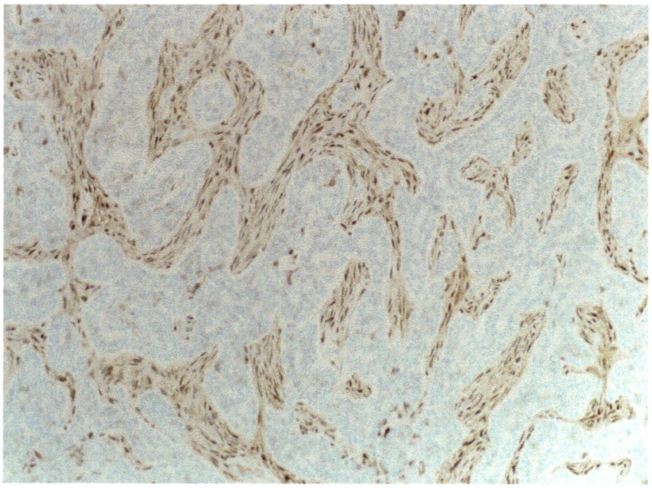

Fig. 9.26 (S-100, 200×) Basal cell adenocarcinoma, focal immunoreactivity

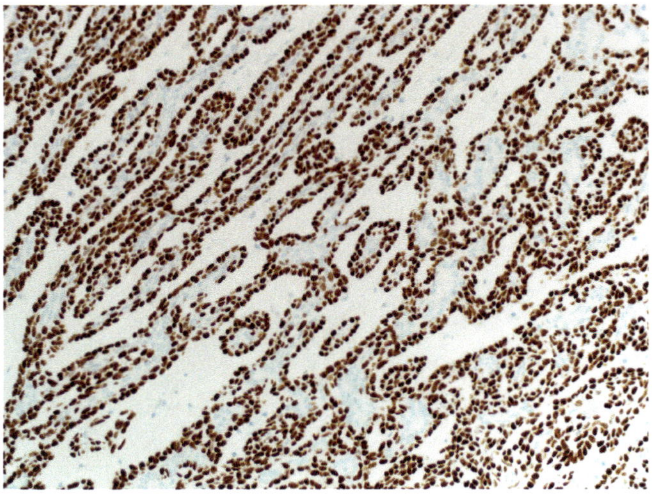

Fig. 9.27 (p63, 200×) Basal cell adenocarcinoma, basal immunoreactivity

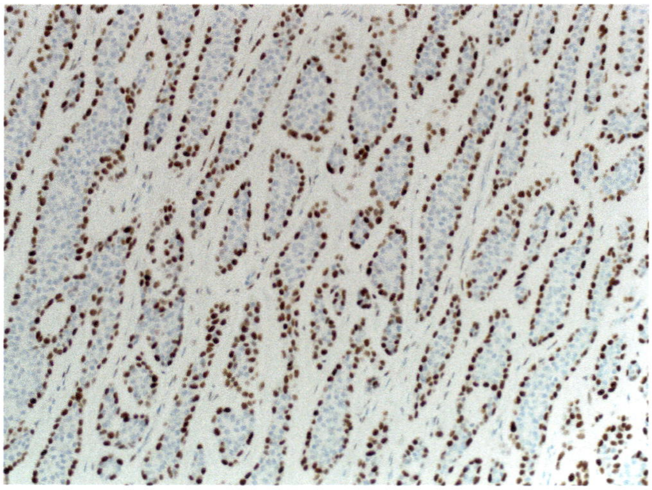

Fig. 9.28 (p63, 200×) Basal cell adenocarcinoma, basal immunoreactivity

Suggested Reading

Chhieng DC, Paulino AF. Basaloid tumors of the salivary glands. Ann Diagn Pathol. 2002;6(6):364–72.

Cuthbertson DW, Raol N, Hicks J, Green L, Parke R. Minor salivary gland basal cell adenocarcinoma: a systematic review and report of a new case. JAMA Otolaryngol Head Neck Surg. 2015;141:276–83.

Ellis GL, Wiscovitch JG. Basal cell adenocarcinomas of the major salivary glands. Oral Surg Oral Med Oral Pathol. 1990;69:461–9.

Hyman BA, Scheithauer BW, Weiland LH, Irons GB. Membranous basal cell adenoma of the parotid gland. Malignant transformation in a patient with multiple dermal cylindromas. Arch Pathol Lab Med. 1988;112:209–11.

Ide F, Kusama K. Sebaceous differentiation in basal cell adenocarcinoma of the submandibular gland. Virchows Arch. 2002;440(5): 547–8.

Klijanienko J, el-Naggar AK, Vielh P. Comparative cytologic and histologic study of fifteen salivary basal-cell tumors: differential diagnostic considerations. Diagn Cytopathol. 1999;21(1):30–4.

Muller S, Barnes L. Basal cell adenocarcinoma of the salivary glands. Report of seven cases and review of the literature. Cancer. 1996;78(12):2471–7.

Nagao T, Sugano I, Ishida Y, Hasegawa M, Matsuzaki O, Konno A, et al. Basal cell adenocarcinoma of the salivary glands: comparison with basal cell adenoma through assessment of cell proliferation, apoptosis, and expression of p53 and bcl-2. Cancer. 1998;82(3):439–47.

Scott AR, Faquin WC, Deschler DG. Parotid mass in a woman with multiple cutaneous cylindromas. Head Neck. 2010;32:684–7.

Williams SB, Ellis GL, Auclair PL. Immunohistochemical analysis of basal cell adenocarcinoma. Oral Surg Oral Med Oral Pathol. 1993;75(1):64–9.

Yu GY, Ubmüller J, Donath K. Membranous basal cell adenoma of the salivary gland: a clinicopathologic study of 12 cases. Acta Otolaryngol. 1998;118:588–93.

Zhan KY, Lentsch EJ. Basal cell adenocarcinomaof the major salivary glands; a population-level stdy of 509 cases. Laryngoscope. 2016;126(5):1086–90.

10 Canalicular Adenoma

Canalicular adenoma affects primarily adults and presents at a mean age of approximately 60 years. Women are involved less than men. The majority of cases involve the upper lip, presenting as single or multiple masses. Canalicular adenoma may be circumscribed or lobulated, comprised of one cell type (ductal), and exhibit a variety of architectural patterns (branching and anastomosing tubules) (Figs. 10.1–10.18).

J. J. García, *Atlas of Salivary Gland Pathology*, https://doi.org/10.1007/978-3-319-09021-4_10

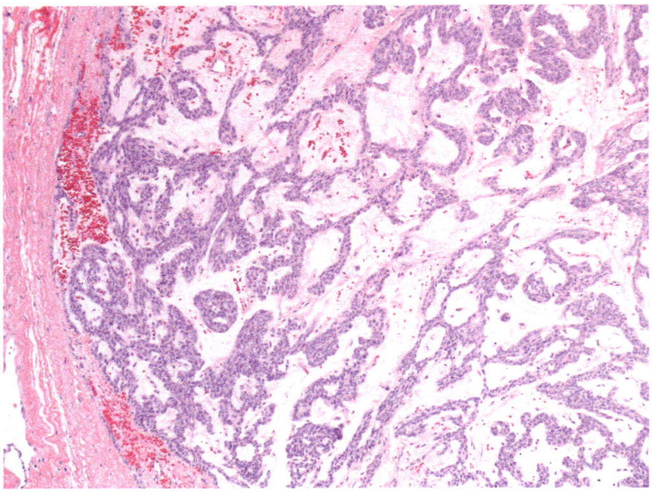

Fig. 10.1 (H&E, 100×) Canalicular adenoma, circumscribed

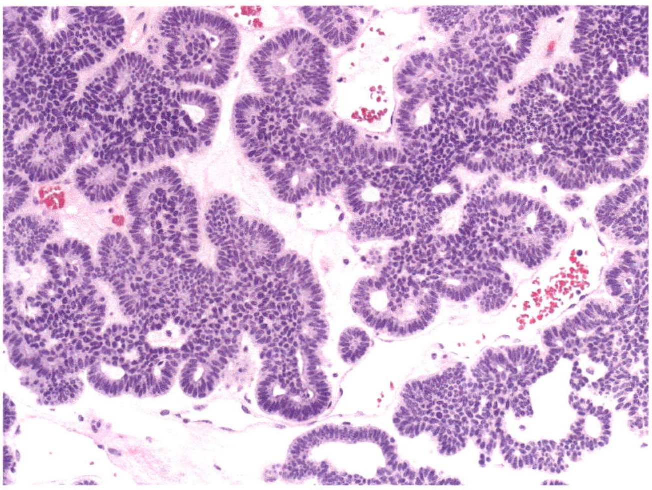

Fig. 10.2 (H&E, 200×) Canalicular adenoma, monophasic

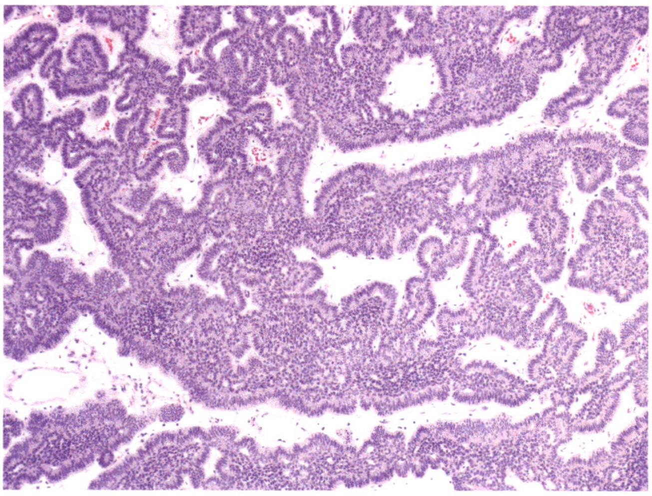

Fig. 10.3 (H&E, 100×) Canalicular adenoma, tubules

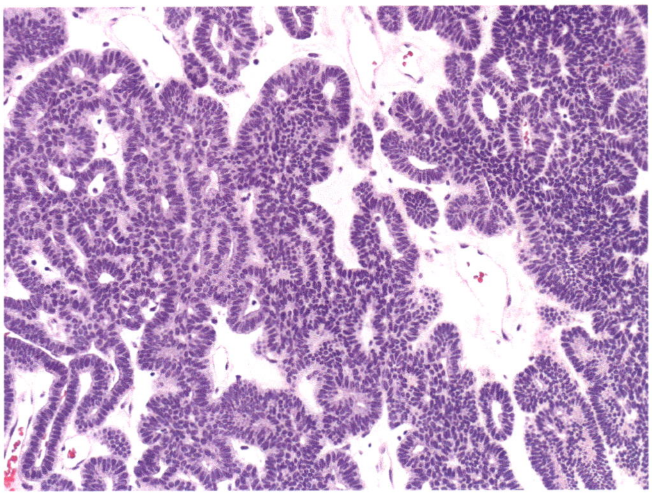

Fig. 10.4 (H&E, 200×) Canalicular adenoma, tubules

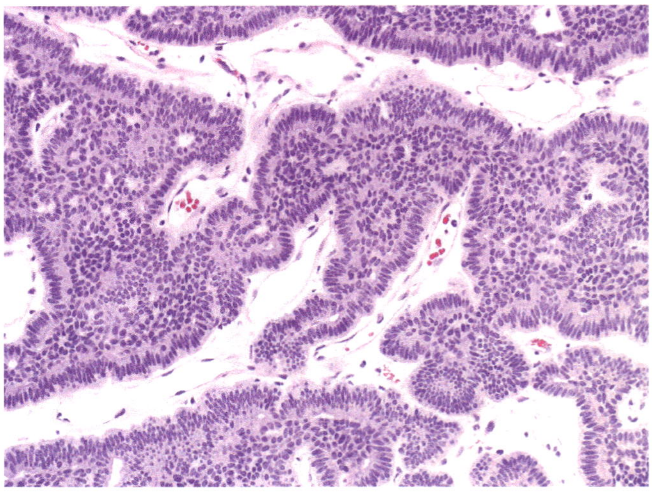

Fig. 10.5 (H&E, 200×) Canalicular adenoma, tubules

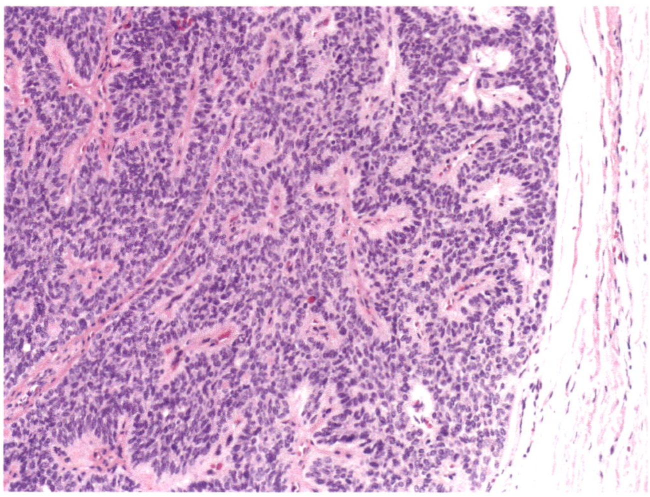

Fig. 10.6 (H&E, 200×) Canalicular adenoma, tubules

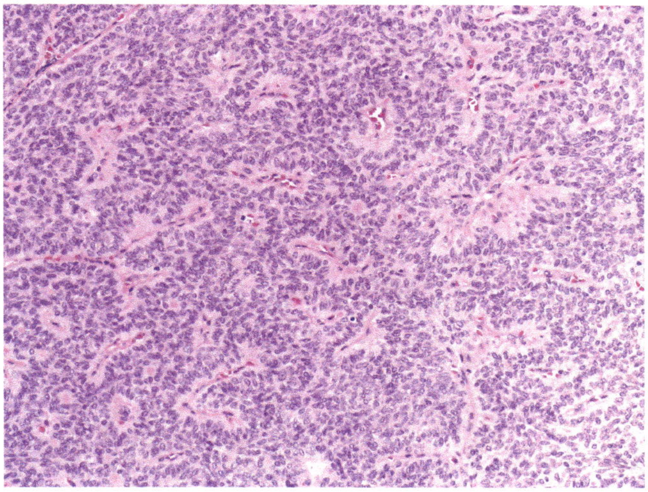

Fig. 10.7 (H&E, 200×) Canalicular adenoma, tubules

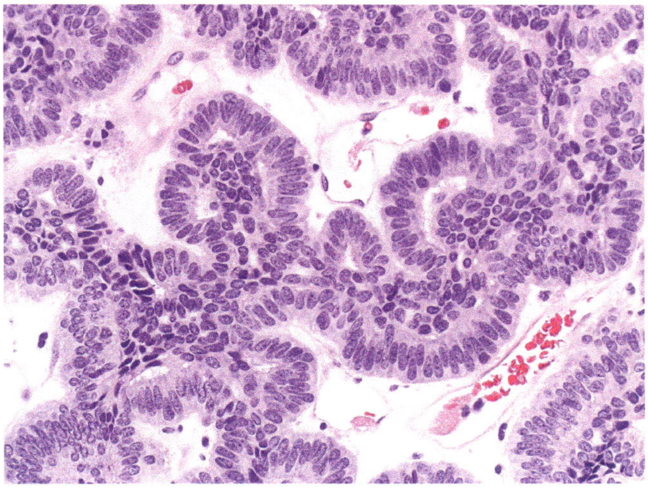

Fig. 10.8 (H&E, 400×) Canalicular adenoma, tubules

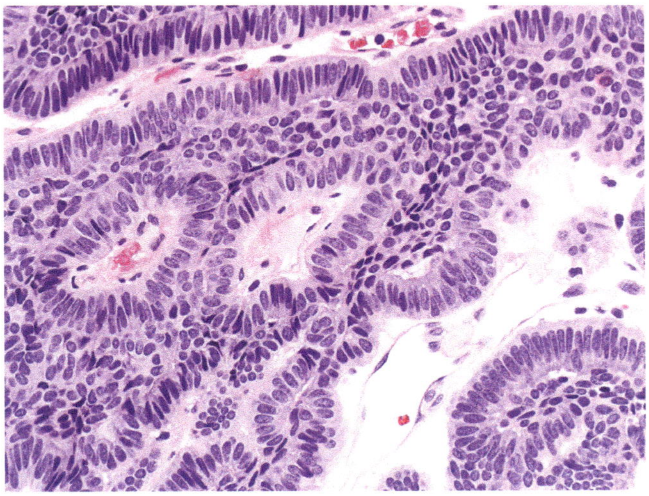

Fig. 10.9 (H&E, 400×) Canalicular adenoma, tubules

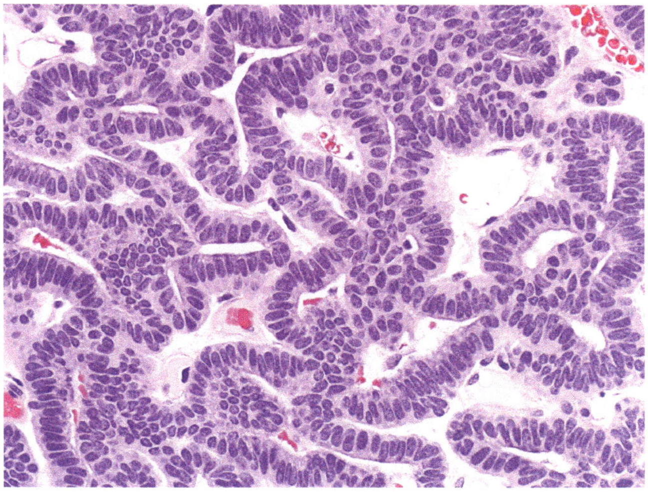

Fig. 10.10 (H&E, 400×) Canalicular adenoma, tubules

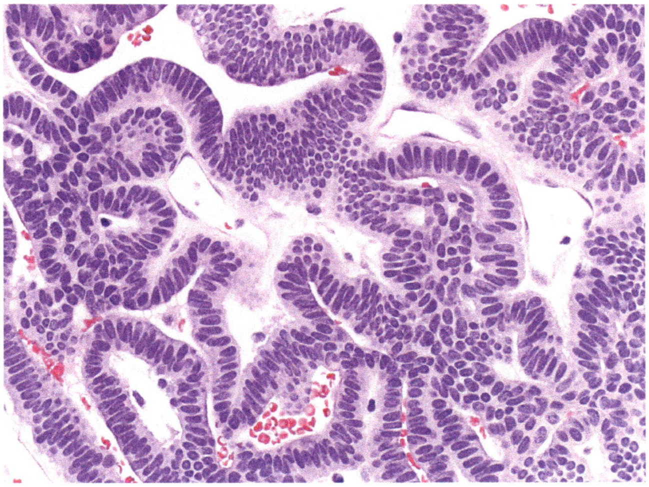

Fig. 10.11 (H&E, 400×) Canalicular adenoma, tubules

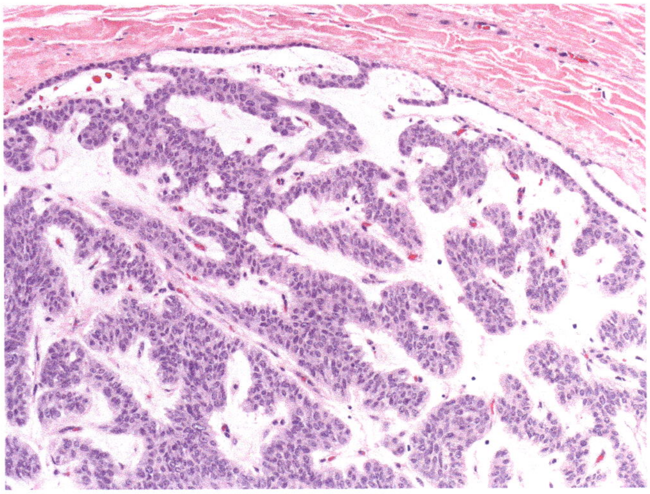

Fig. 10.12 (H&E, 200×) Canalicular adenoma, myxoid

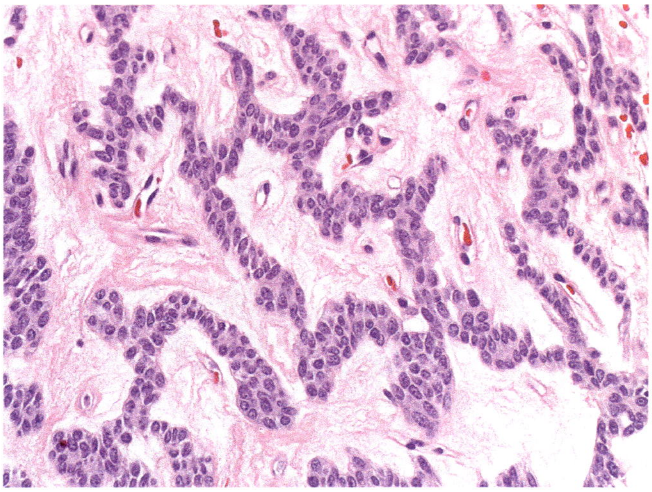

Fig. 10.13 (H&E, 400×) Canalicular adenoma, myxoid

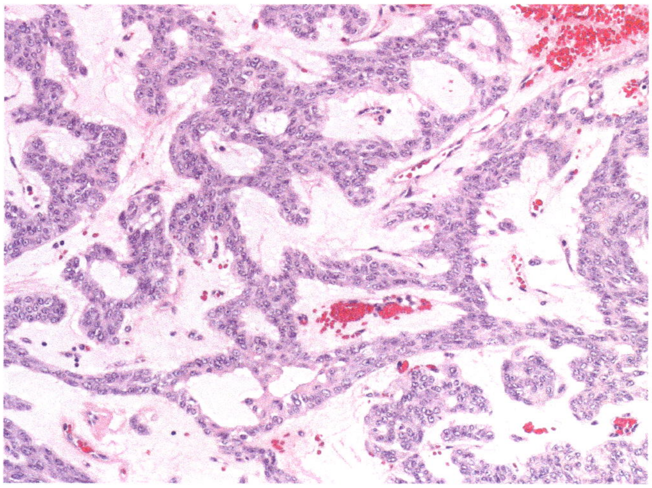

Fig. 10.14 (H&E, 200×) Canalicular adenoma, vascular

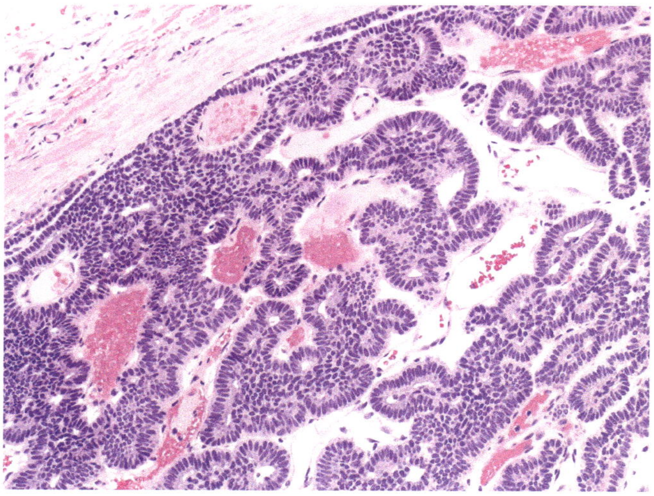

Fig. 10.15 (H&E, 200×) Canalicular adenoma, vascular

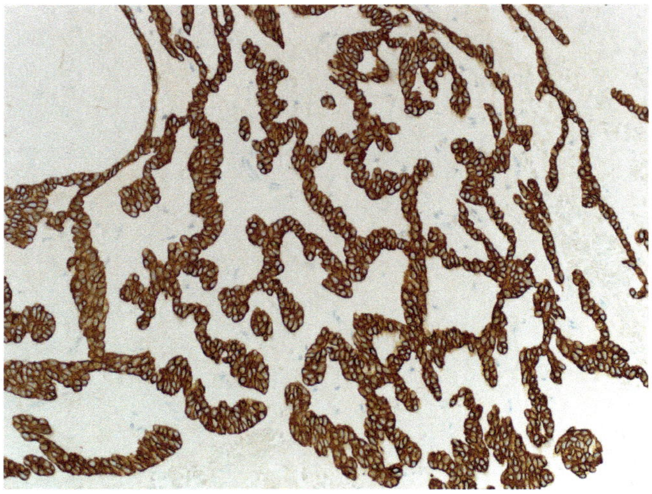

Fig. 10.16 (AE1/AE3, 200×) Canalicular adenoma, diffuse immunoreactivity

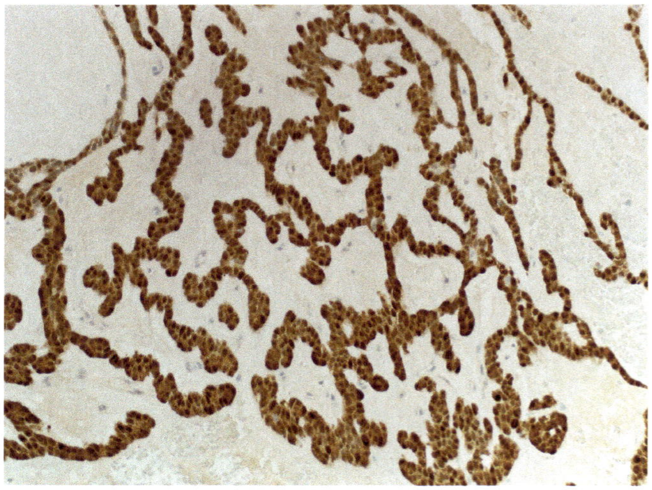

Fig. 10.17 (S-100, 200×) Canalicular adenoma, diffuse immunoreactivity

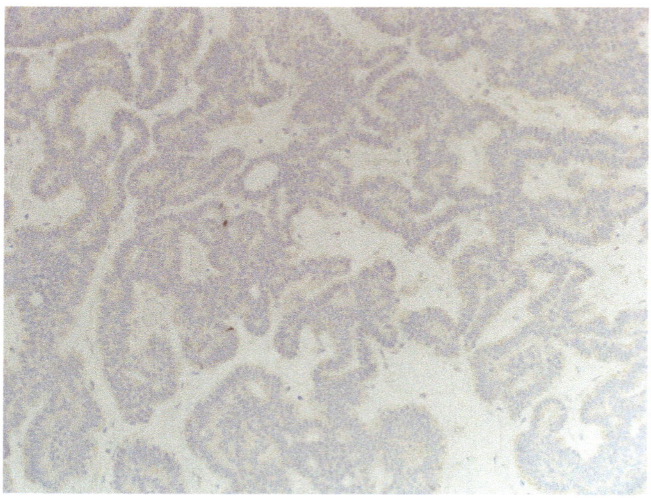

Fig. 10.18 (p63, 200×) Canalicular adenoma, rare immunoreactivity

Suggested Reading

Daley TD. The canalicular adenoma: considerations on differential diagnosis and treatment. J Oral Maxillofac Surg. 1984;42(11):728–30.

Daley TD, Gardner DG, Smout MS. Canalicular adenoma: not a basal cell adenoma. Oral Surg Oral Med Oral Pathol. 1984;57(2):181–8.

Edwards PC, Bhuiya T, Kelsch RD. Assessment of p63 expression in the salivary gland neoplasms adenoid cystic carcinoma, polymorphous low-grade adenocarcinoma, and basal cell and canalicular adenomas. Oral Surg Oral Med Oral Pathol Oral Radiol Endod. 2004;97(5):613–9.

Gardner DG, Daley TD. The use of the terms monomorphic adenoma, basal cell adenoma, and canalicular adenoma as applied to salivary gland tumors. Oral Surg Oral Med Oral Pathol. 1983;56(6):608–15.

Machado de Sousa SO, Soares de Araújo N, Corrêa L, Pires Soubhia AM, Cavalcanti de Araújo V. Immunohistochemical aspects of basal cell adenoma and canalicular adenoma of salivary glands. Oral Oncol. 2001;37(4):365–8.

Pires FR, Pringle GA, de Almeida OP, Chen SY. Intra-oral minor salivary gland tumors: a clinicopathological study of 546 cases. Oral Oncol. 2007;43:463–70.

Samar ME, Avila RE, Fonseca IB, Anderson W, Fonseca GM, Cantin M. Multifocal canalicular adenoma of the minor labial salivary glands. Int J Clin Exp Pathol. 2014;7:8205–10.

Thompson LD, Bauer JL, Chiosea S, McHugh JB, Seethala RR, Miettinen M, et al. Canalicular adenoma: a clinicopathologic and immunohistochemical analysis of 67 cases with a review of the literature. Head Neck Pathol. 2015;9:181–95.

Waldron CA, El-Mofty SK, Gnepp DR. Tumors of the intraoral minor salivary glands: a demographic and histologic study of 426 cases. Oral Surg Oral Med Oral Pathol. 1988;66:323–33.

Wang D, Li Y, He H, Liu L, Wu L, He Z. Intraoral minor salivary gland tumors in a Chinese population: a retrospective study on 737 cases. Oral Surg Oral Med Oral Pathol Oral Radiol Endod. 2007;104:94–100.

11 Carcinosarcoma

Carcinosarcoma is an exceedingly rare malignancy that affects adults and presents at a mean age of approximately 60 years. Women are involved less than men. The majority of cases involve major salivary glands, presenting as single or multiple masses. Most cases of carcinosarcoma behave as high-grade malignancies. Carcinosarcoma may be circumscribed or infiltrative and comprised of malignant epithelial and mesenchymal elements (Figs. 11.1–11.18).

J. J. García, *Atlas of Salivary Gland Pathology*, https://doi.org/10.1007/978-3-319-09021-4_11

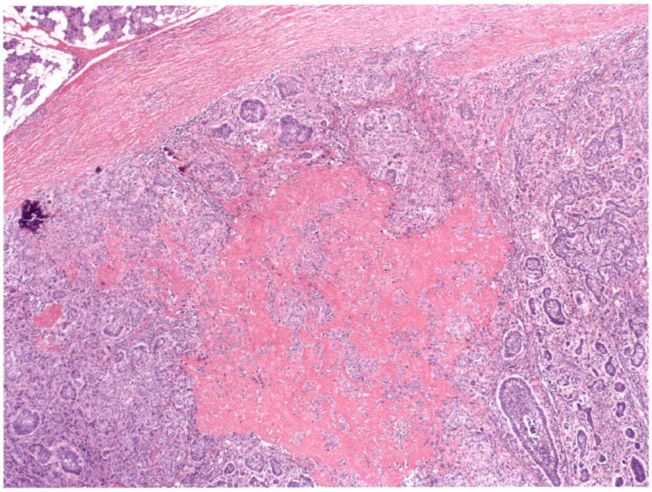

Fig. 11.1 (H&E, 40×) Carcinosarcoma, circumscribed

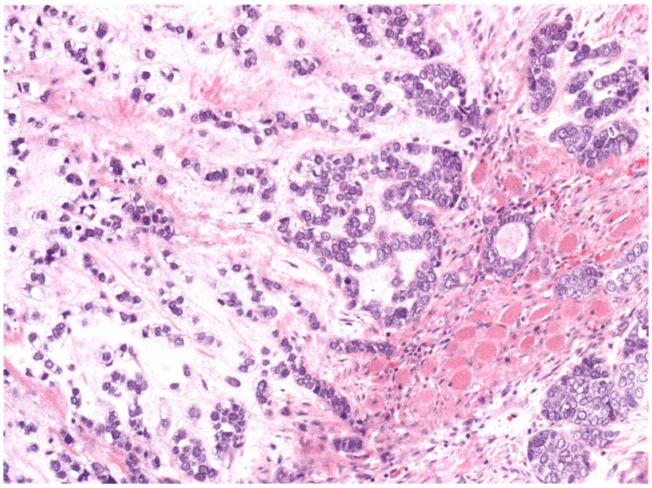

Fig. 11.2 (H&E, 200×) Carcinosarcoma, infiltrative

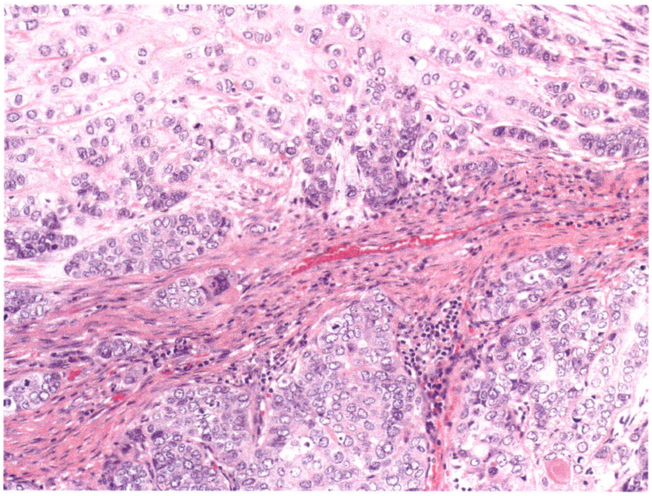

Fig. 11.3 (H&E, 200×) Carcinosarcoma, biphasic

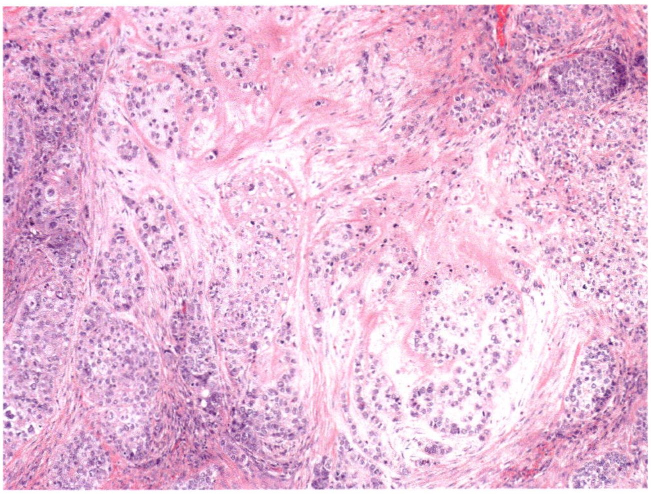

Fig. 11.4 (H&E, 100×) Carcinosarcoma, malignant epithelial and mesenchymal elements

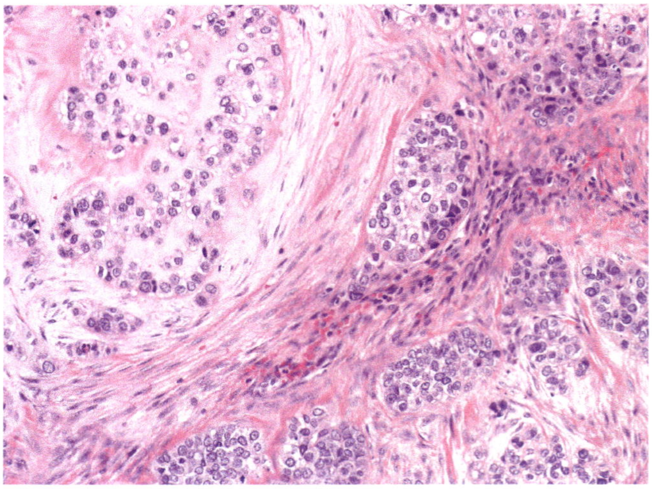

Fig. 11.5 (H&E, 200×) Carcinosarcoma, malignant epithelial and mesenchymal elements

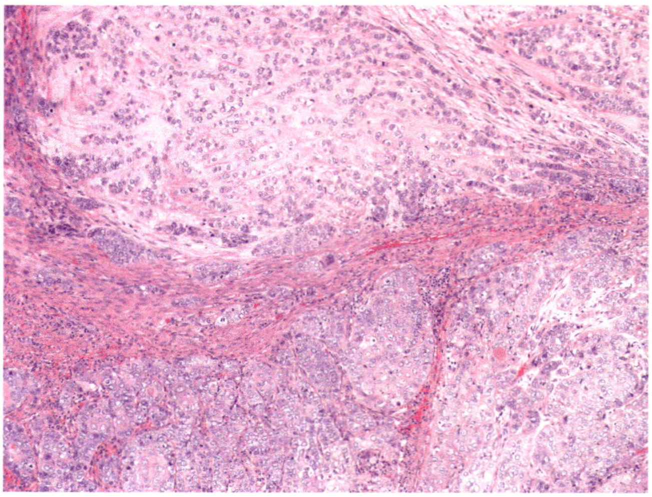

Fig. 11.6 (H&E, 100×) Carcinosarcoma, malignant epithelial and mesenchymal elements

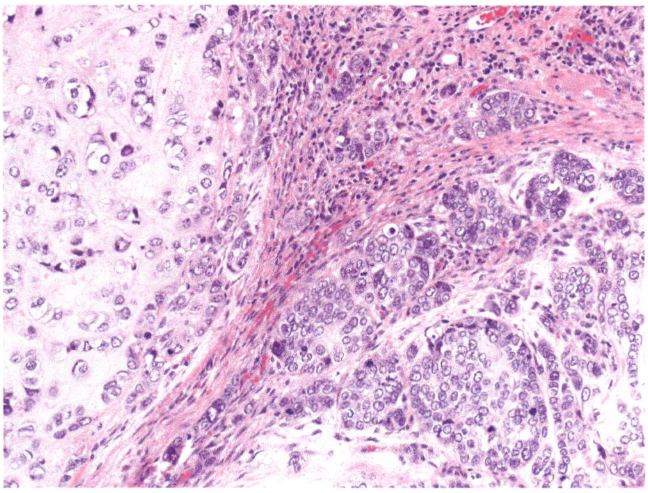

Fig. 11.7 (H&E, 200×) Carcinosarcoma, malignant epithelial and mesenchymal elements

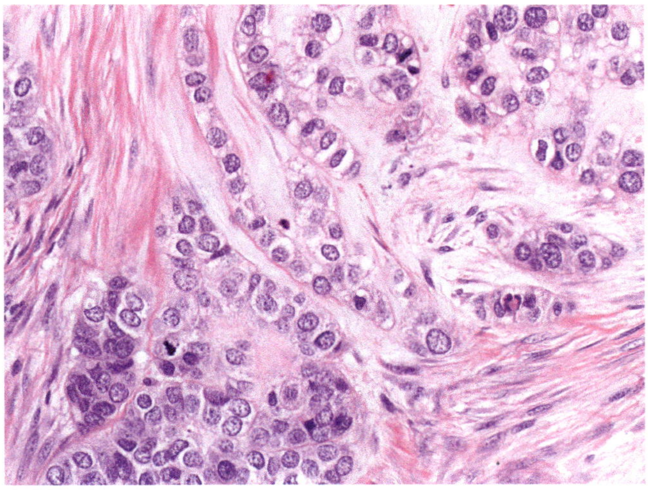

Fig. 11.8 (H&E, 400×) Carcinosarcoma, malignant epithelial and mesenchymal elements

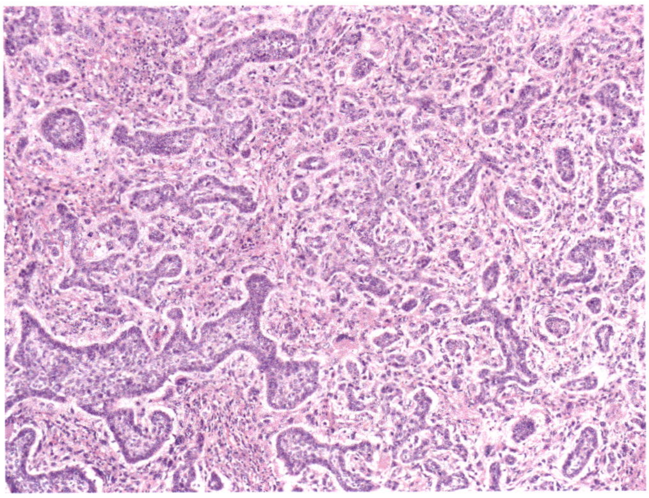

Fig. 11.9 (H&E, 100×) Carcinosarcoma, malignant epithelial and mesenchymal elements

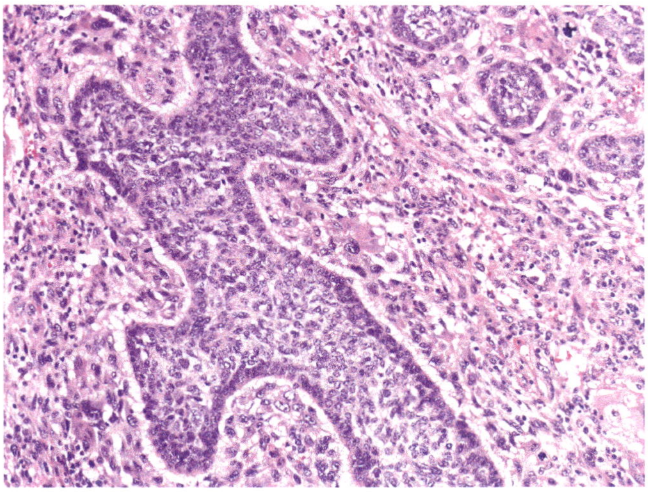

Fig. 11.10 (H&E, 200×) Carcinosarcoma, cytomorphologic atypia

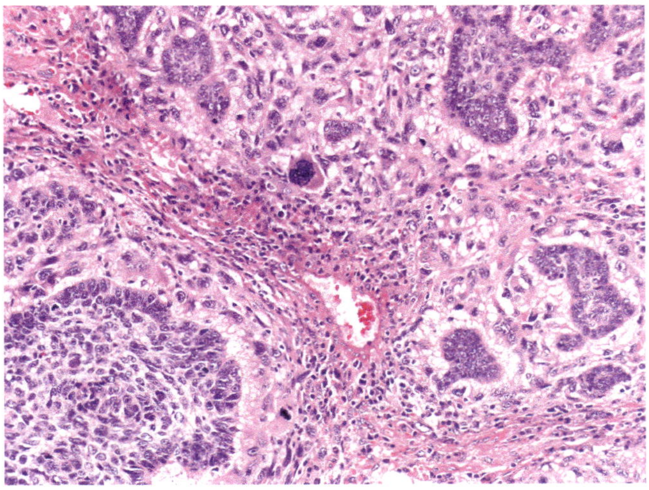

Fig. 11.11 (H&E, 400×) Carcinosarcoma, cytomorphologic atypia

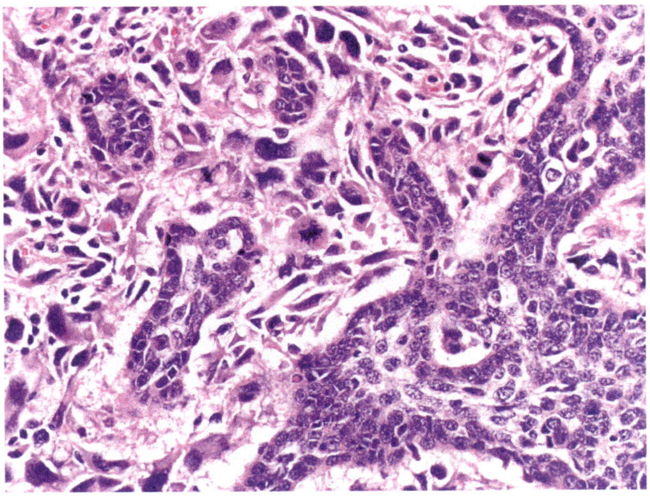

Fig. 11.12 (H&E, 400×) Carcinosarcoma, mitotic activity

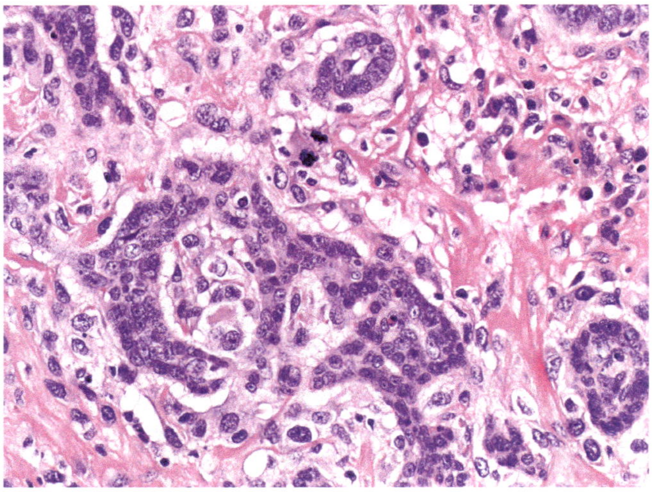

Fig. 11.13 (H&E, 400×) Carcinosarcoma, mitotic activity

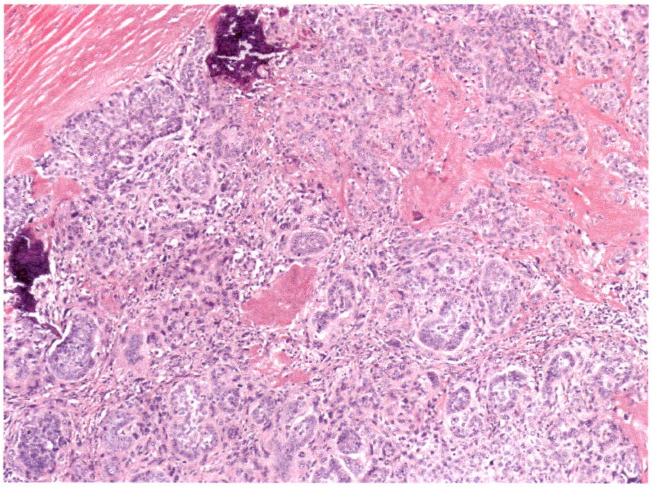

Fig. 11.14 (H&E, 100×) Carcinosarcoma, microcalcifications

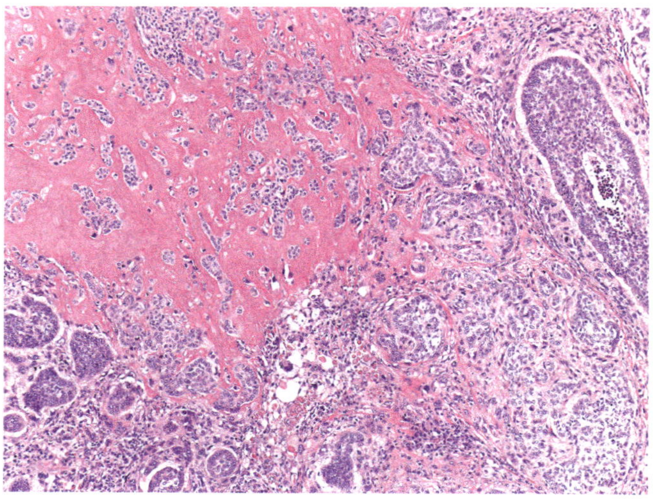

Fig. 11.15 (H&E, 100×) Carcinosarcoma, osteoid

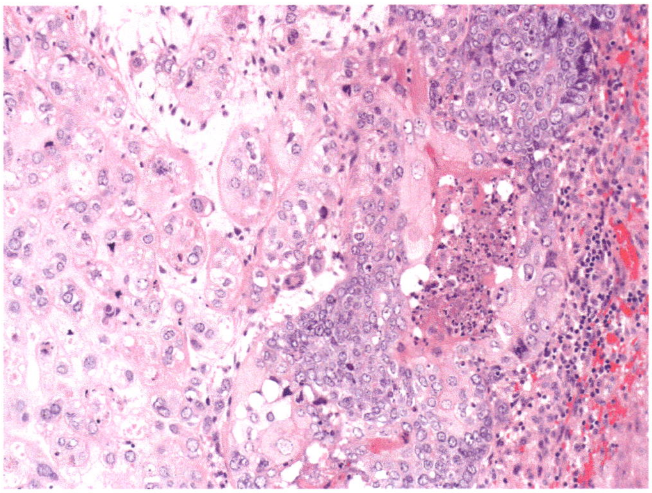

Fig. 11.16 (H&E, 200×) Carcinosarcoma, necrosis

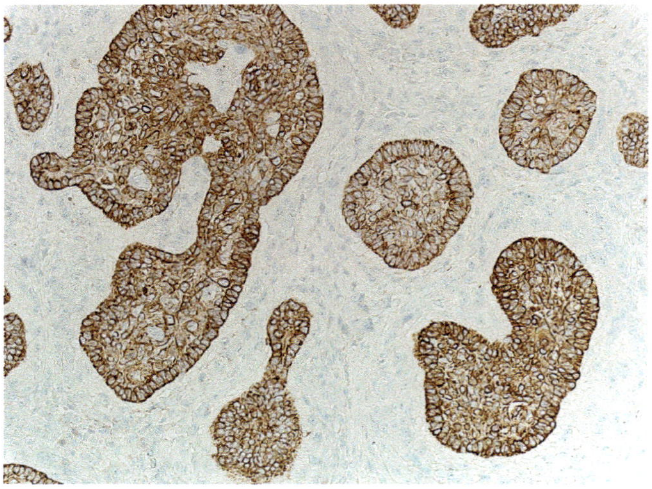

Fig. 11.17 (AE1/AE3, 200×) Carcinosarcoma, focal immunoreactivity

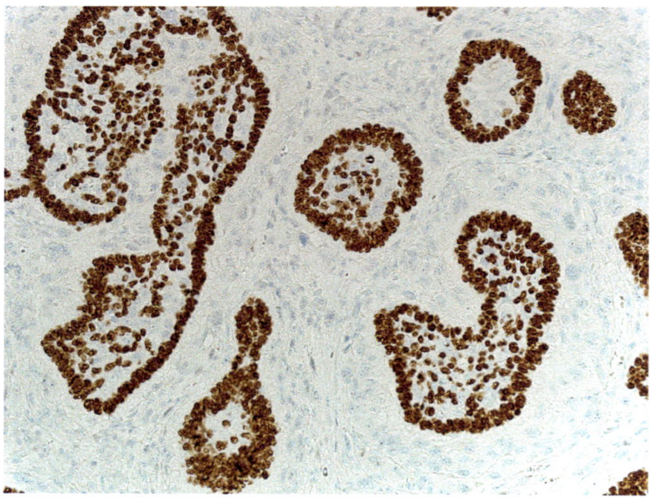

Fig. 11.18 (p63, 200×) Carcinosarcoma, focal immunoreactivity

Suggested Reading

Alvarez-Cañas C, Rodilla IG. True malignant mixed tumor (carcinosarcoma) of the parotid gland. Report of a case with immunohistochemical study. Oral Surg Oral Med Oral Pathol Oral Radiol Endod. 1996;81:454–8.

Bhalla RK, Jones TM, Taylor W, Roland NJ. Carcinosarcoma (malignant mixed tumor) of the submandibular gland: a case report and review of the literature. J Oral Maxillofac Surg. 2002;60(9): 1067–9.

Götte K, Riedel F, Coy JF, Spahn V, Hörmann K. Salivary gland carcinosarcoma: immunohistochemical, molecular genetic and electron microscopic findings. Oral Oncol. 2000;36(4):360–4.

Gnepp DR. Malignant mixed tumors of the salivary glands: a review. Pathol Annu. 1993;28:279–328.

Harada H. Histomorphological investigation regarding to malignant transformation of pleomorphic adenoma (so-called malignant mixed tumor) of the salivary gland origin; special reference to carcinosarcoma. Kurume Med J. 2000;47:307–23.

Kwon MY, Gu M. True malignant mixed tumor (carcinosarcoma) of parotid gland with unusual mesenchymal component: a case report and review of the literature. Arch Pathol Lab Med. 2001;125(6):812–5.

Stephen J, Batsakis JG, Luna MA, von der Heyden U, Byers RM. True malignant mixed tumors (carcinosarcoma) of salivary glands. Oral Surg Oral Med Oral Pathol. 1986;61:597–602.

Taki NH, Laver N, Quinto T, Wein RO. Carcinosarcoma de novo of the parotid gland: case report. Head Neck. 2013;35:E161–3.

12 Clear Cell Carcinoma

Clear cell carcinoma affects primarily adults and presents at a mean age of approximately 60 years. Women are involved more than men. The majority of cases involve minor salivary glands in the oral cavity, presenting as single or multiple masses. Most cases of clear cell carcinoma behave as low-grade malignancies. Clear cell carcinoma is infiltrative, comprised of one cell type (clear and/or eosinophilic), and may exhibit a variety of architectural patterns (solid, trabecular, and single cells) with or without hyalinized stroma (Figs. 12.1–12.20).

J. J. García, *Atlas of Salivary Gland Pathology*, https://doi.org/10.1007/978-3-319-09021-4_12

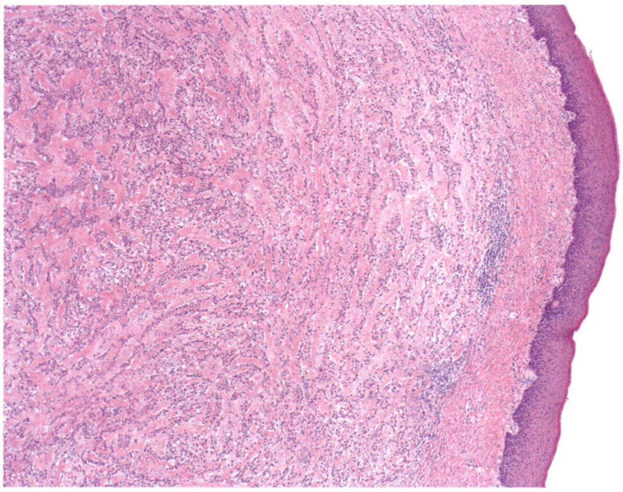

Fig. 12.1 (H&E, 40×) Clear cell carcinoma, circumscribed

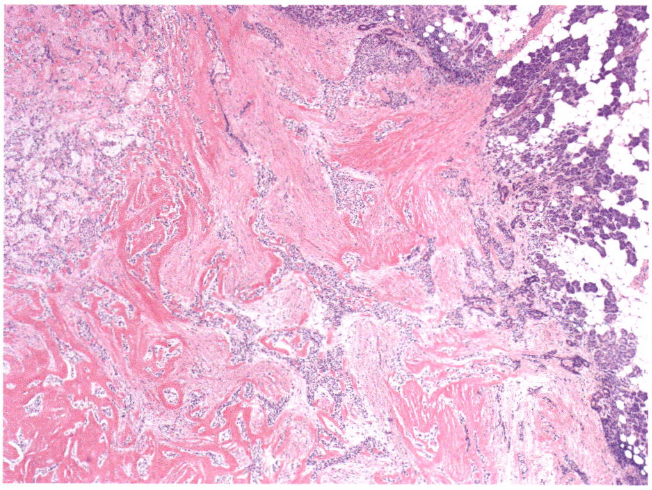

Fig. 12.2 (H&E, 40×) Clear cell carcinoma, infiltrative

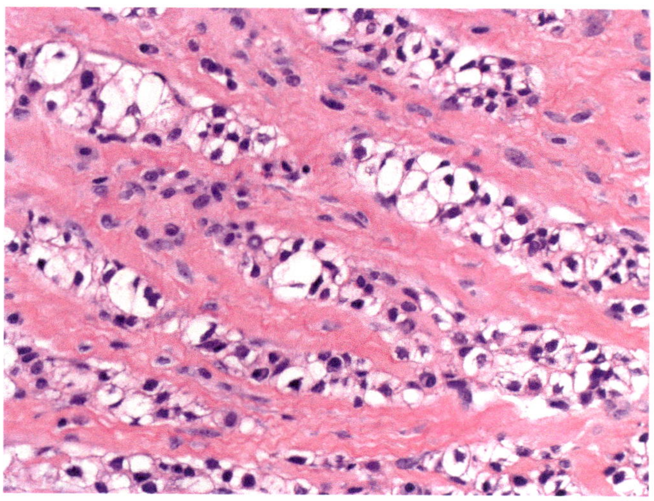

Fig. 12.3 (H&E, 400×) Clear cell carcinoma, monophasic

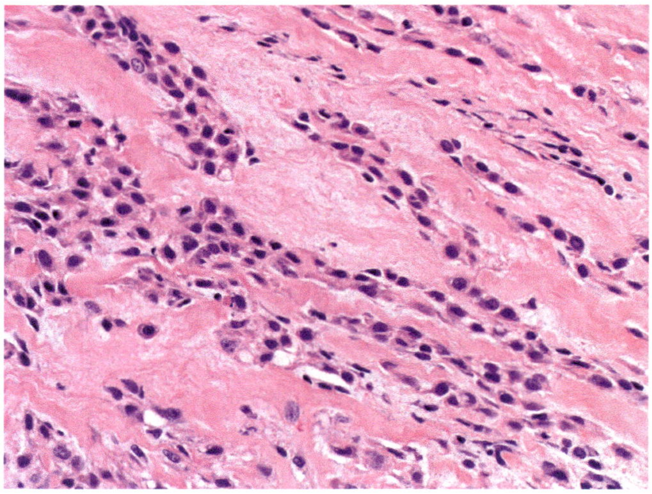

Fig. 12.4 (H&E, 400×) Clear cell carcinoma, eosinophilic

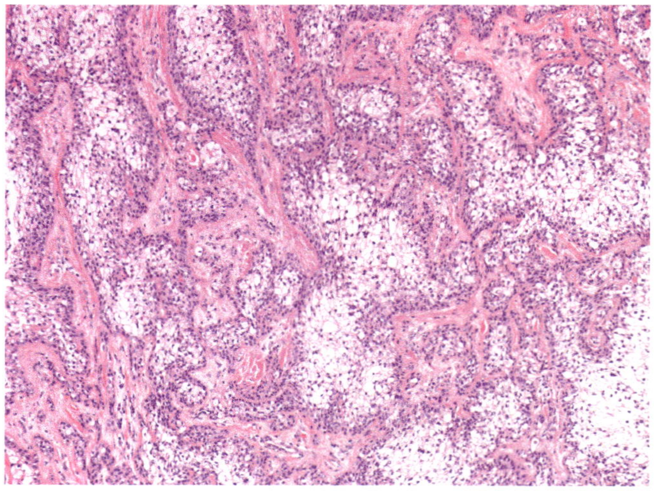

Fig. 12.5 (H&E, 100×) Clear cell carcinoma, eosinophilic and clear

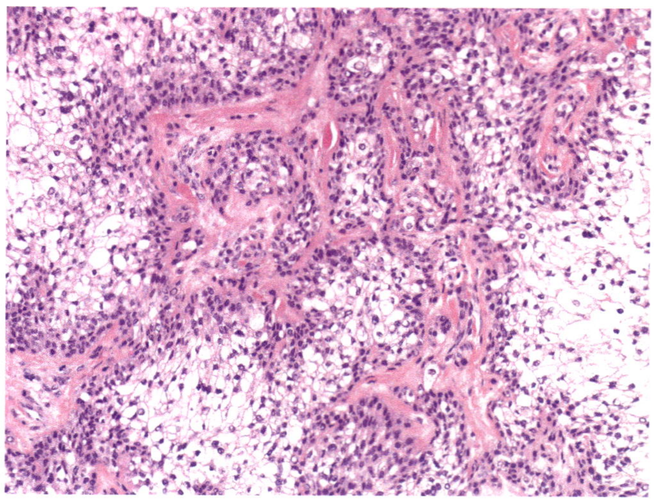

Fig. 12.6 (H&E, 200×) Clear cell carcinoma, eosinophilic and clear

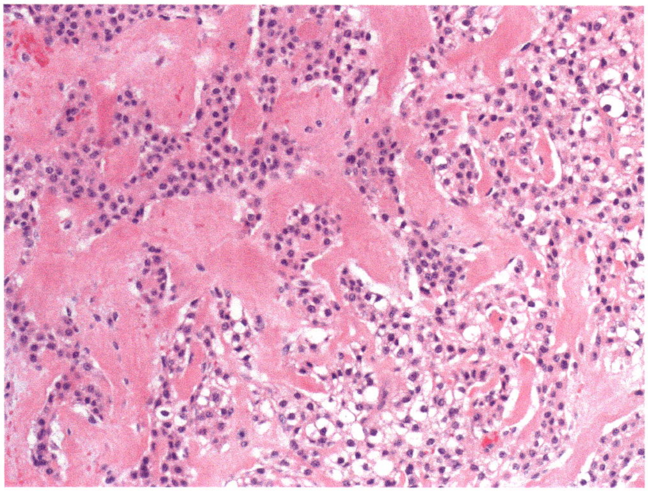

Fig. 12.7 (H&E, 200×) Clear cell carcinoma, eosinophilic and clear

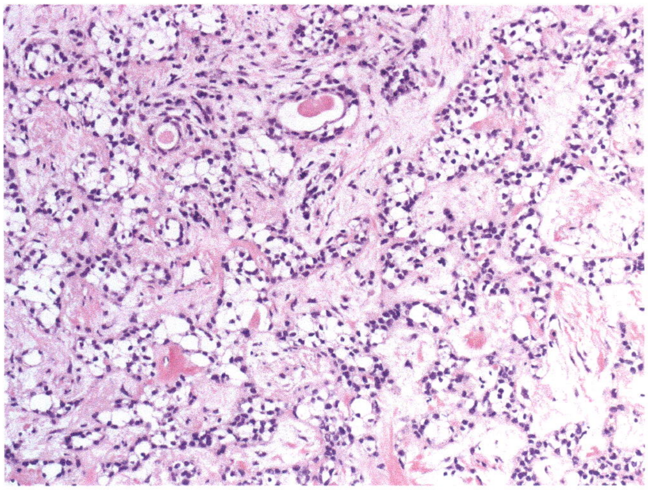

Fig. 12.8 (H&E, 200×) Clear cell carcinoma, clear

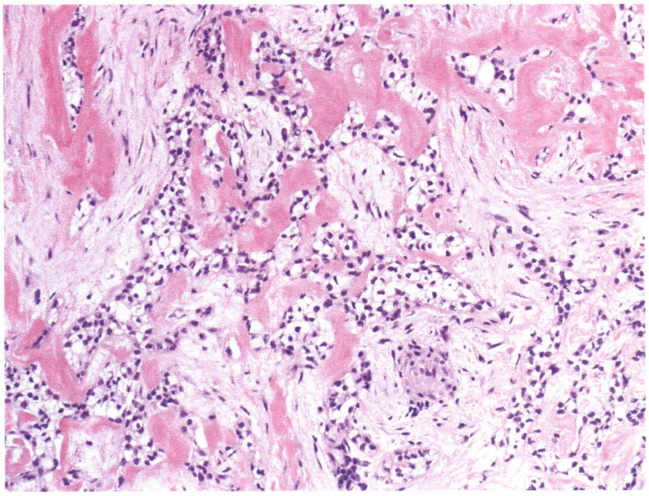

Fig. 12.9 (H&E, 200×) Clear cell carcinoma, clear

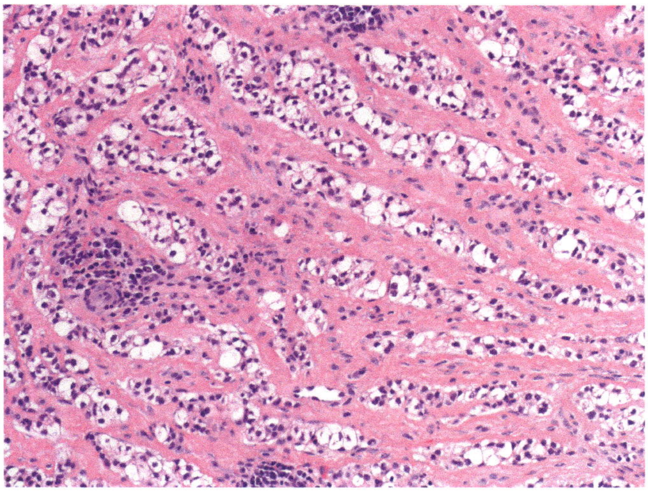

Fig. 12.10 (H&E, 200×) Clear cell carcinoma, clear

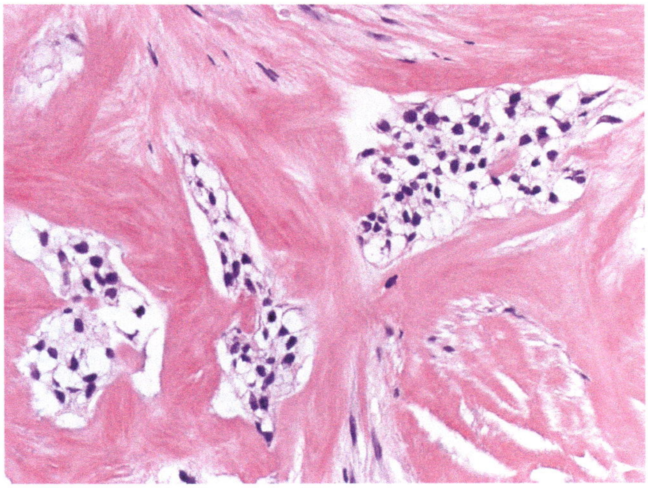

Fig. 12.11 (H&E, 400×) Clear cell carcinoma, clear

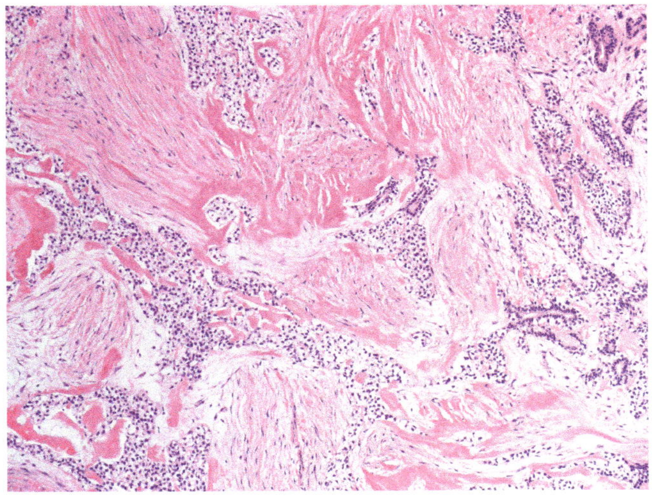

Fig. 12.12 (H&E, 100×) Clear cell carcinoma, hyalinizing

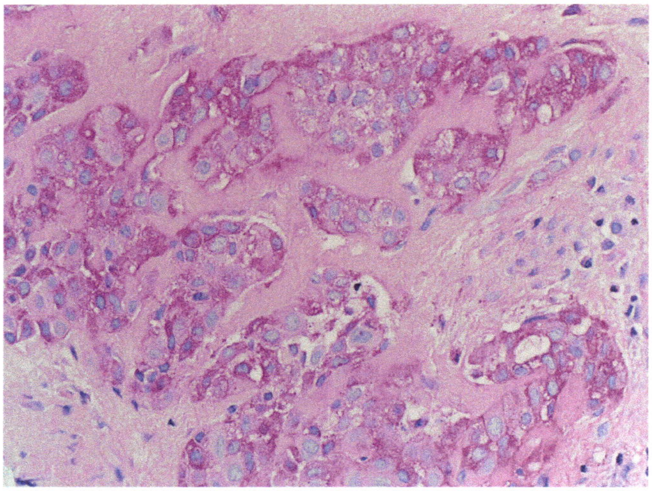

Fig. 12.13 (PAS, 400×) Clear cell carcinoma, intracytoplasmic reactivity

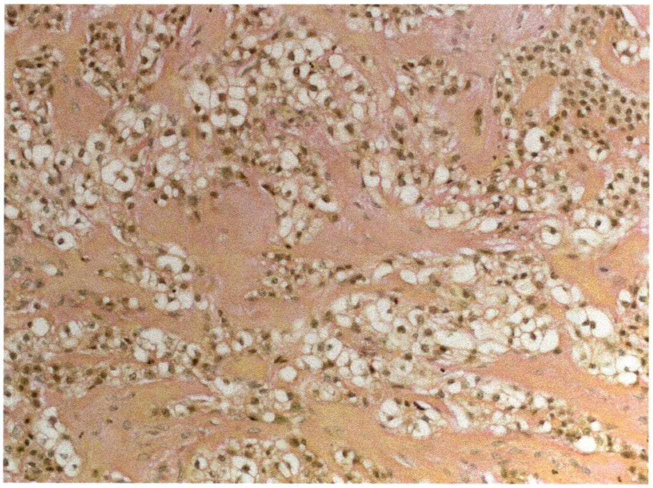

Fig. 12.14 (Mucicarmine, 200×) Clear cell carcinoma, negative reactivity

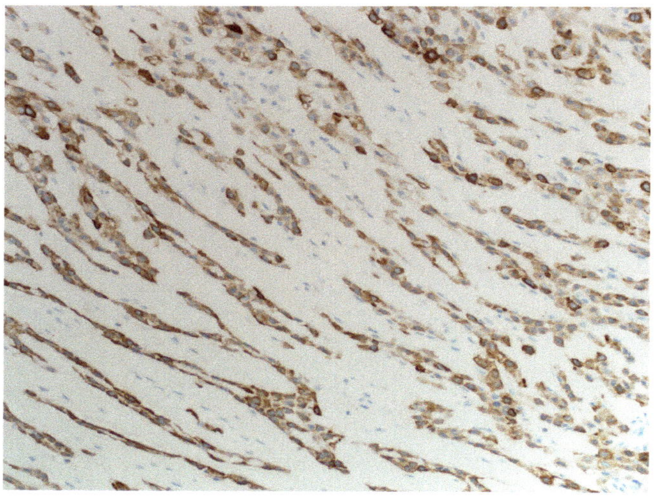

Fig. 12.15 (AE1/AE3, 200×) Clear cell carcinoma, diffuse immunoreactivity

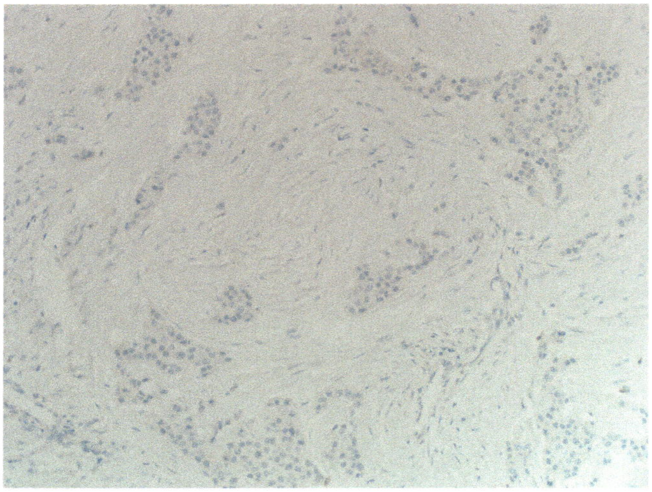

Fig. 12.16 (S-100, 200×) Clear cell carcinoma, negative immunoreactivity

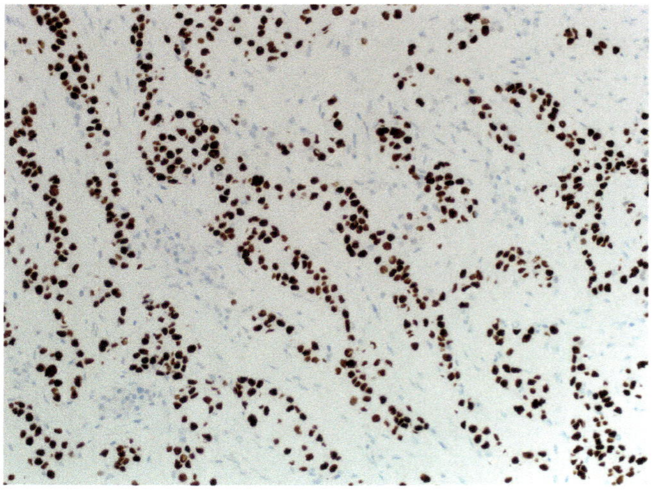

Fig. 12.17 (p63, 200×) Clear cell carcinoma, diffuse immunoreactivity

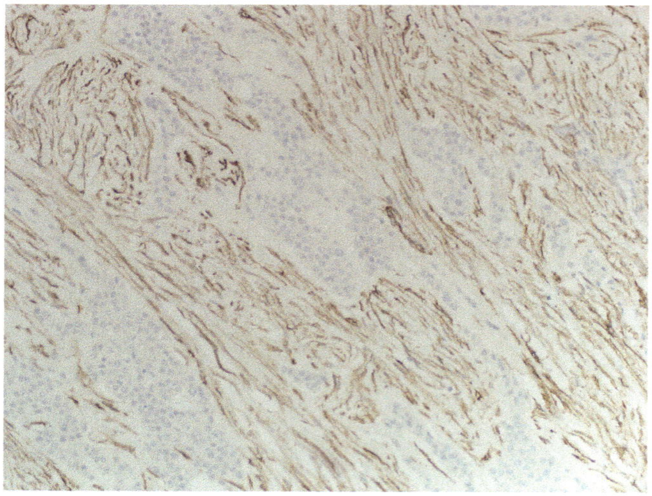

Fig. 12.18 (SMA, 200×) Clear cell carcinoma, negative immunoreactivity

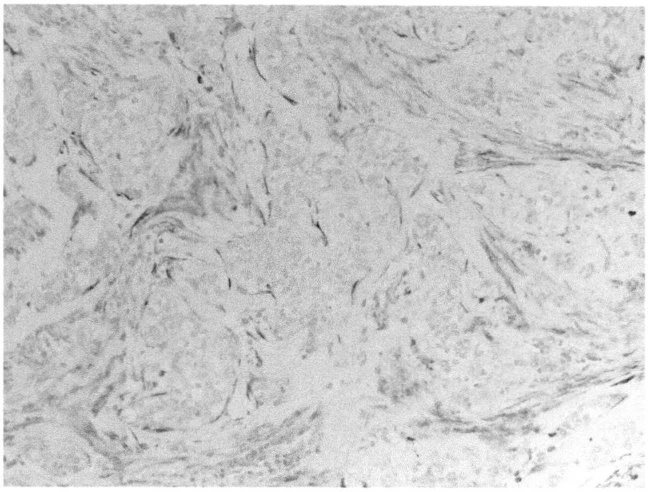

Fig. 12.19 (Calponin, 200×) Clear cell carcinoma, negative immunoreactivity

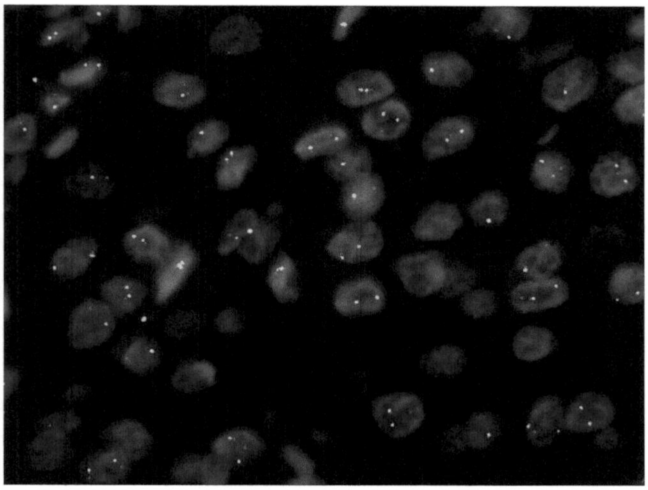

Fig. 12.20 (Fluorescent in situ hybridization, 600×) Clear cell carcinoma, *EWSR1* rearrangement

Suggested Reading

Antonescu CR, Katabi N, Zhang L, Sung YS, Seethala RR, Jordan RC, et al. EWSR1-ATF1 fusion is a novel and consistent finding in hyalinizing clear-cell carcinoma of salivary gland. Genes Chromosomes Cancer. 2011;50(7):559–70.

Jin R, Craddock KJ, Irish JC, Perez-Ordonez B, Weinreb I. Recurrent hyalinizing clear cell carcinoma of the base of tongue with high-grade transformation and EWSR1 gene rearrangement by FISH. Head Neck Pathol. 2012;6(3):389–94.

Lai G, Nemolato S, Lecca S, Parodo G, Medda C, Faa G. The role of immunohistochemistry in the diagnosis of hyalinizing clear cell carcinoma of the minor salivary gland: a case report. Eur J Histochem. 2008;52:251–4.

Milchgrub S, Gnepp DR, Vuitch F, Delgado R, Albores-Saavedra J. Hyalinizing clear cell carcinoma of salivary gland. Am J Surg Pathol. 1994;18(1):74–82.

Milchgrub S, Vuitch F, Saboorian MH, Hameed A, Wu H, Albores-Saavedra J. Hyalinizing clear-cell carcinoma of salivary glands in fine-needle aspiration. Diagn Cytopathol. 2000;23(5):333–7.

O'Sullivan-Mejia ED, Massey HD, Faquin WC, Powers CN. Hyalinizing clear cell carcinoma: report of eight cases and a review of literature. Head Neck Pathol. 2009;3:179–85.

Shah AA, LeGallo RD, van Zante A, Frierson HF Jr, Mills SE, Berean KW, et al. EWSR1 genetic rearrangements in salivary gland tumors: a specific and very common feature of hyalinizing clear cell carcinoma. Am J Surg Pathol. 2013;37(4):571–8.

Simpson RH, Sarsfield PT, Clarke T, Babajews AV. Clear cell carcinoma of minor salivary glands. Histopathology. 1990;17(5):433–8.

Solar AA, Schmidt BL, Jordan RC. Hyalinizing clear cell carcinoma: case series and comprehensive review of the literature. Cancer. 2009;115(1):75–83.

Tanguay J, Weinreb I. What the EWSR1-ATF1 fusion has taught us about hyalinizing clear cell carcinoma. Head Neck Pathol. 2013;7:28–34.

Wang B, Brandwein M, Gordon R, Robinson R, Urken M, Zarbo RJ. Primary salivary clear cell tumors—a diagnostic approach: a clinicopathologic and immunohistochemical study of 20 patients with clear cell carcinoma, clear cell myoepithelial carcinoma, and epithelial-myoepithelial carcinoma. Arch Pathol Lab Med. 2002;126(6):676–85.

Weinreb I. Hyalinizing clear cell carcinoma of salivary gland: a review and update. Head Neck Pathol. 2013;7(Suppl 1):S20–9.

13 Epithelial-Myoepithelial Carcinoma

Epithelial-myoepithelial carcinoma affects children and adults and presents at a mean age of approximately 60 years. Women are involved slightly more than men. The majority of cases involve the parotid gland, presenting as single or multiple masses. Most cases of epithelial-myoepithelial carcinoma behave as low to intermediate grade malignancies; however, a subset of cases with high-grade transformation (necrosis, elevated mitotic activity, and cytomorphologic atypia) are predisposed to recurrence, lymph node involvement, and distant metastasis. Epithelial-myoepithelial carcinoma may be circumscribed or infiltrative, comprised of multiple cell types (ductal and myoepithelial), and exhibit a variety of architectural patterns (tubular, cystic, and solid) (Figs. 13.1–13.36).

J. J. García, *Atlas of Salivary Gland Pathology*, https://doi.org/10.1007/978-3-319-09021-4_13

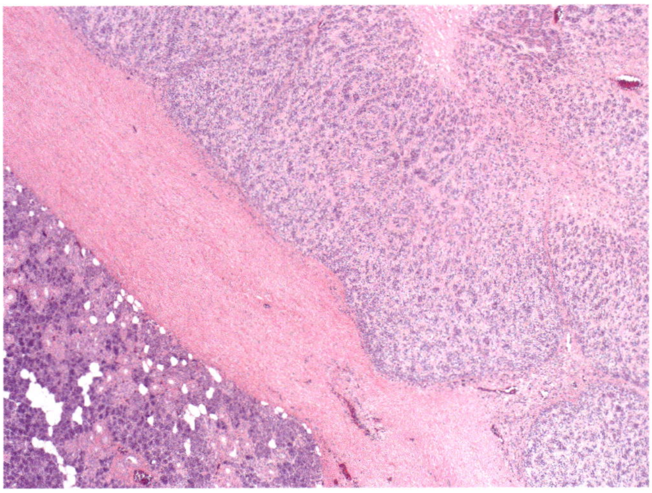

Fig. 13.1 (H&E, 40×) Epithelial-myoepithelial carcinoma, encapsulated

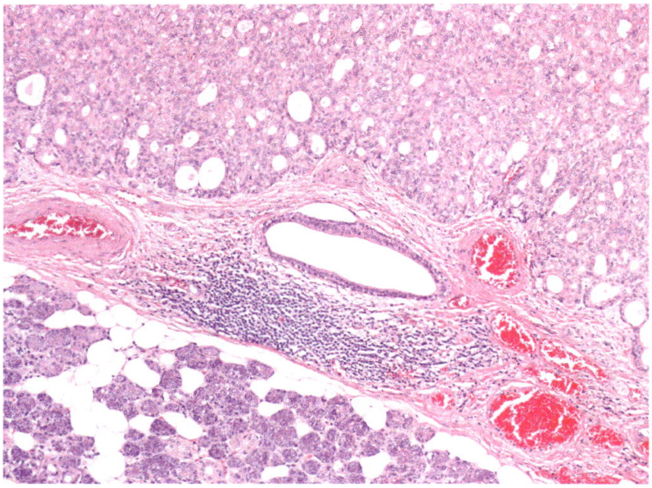

Fig. 13.2 (H&E, 100×) Epithelial-myoepithelial carcinoma, circumscribed

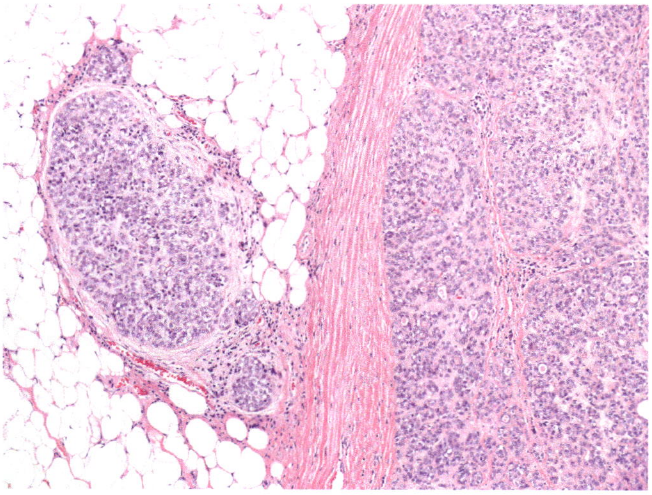

Fig. 13.3 (H&E, 100×) Epithelial-myoepithelial carcinoma, infiltrative

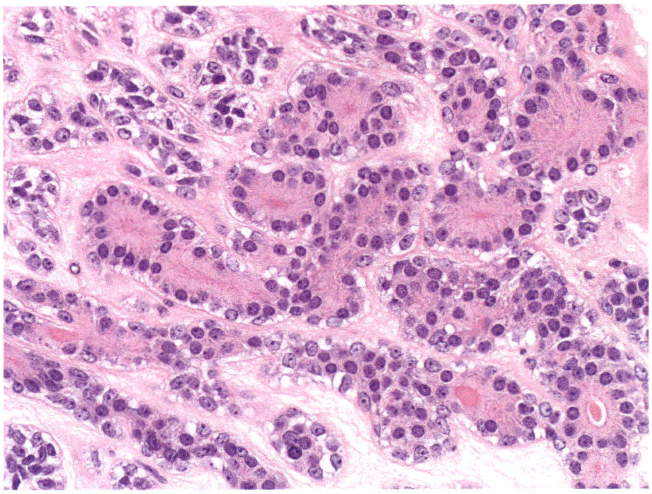

Fig. 13.4 (H&E, 400×) Epithelial-myoepithelial carcinoma, biphasic

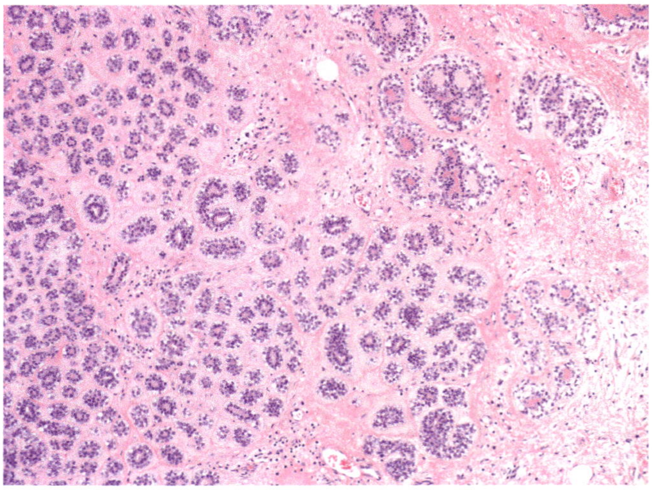

Fig. 13.5 (H&E, 100×) Epithelial-myoepithelial carcinoma, tubular

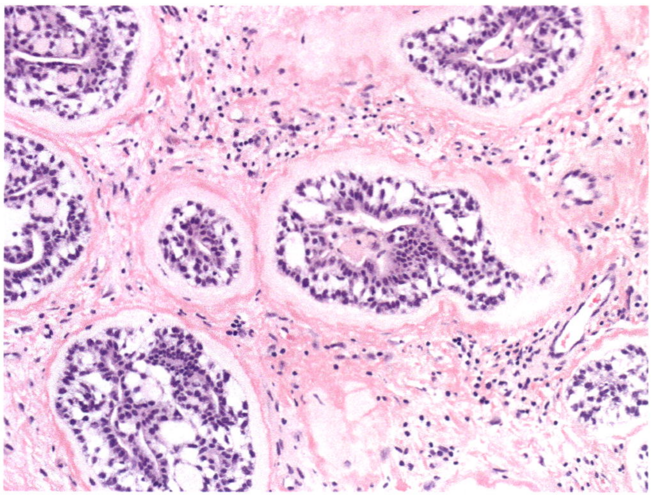

Fig. 13.6 (H&E, 200×) Epithelial-myoepithelial carcinoma, tubular

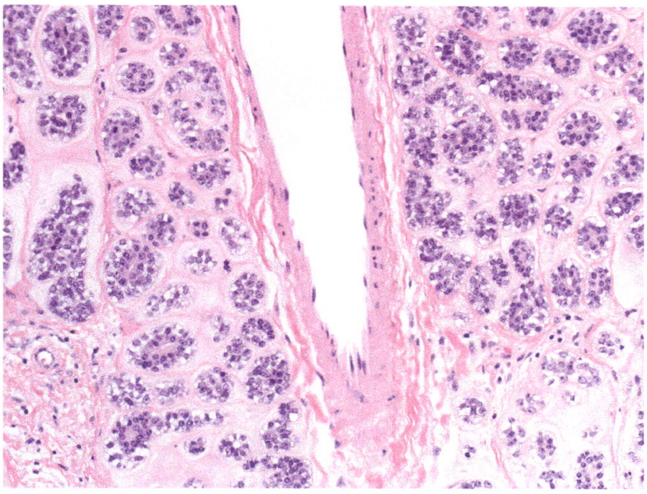

Fig. 13.7 (H&E, 200×) Epithelial-myoepithelial carcinoma, tubular

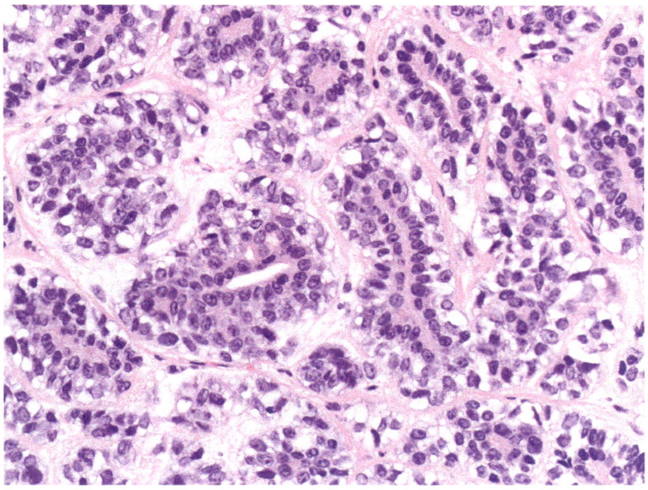

Fig. 13.8 (H&E, 400×) Epithelial-myoepithelial carcinoma, tubular

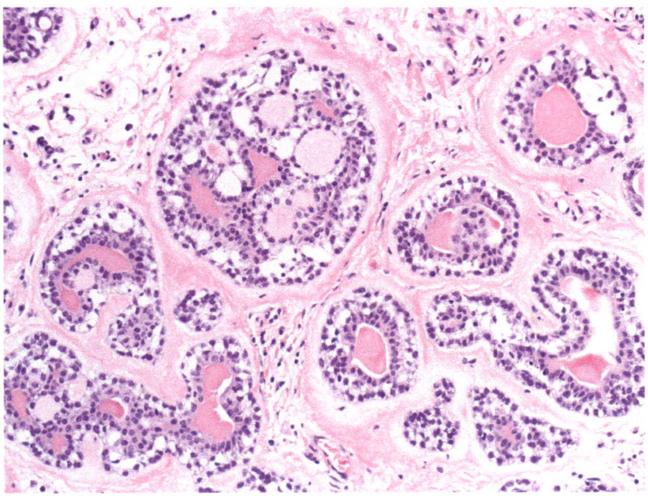

Fig. 13.9 (H&E, 200×) Epithelial-myoepithelial carcinoma, tubular and cribriform

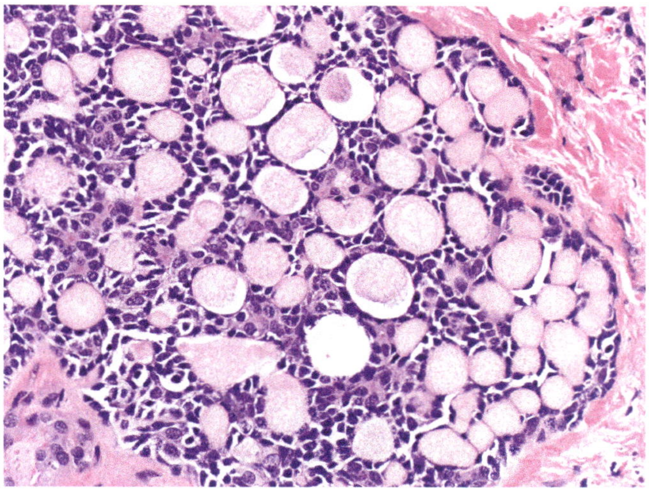

Fig. 13.10 (H&E, 400×) Epithelial-myoepithelial carcinoma, cribriform

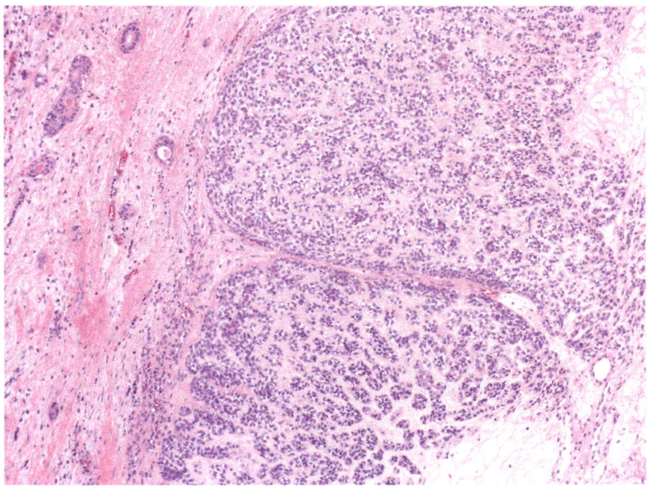

Fig. 13.11 (H&E, 100×) Epithelial-myoepithelial carcinoma, solid

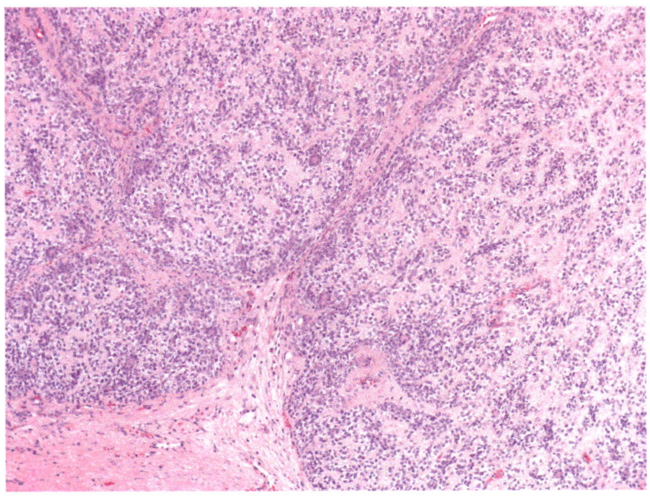

Fig. 13.12 (H&E, 100×) Epithelial-myoepithelial carcinoma, solid

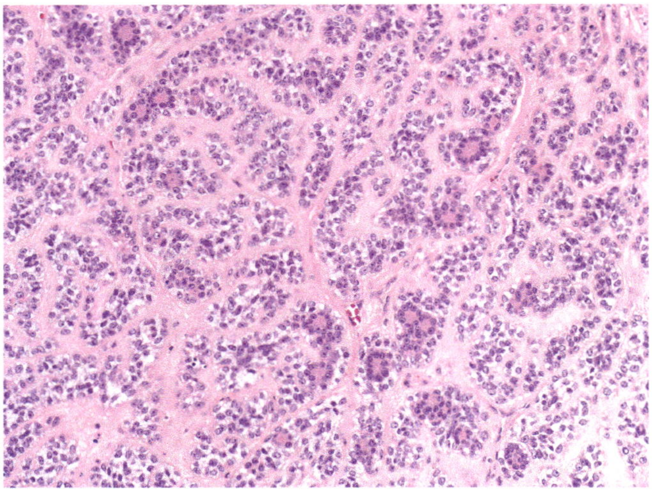

Fig. 13.13 (H&E, 200×) Epithelial-myoepithelial carcinoma, solid

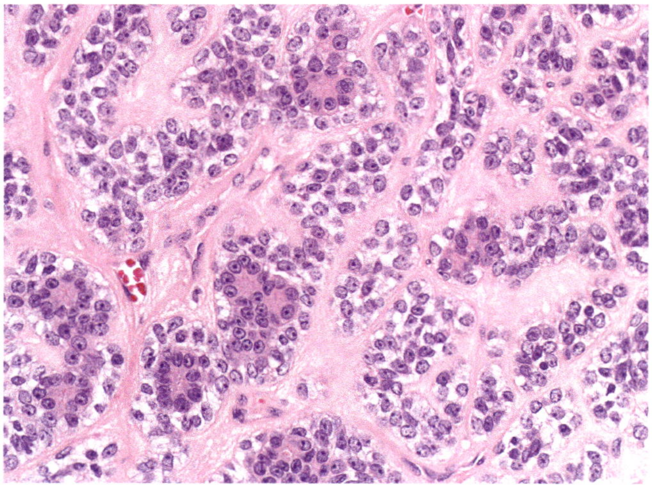

Fig. 13.14 (H&E, 400×) Epithelial-myoepithelial carcinoma, solid

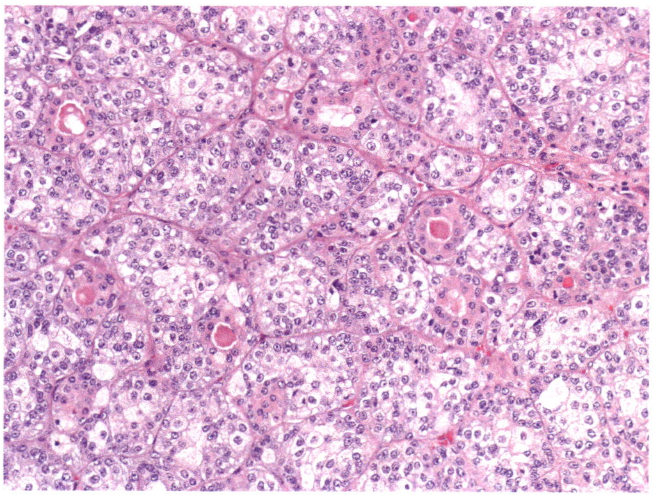

Fig. 13.15 (H&E, 200×) Epithelial-myoepithelial carcinoma, sebaceous

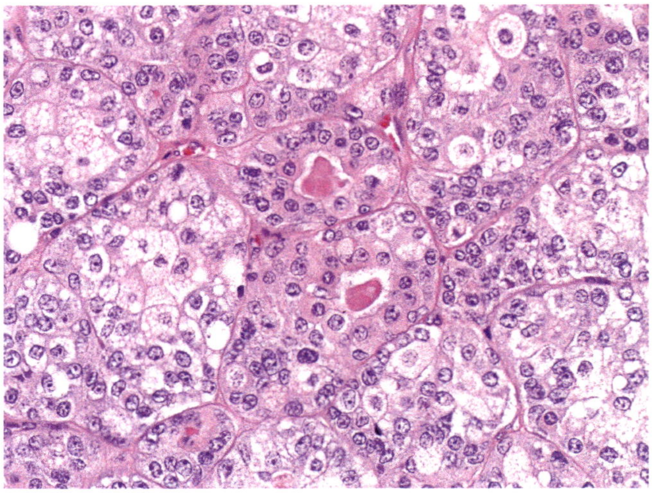

Fig. 13.16 (H&E, 400×) Epithelial-myoepithelial carcinoma, sebaceous

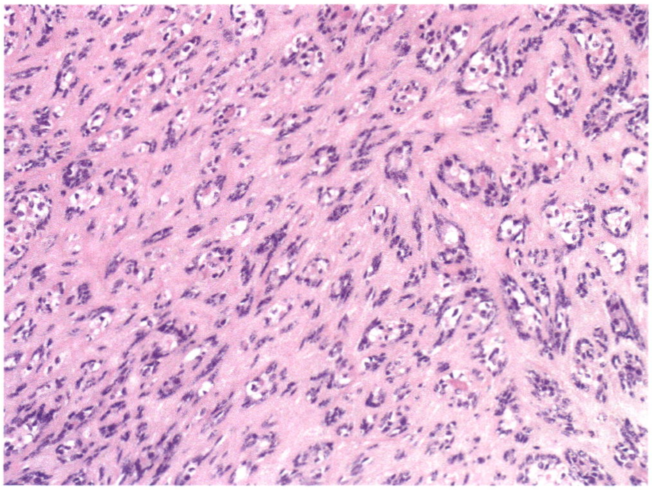

Fig. 13.17 (H&E, 200×) Epithelial-myoepithelial carcinoma, spindled

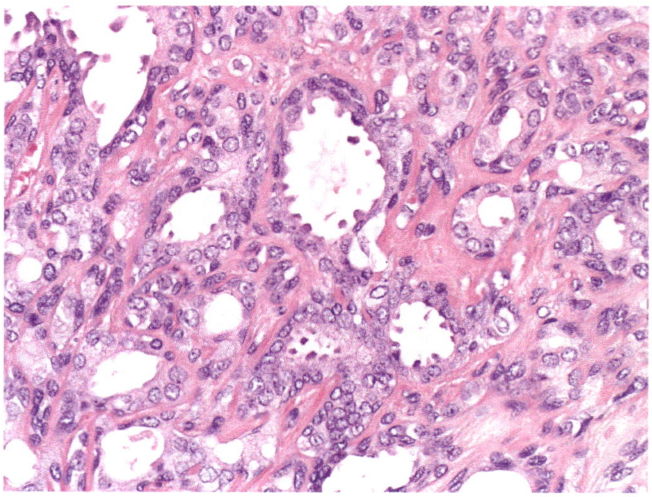

Fig. 13.18 (H&E, 400×) Epithelial-myoepithelial carcinoma, apocrine

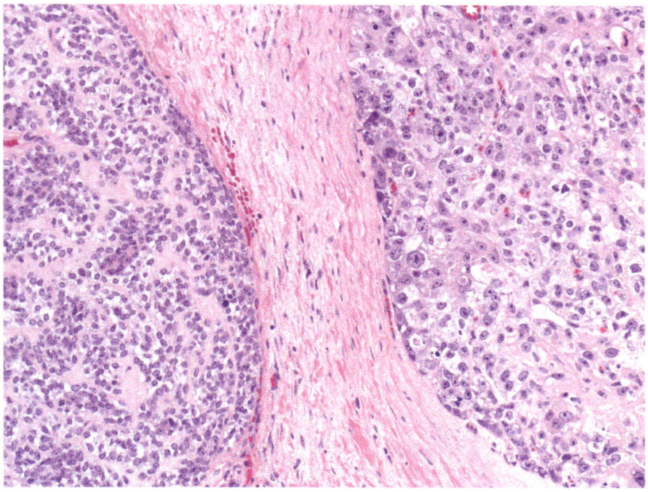

Fig. 13.19 (H&E, 200×) Epithelial-myoepithelial carcinoma, high-grade transformation, cytomorphologic atypia

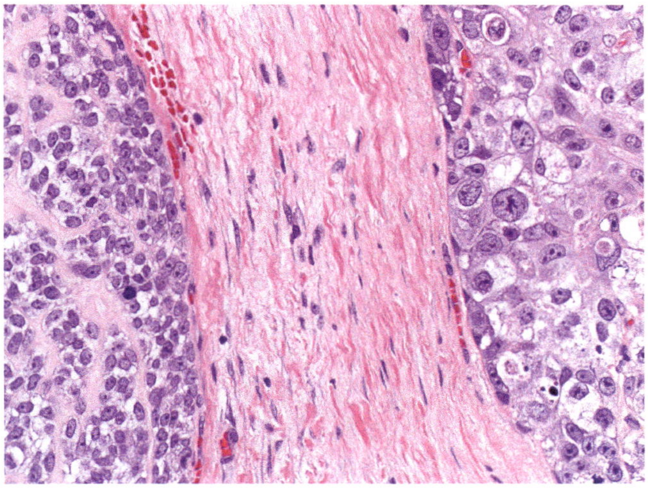

Fig. 13.20 (H&E, 400×) Epithelial-myoepithelial carcinoma, high-grade transformation, cytomorphologic atypia

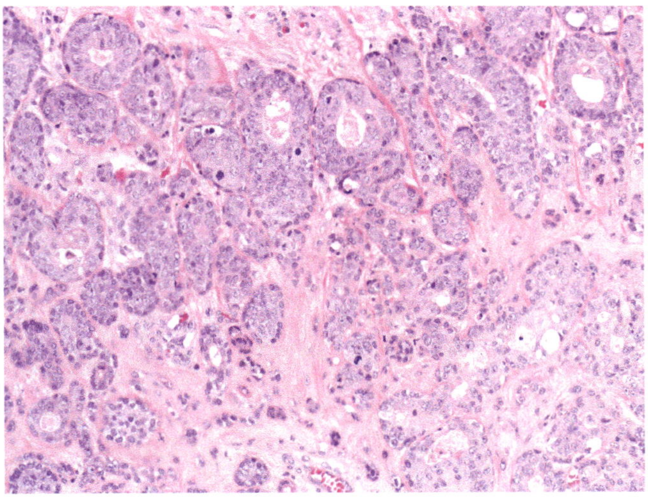

Fig. 13.21 (H&E, 200×) Epithelial-myoepithelial carcinoma, high-grade transformation, cytomorphologic atypia

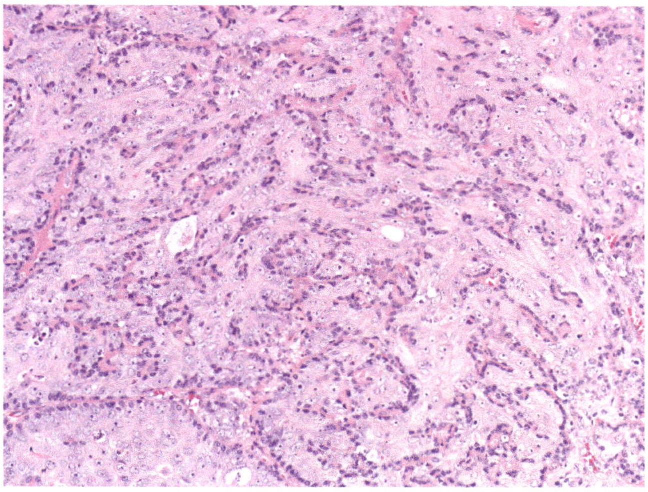

Fig. 13.22 (H&E, 200×) Epithelial-myoepithelial carcinoma, high-grade transformation, cytomorphologic atypia

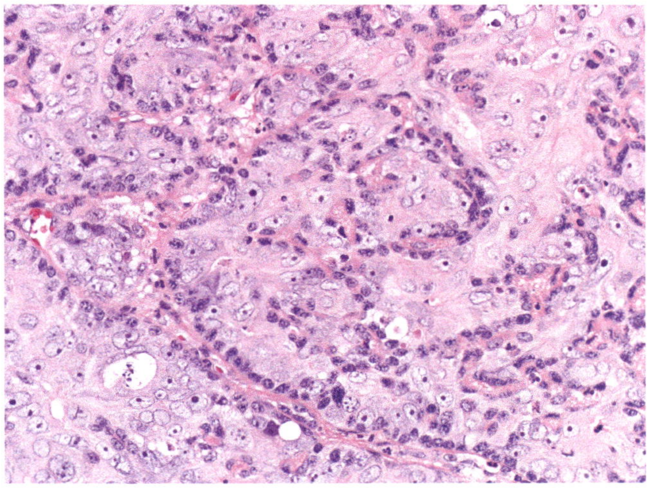

Fig. 13.23 (H&E, 400×) Epithelial-myoepithelial carcinoma, high-grade transformation, cytomorphologic atypia

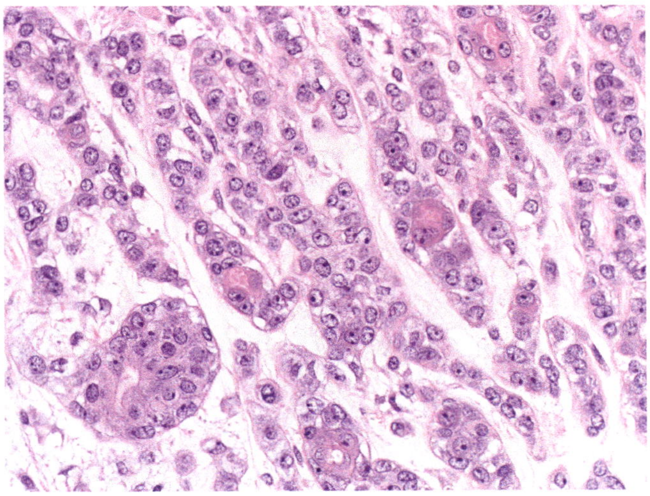

Fig. 13.24 (H&E, 400×) Epithelial-myoepithelial carcinoma, high-grade transformation, cytomorphologic atypia

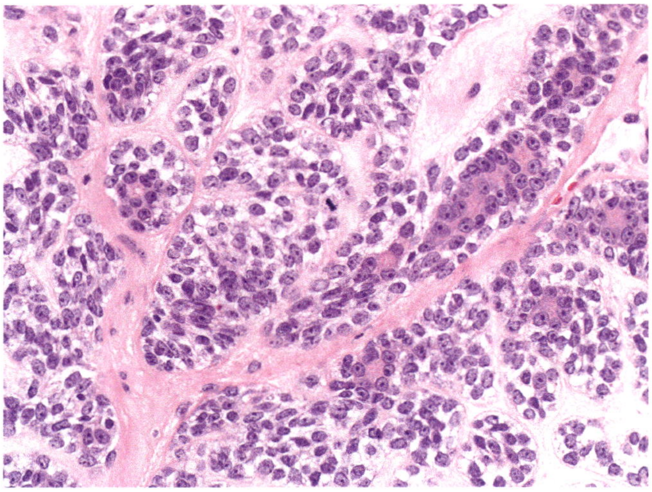

Fig. 13.25 (H&E, 400×) Epithelial-myoepithelial carcinoma, high-grade transformation, mitotic activity

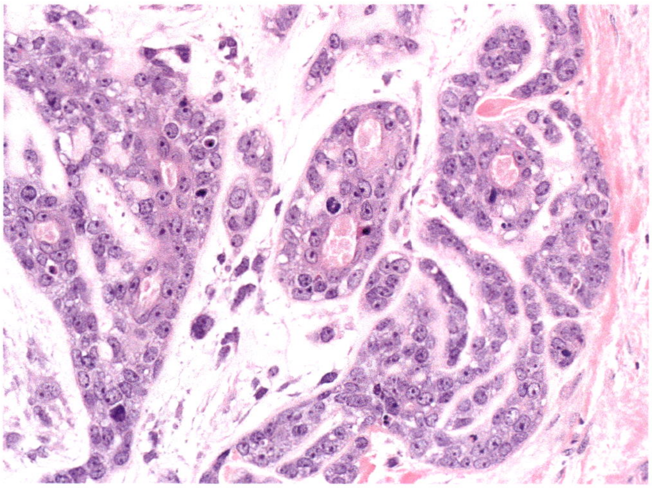

Fig. 13.26 (H&E, 400×) Epithelial-myoepithelial carcinoma, high-grade transformation, mitotic activity

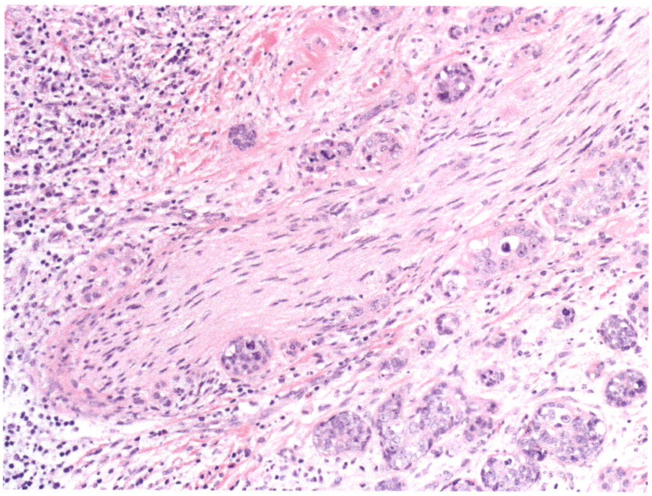

Fig. 13.27 (H&E, 200×) Epithelial-myoepithelial carcinoma, high-grade transformation, perineural invasion

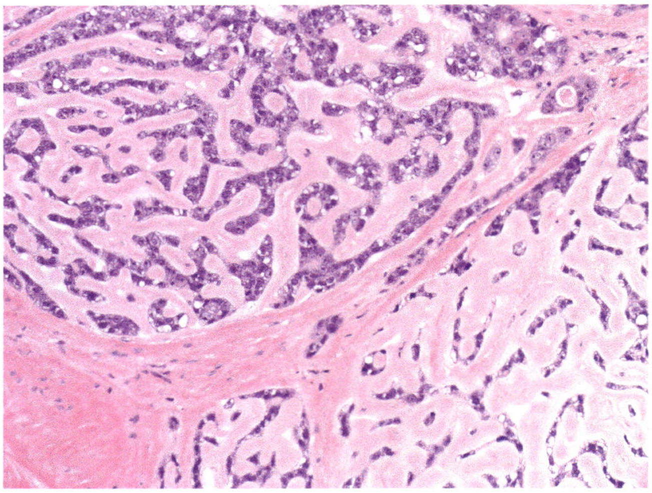

Fig. 13.28 (H&E, 200×) Epithelial-myoepithelial carcinoma, basement membrane-like material

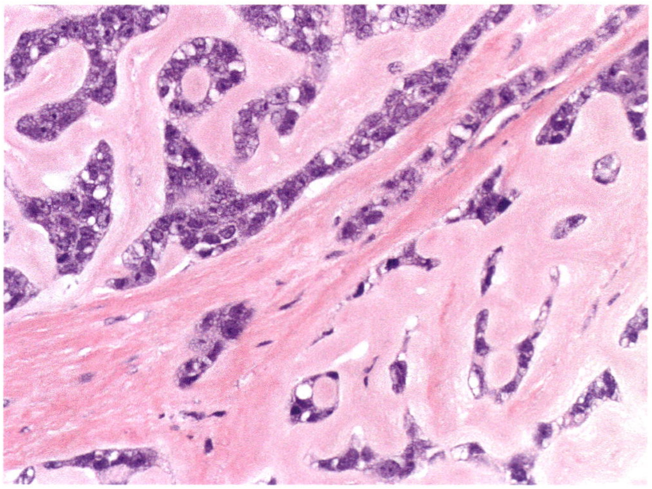

Fig. 13.29 (H&E, 400×) Epithelial-myoepithelial carcinoma, basement membrane-like material

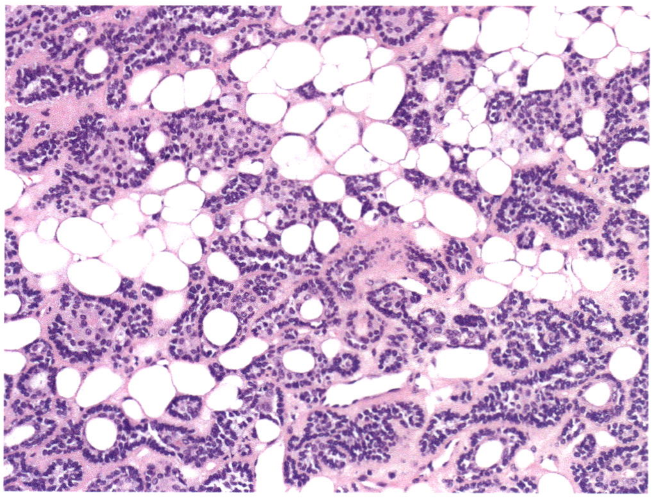

Fig. 13.30 (H&E, 200×) Epithelial-myoepithelial carcinoma, adipocytic metaplasia

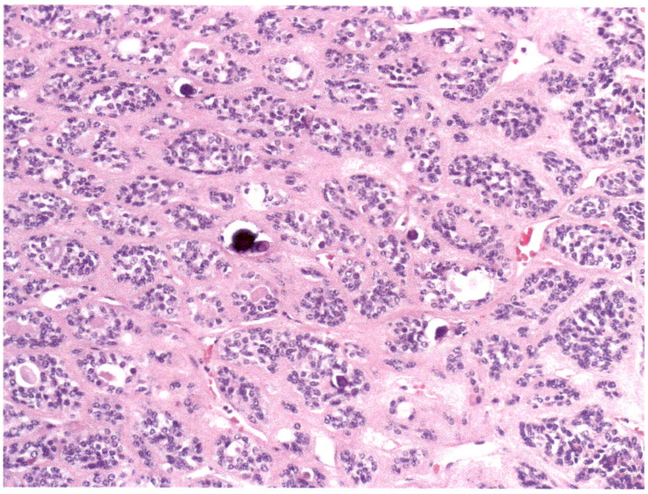

Fig. 13.31 (H&E, 200×) Epithelial-myoepithelial carcinoma, microcalcifications

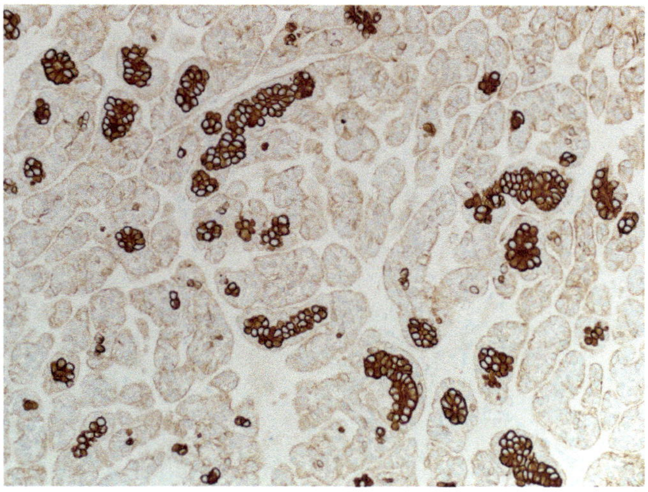

Fig. 13.32 (AE1/AE3, 200×) Epithelial-myoepithelial carcinoma, ductal immunoreactivity

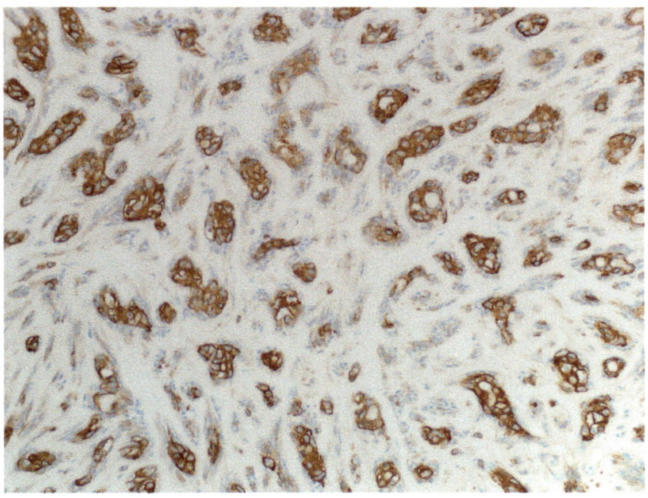

Fig. 13.33 (AE1/AE3, 200×) Epithelial-myoepithelial carcinoma, ductal immunoreactivity

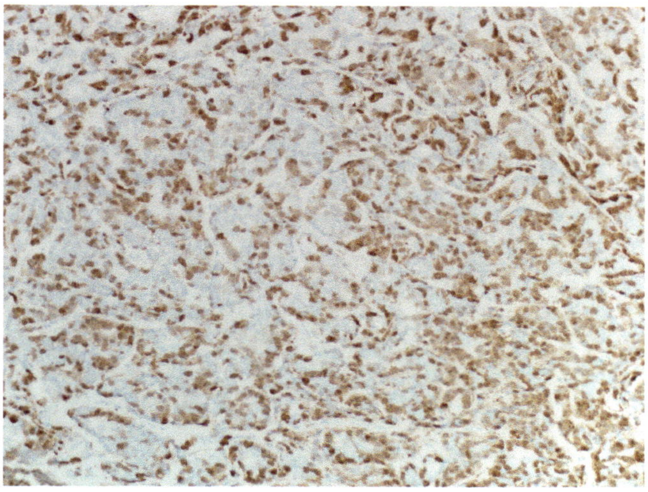

Fig. 13.34 (S-100, 200×) Epithelial-myoepithelial carcinoma, myoepithelial immunoreactivity

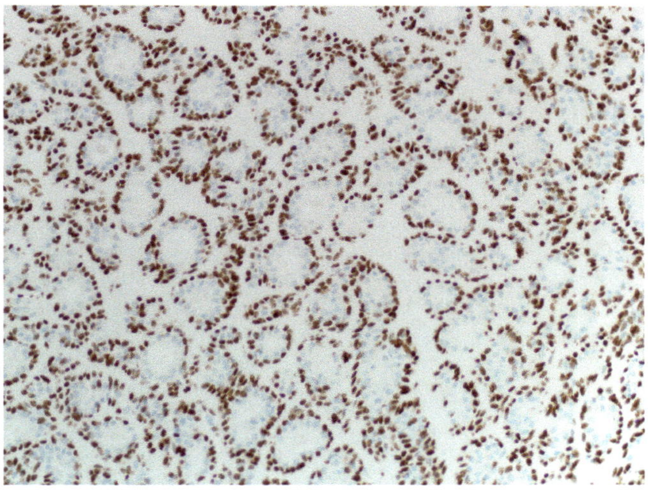

Fig. 13.35 (p63, 200×) Epithelial-myoepithelial carcinoma, myoepithelial immunoreactivity

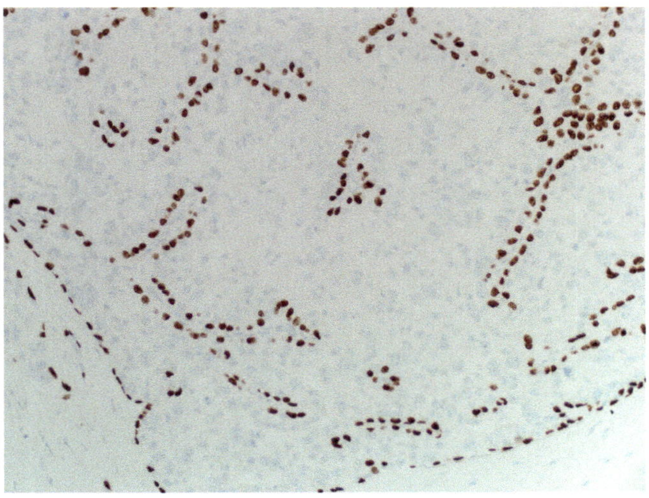

Fig. 13.36 (p63, 200×) Epithelial-myoepithelial carcinoma, myoepithelial immunoreactivity

Suggested Reading

Alos L, Carrillo R, Ramos J, Baez JM, Mallofre C, Fernandez PL, et al. High-grade carcinoma component in epithelial-myoepithelial carcinoma of salivary glands clinicopathological, immunohistochemical and flow-cytometric study of three cases. Virchows Arch. 1999;434(4):291–9.

Fonseca I, Soares J. Epithelial-myoepithelial carcinoma of the salivary glands: a study of 22 cases. Virchows Arch A Pathol Anat Histopathol. 1993;422:389–96.

Roy P, Bullock MJ, Perez-Ordonez B, Dardick I, Weinreb I. Epithelial-myoepithelial carcinoma with high-grade transformation. Am J Surg Pathol. 2010;34(9):1258–65.

Seethala RR. Oncocytic and apocrine epithelial-myoepithelial carcinoma: novel variants of a challenging tumor. Head Neck Pathol. 2013;7(Suppl 1):S77–84.

Seethala RR, Barnes EL, Hunt JL. Epithelial-myoepithelial carcinoma: a review of the clinicopathologic spectrum and immunophenotypic characteristics in 61 tumors of the salivary glands and upper aerodigestive tract. Am J Surg Pathol. 2007;31(1):44–57.

Seethala RR, Richmond JA, Hoschar AP, Barnes EL. New variants of epithelial-myoepithelial carcinoma: oncocytic-sebaceous and apocrine. Arch Pathol Lab Med. 2009;133:950.

Shinozaki A, Nagao T, Endo H, Kato N, Hirokawa M, Mizobuchi K, et al. Sebaceous epithelial-myoepithelial carcinoma of the salivary gland: clinicopathologic and immunohistochemical analysis of 6 cases of a new histologic variant. Am J Surg Pathol. 2008;32(6):913–23.

Vazquez A, Patel TD, D'Aguillo CM, Abdou RY, Farver W, Baredes S, et al. Epithelial-myoepithelial carcinoma of the salivary glands: an analysis of 246 cases. Otolaryngol Head Neck Surg. 2015;153:569–74.

Wang B, Brandwein M, Gordon R, Robinson R, Urken M, Zarbo RJ. Primary salivary clear cell tumors--a diagnostic approach: a clinicopathologic and immunohistochemical study of 20 patients with clear cell carcinoma, clear cell myoepithelial carcinoma, and epithelial-myoepithelial carcinoma.[see comment]. Arch Pathol Lab Med. 2002;126(6):676–85.

14 Intraductal Carcinoma

Intraductal carcinoma affects children and adults. The majority of cases involve major salivary glands, presenting as single or multiple masses. Most cases of intraductal carcinoma behave as low to intermediate-grade malignancies. Intraductal carcinoma may be circumscribed or infiltrative, comprised of multiple cell types (ductal and myoepithelial), and exhibit a variety of architectural patterns (cribriform and papillary) (Figs. 14.1–14.30).

J. J. García, *Atlas of Salivary Gland Pathology*, https://doi.org/10.1007/978-3-319-09021-4_14

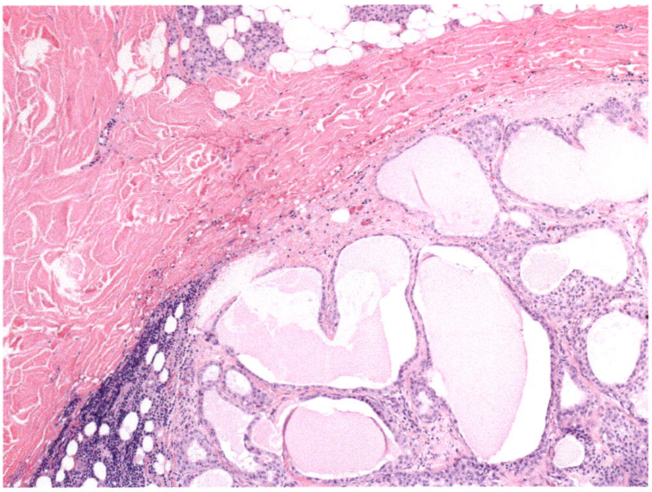

Fig. 14.1 (H&E, 100×) Intraductal carcinoma, circumscribed

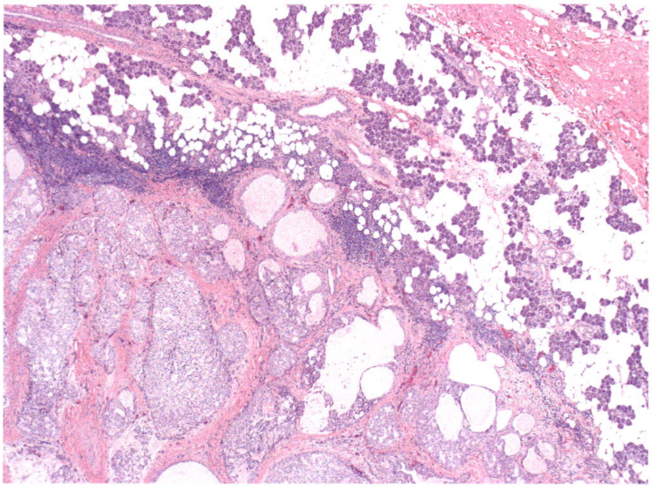

Fig. 14.2 (H&E, 40×) Intraductal carcinoma, infiltrative

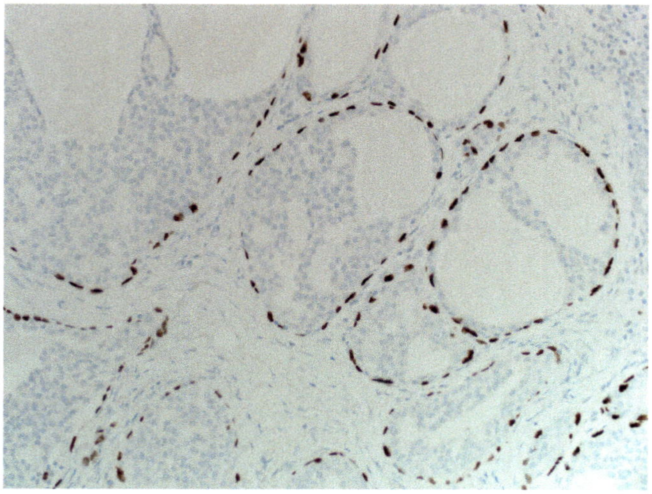

Fig. 14.3 (p63, 200×) Intraductal carcinoma, biphasic

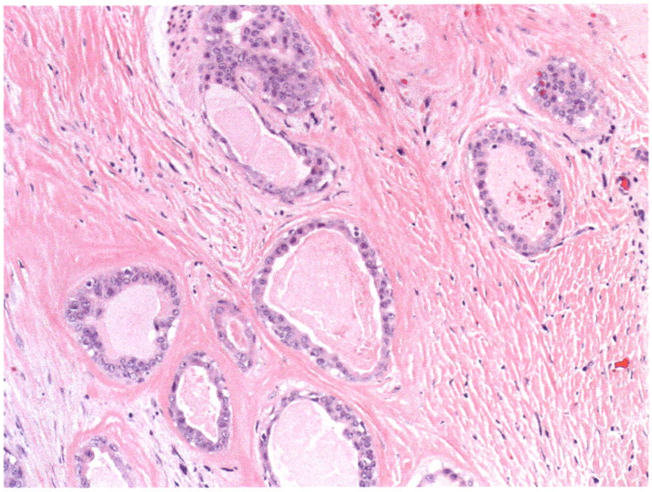

Fig. 14.4 (H&E, 200×) Intraductal carcinoma, cribriform

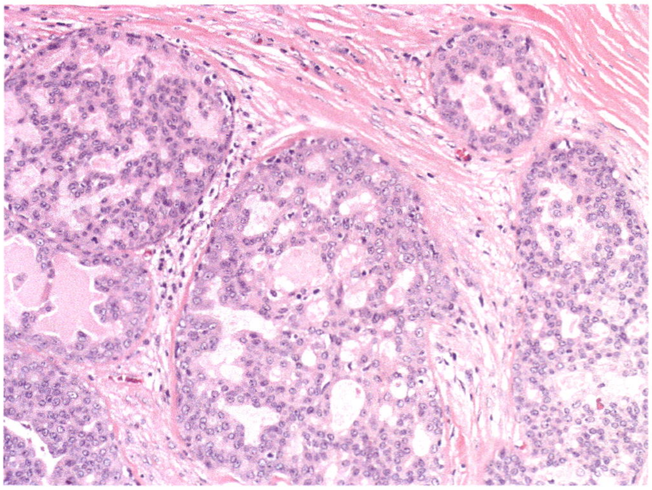

Fig. 14.5 (H&E, 200×) Intraductal carcinoma, cribriform

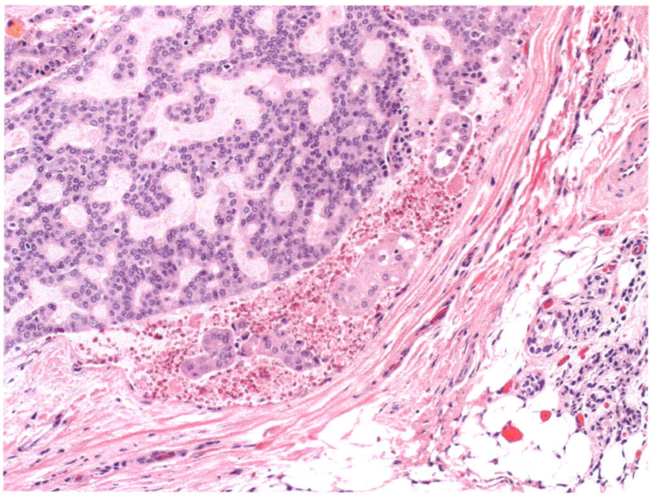

Fig. 14.6 (H&E, 200×) Intraductal carcinoma, cribriform

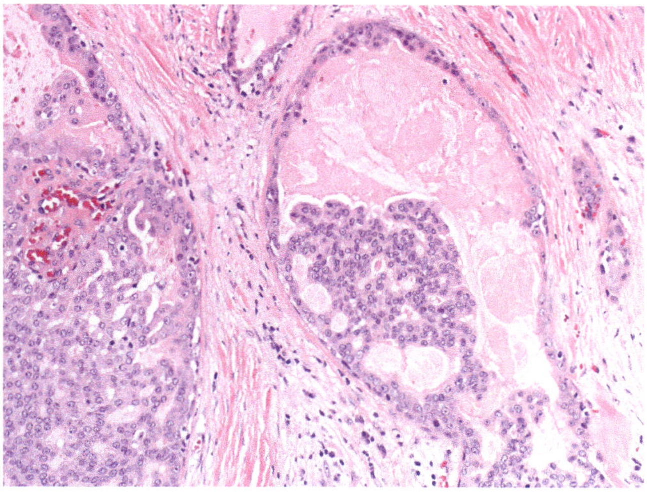

Fig. 14.7 (H&E, 200×) Intraductal carcinoma, cribriform

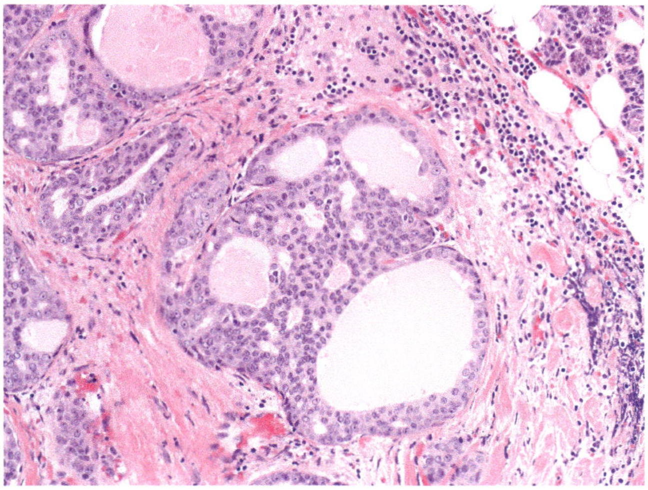

Fig. 14.8 (H&E, 200×) Intraductal carcinoma, cribriform

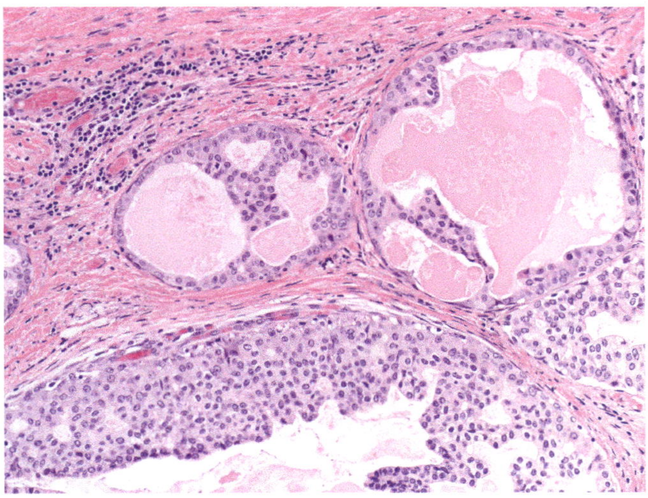

Fig. 14.9 (H&E, 200×) Intraductal carcinoma, cribriform

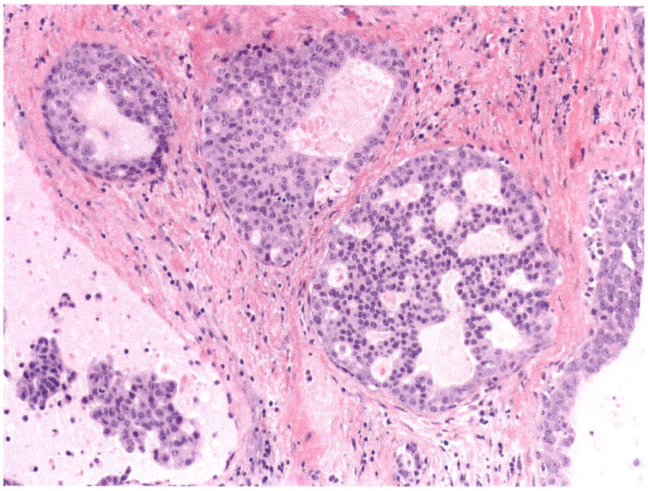

Fig. 14.10 (H&E, 200×) Intraductal carcinoma, cribriform

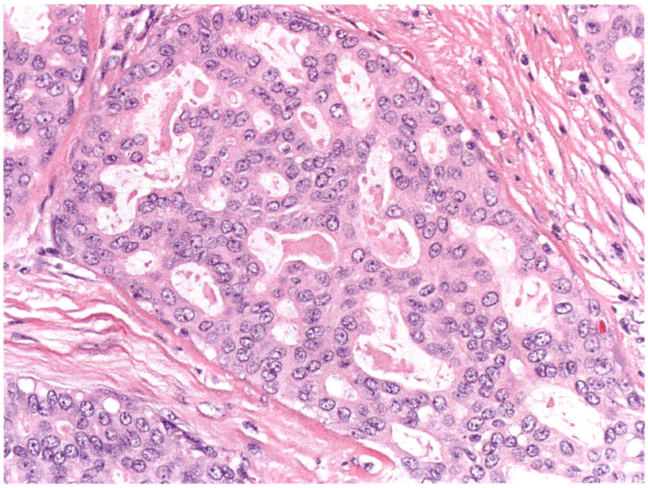

Fig. 14.11 (H&E, 400×) Intraductal carcinoma, cribriform

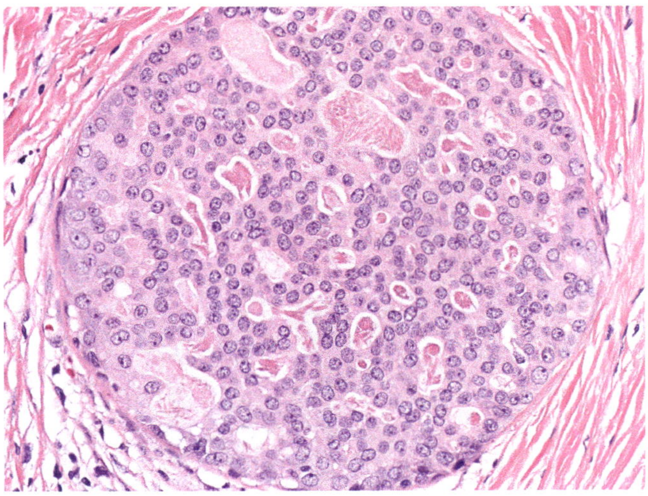

Fig. 14.12 (H&E, 400×) Intraductal carcinoma, cribriform

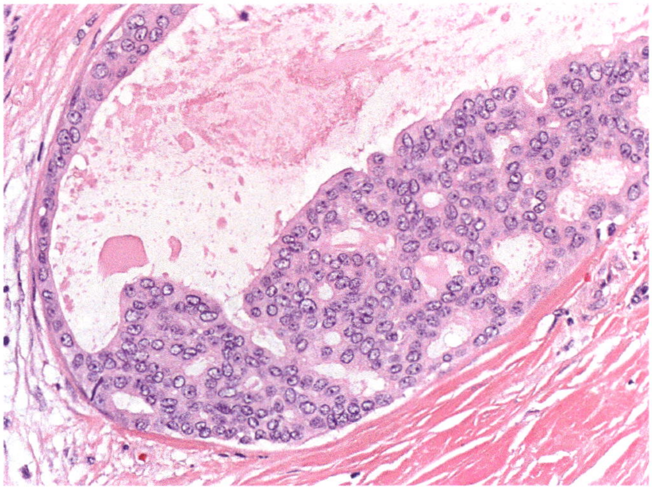

Fig. 14.13 (H&E, 400×) Intraductal carcinoma, cribriform

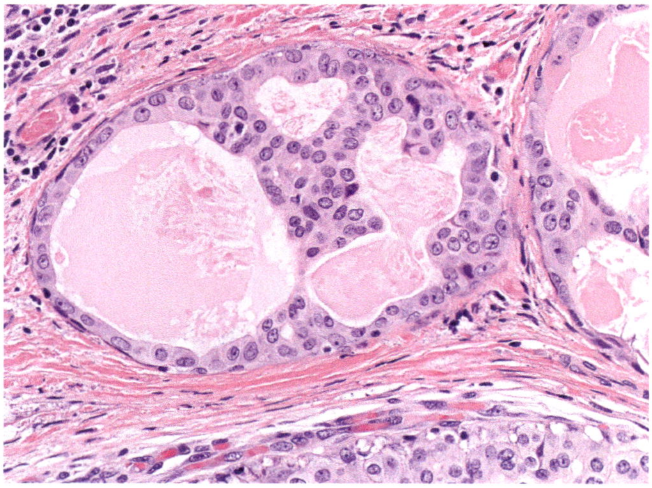

Fig. 14.14 (H&E, 400×) Intraductal carcinoma, cribriform

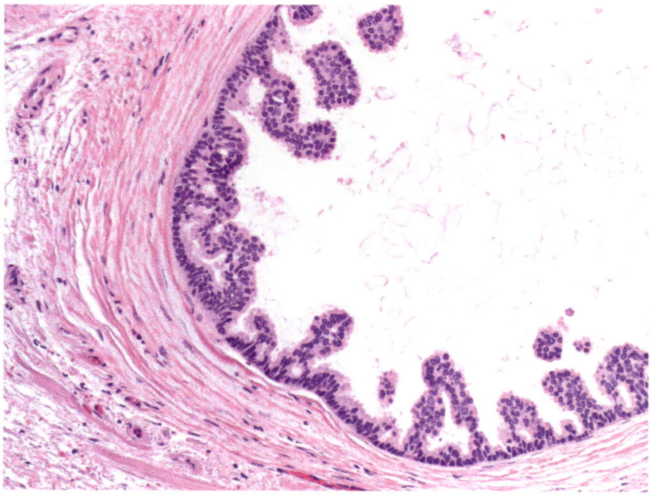

Fig. 14.15 (H&E, 200×) Intraductal carcinoma, papillary

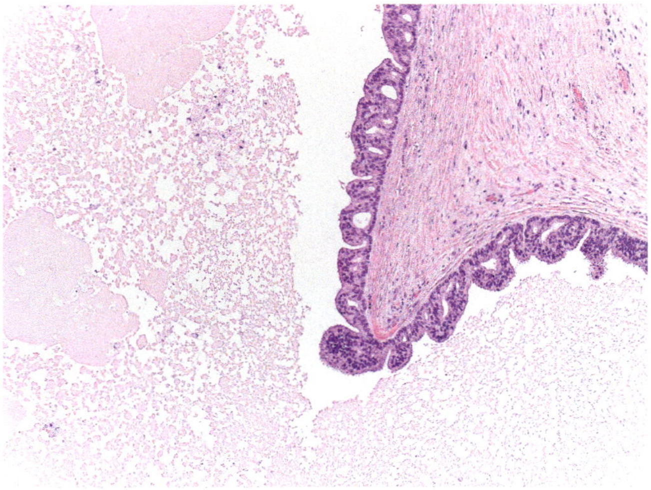

Fig. 14.16 (H&E, 100×) Intraductal carcinoma, papillary

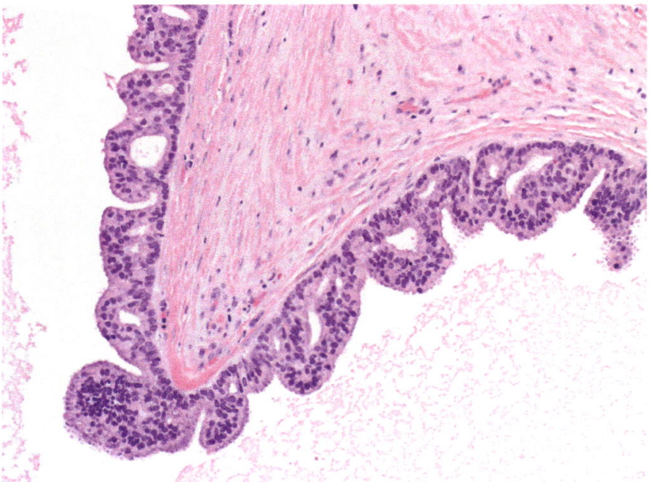

Fig. 14.17 (H&E, 200×) Intraductal carcinoma, papillary

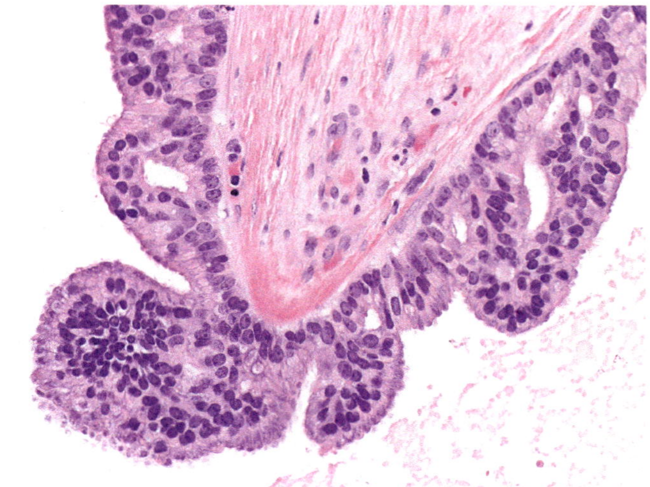

Fig. 14.18 (H&E, 400×) Intraductal carcinoma, papillary

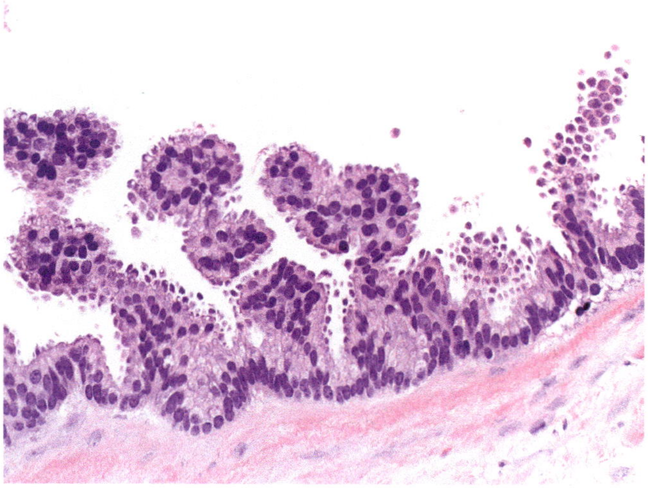

Fig. 14.19 (H&E, 400×) Intraductal carcinoma, papillary

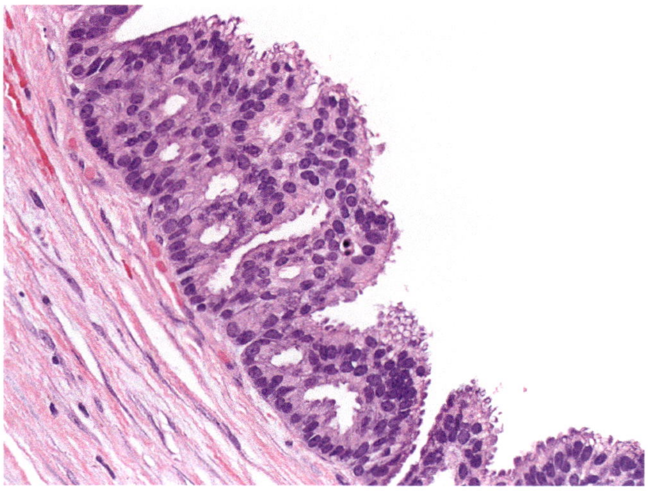

Fig. 14.20 (H&E, 400×) Intraductal carcinoma, papillary

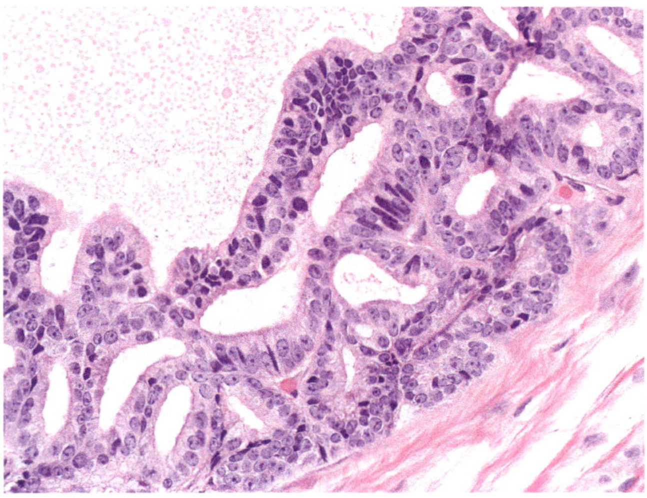

Fig. 14.21 (H&E, 400×) Intraductal carcinoma, papillary

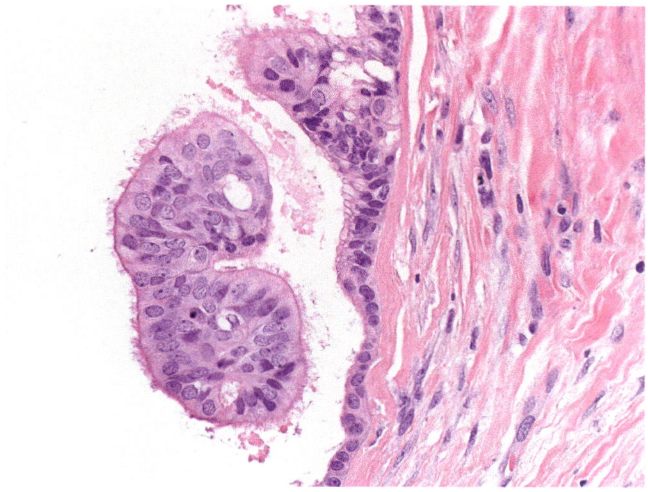

Fig. 14.22 (H&E, 400×) Intraductal carcinoma, ciliated

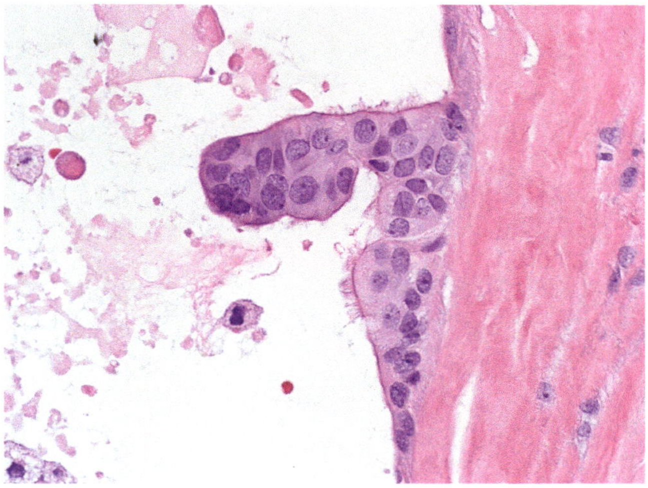

Fig. 14.23 (H&E, 600×) Intraductal carcinoma, ciliated

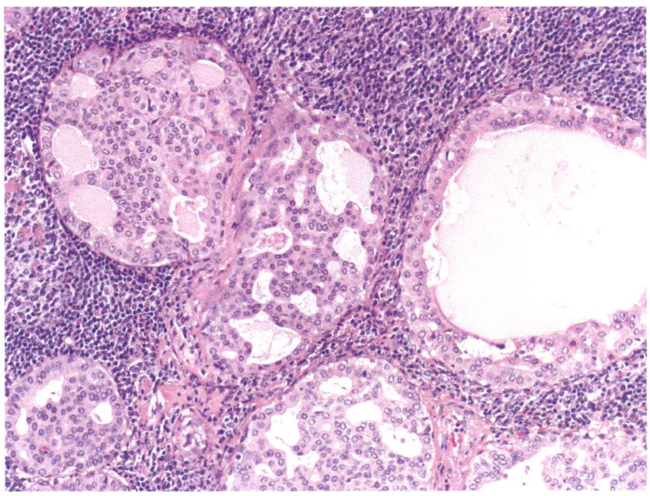

Fig. 14.24 (H&E, 200×) Intraductal carcinoma, tumor-associated lymphoid proliferation

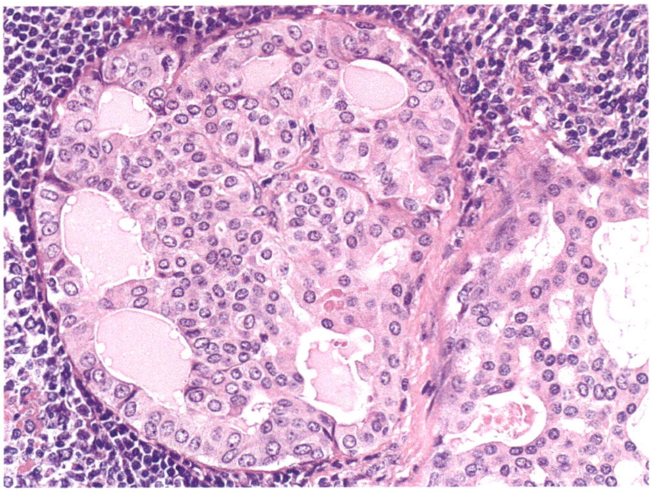

Fig. 14.25 (H&E, 400×) Intraductal carcinoma, tumor-associated lymphoid proliferation

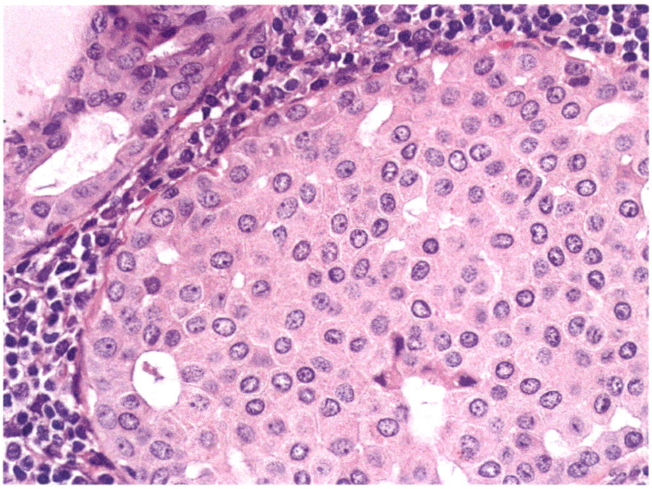

Fig. 14.26 (H&E, 600×) Intraductal carcinoma, tumor-associated lymphoid proliferation

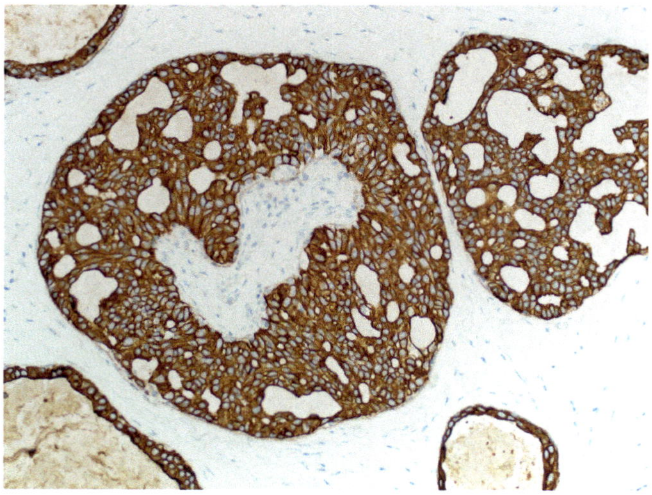

Fig. 14.27 (AE1/AE3, 200×) Intraductal carcinoma, diffuse immunoreactivity

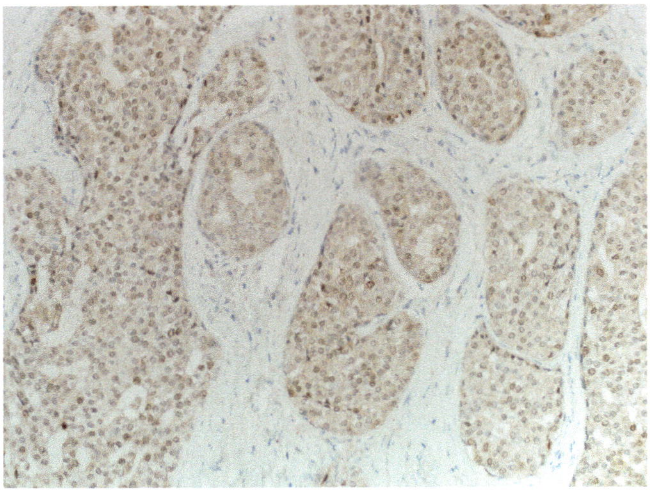

Fig. 14.28 (S-100, 200×) Intraductal carcinoma, diffuse immunoreactivity

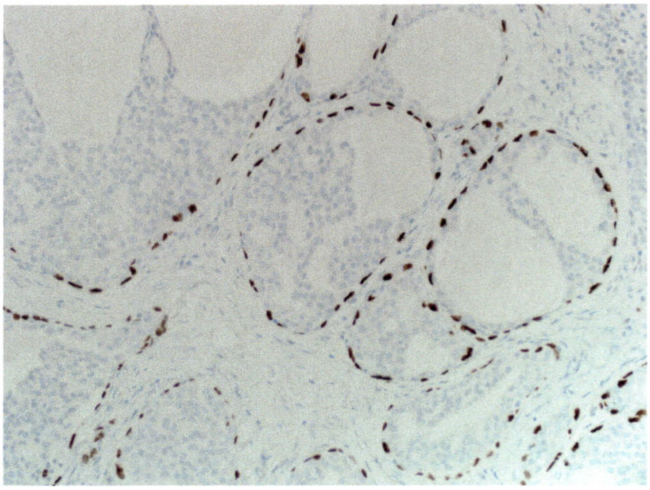

Fig. 14.29 (p63, 200×) Intraductal carcinoma, basal immunoreactivity

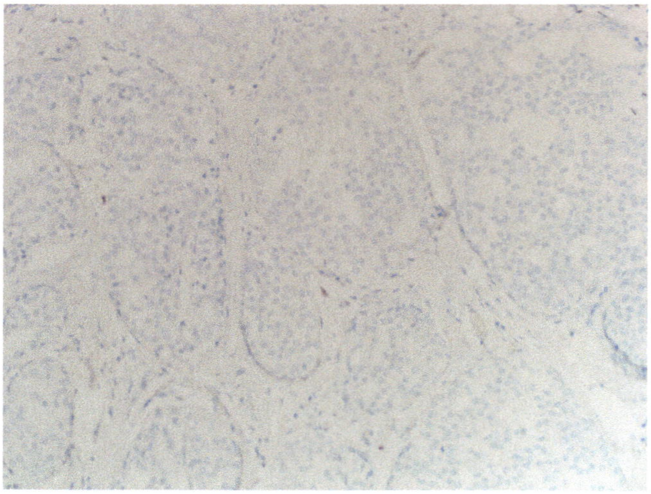

Fig. 14.30 (Androgen receptor, 200×) Intraductal carcinoma, negative immunoreactivity

Suggested Reading

Brandwein-Gensler M, Hille J, Wang BY, Urken M, Gordon R, Wang LJ, et al. Low-grade salivary duct carcinoma: description of 16 cases. Am J Surg Pathol. 2004;28:1040–4.

Croitoru CM, Mooney JE, Luna MA. Sebaceous lymphadenocarcinoma of salivary glands. Ann Diagn Pathol. 2003;7(4):236–9.

Delgado R, Klimstra D, Albores-Saavedra J. Low-grade salivary duct carcinoma: a distinctive variant with a low-grade histology and a predominant intraductal growth pattern. Cancer. 1996;78:958–67.

Gallego L, Junquera L, Fresno MF. Non-sebaceous lymphadenoma of the parotid gland: immunohistochemical study and DNA ploidy analysis. Oral Surg Oral Med Oral Pathol Oral Radiol Endod. 2009;107(4):555–8.

Ide F, Mishima K, Saito I. Circumscribed salivary duct carcinoma of the palate: a non-threatening variant. Histopathology. 2004;45:89–91.

Kuo YJ, Weinreb I, Perez-Ordonez B. Low-grade salivary duct carcinoma or low-grade intraductal carcinoma? Review of the literature. Head Neck Pathol. 2013;7(Suppl 1):S59–67.

Kusafuka K, Itoh H, Sugiyama C, Nakajima T. Low-grade salivary duct carcinoma of the parotid gland: report of a case with immunohistochemical analysis. Med Mol Morphol. 2010;43:178–84.

Laco J, Podhola M, Dolezalova H. Low-grade cribriform cystadenocarcinoma of the parotid gland: a neoplasm with favorable prognosis, distinct from salivary duct carcinoma. Int J Surg Pathol. 2010;18:369–73.

Nakatsuka S, Harada H, Fujiyama H, Takeda K, Kitamura K, Kimura H, et al. An invasive adenocarijoma of the accessory parotid gland: a rare example developing from a low-grade cribriform cystadenocarcinoma? Diagn Pathol. 2011;6:122.

Simpson RH. Salivary duct carcinoma: new developments-morphological variants including pure in situ high-grade lesions; proposed molecular classification. Head Neck Pathol. 2013;7(Suppl 1):S48–58.

Tatemoto Y, Ohno A, Osaki T. Low malignant intraductal carcinoma on the hard palate: a variant of salivary duct carcinoma? Eur J Cancer B Oral Oncol. 1996;32B(4):275–7.

Weinreb I, Tabanda-Lichauco R, Van der Kwast T, Perez-Ordonez B. Low-grade intraductal carcinoma of salivary gland: report of 3 cases with marked apocrine differentiation. Am J Surg Pathol. 2006;30:1014–21.

15 Lymphadenoma

Lymphadenoma affects children and adults and presents at a mean age of approximately 65 years. Women and men are involved with similar frequency. The majority of cases involve the parotid gland, presenting as a single mass. Lymphadenoma is circumscribed, comprised of multiple cell types (ductal and basal), and may exhibit a variety of architectural patterns (nests and cysts) in a background of reactive lymphoid tissue. Sebaceous cells may or may not be present (sebaceous and non-sebaceous) (Figs. 15.1–15.16).

J. J. García, *Atlas of Salivary Gland Pathology*, https://doi.org/10.1007/978-3-319-09021-4_15

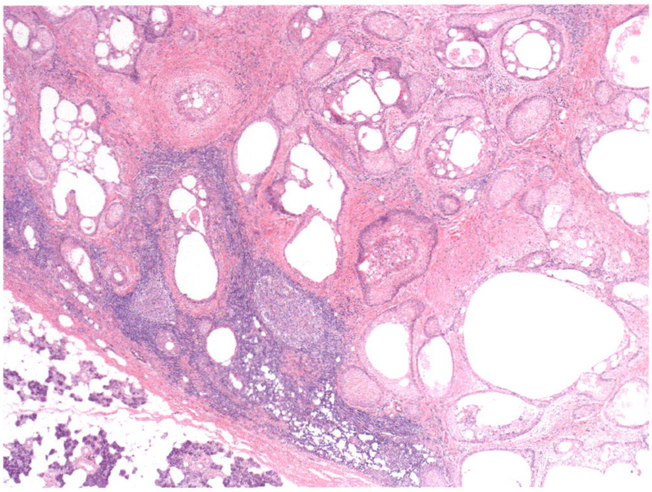

Fig. 15.1 (H&E, 40×) Lymphadenoma, circumscribed

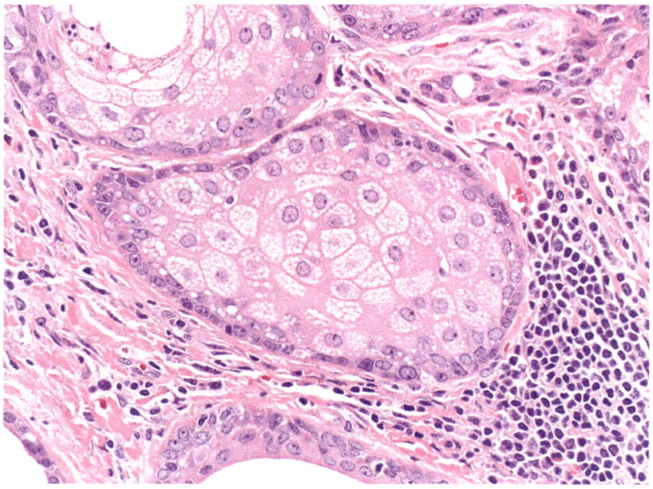

Fig. 15.2 (H&E, 400×) Lymphadenoma, biphasic

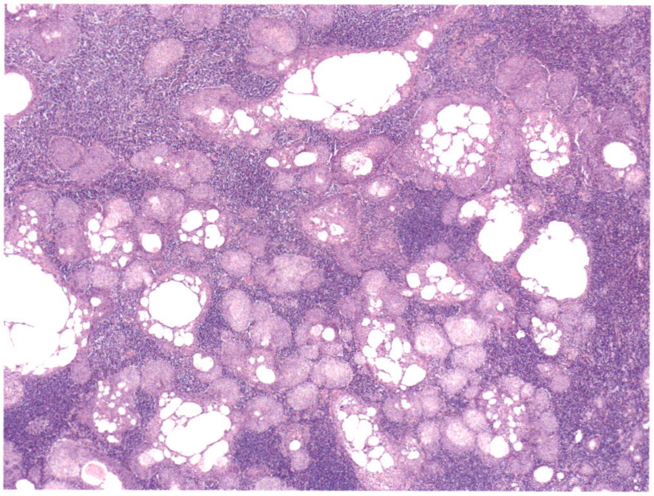

Fig. 15.3 (H&E, 40×) Lymphadenoma, sebaceous

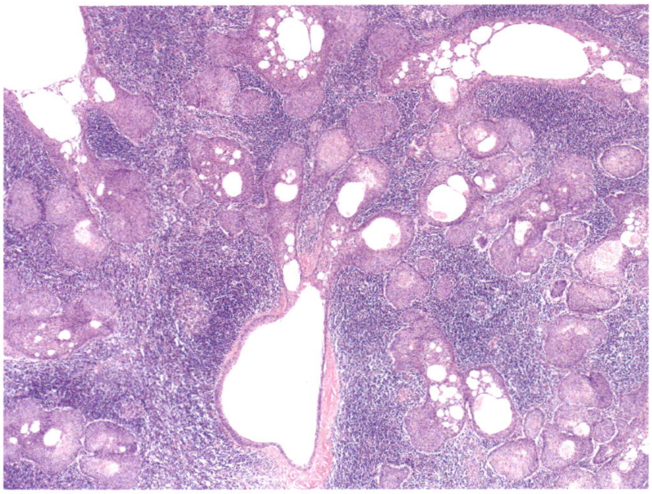

Fig. 15.4 (H&E, 40×) Lymphadenoma, sebaceous

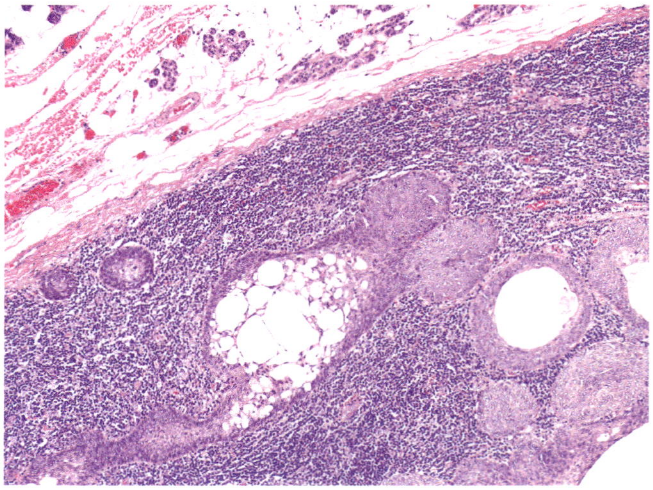

Fig. 15.5 (H&E, 100×) Lymphadenoma, sebaceous

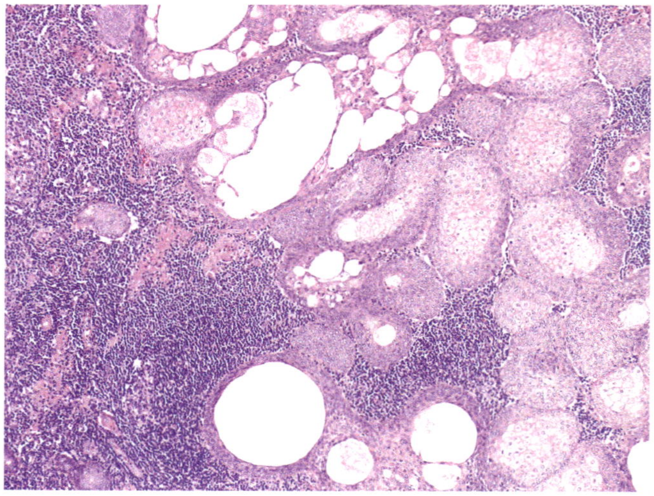

Fig. 15.6 (H&E, 100×) Lymphadenoma, sebaceous

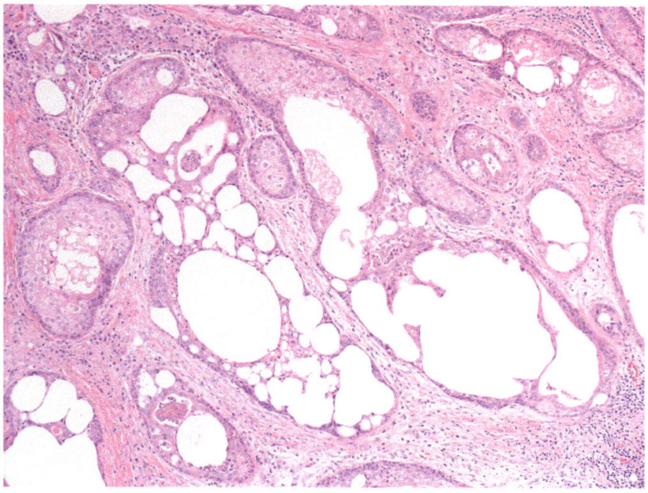

Fig. 15.7 (H&E, 100×) Lymphadenoma, sebaceous

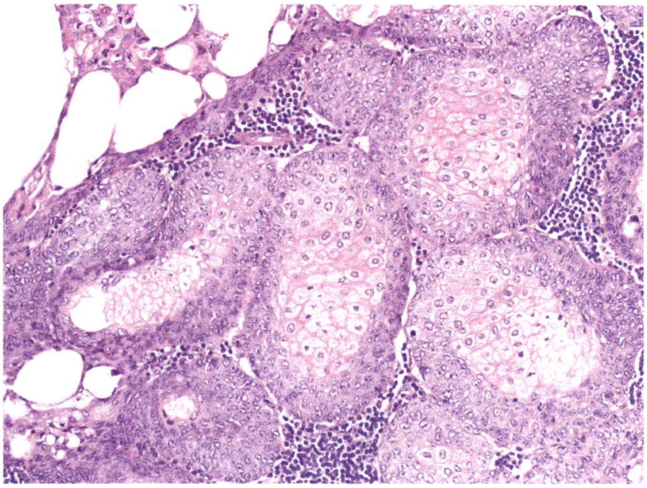

Fig. 15.8 (H&E, 200×) Lymphadenoma, sebaceous

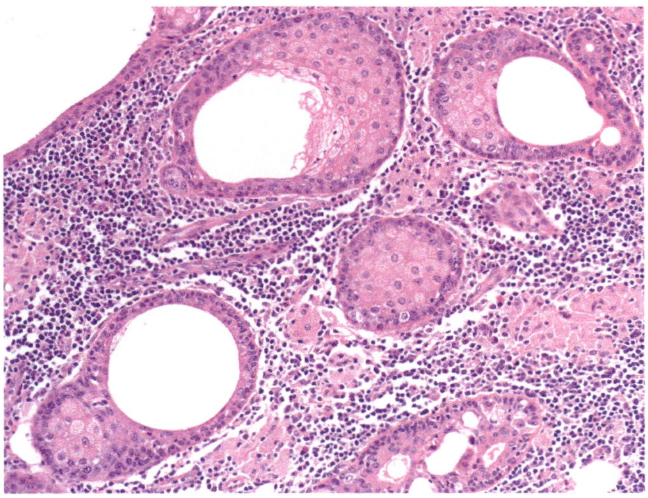

Fig. 15.9 (H&E, 200×) Lymphadenoma, sebaceous

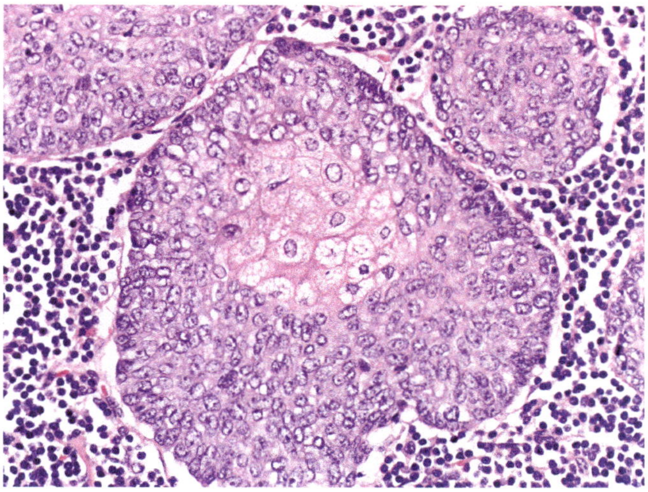

Fig. 15.10 (H&E, 400×) Lymphadenoma, sebaceous

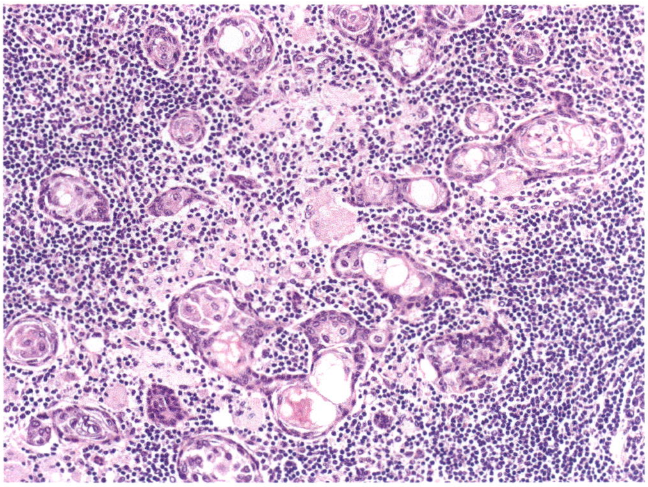

Fig. 15.11 (H&E, 200×) Lymphadenoma, sebaceous, histiocytic reaction

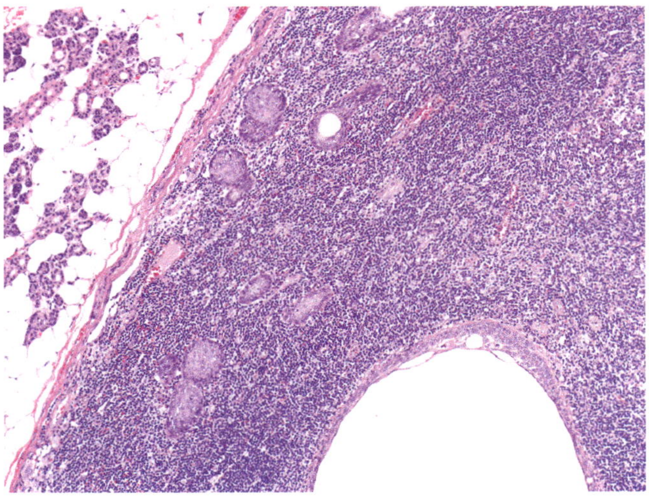

Fig. 15.12 (H&E, 100×) Lymphadenoma, non-sebaceous

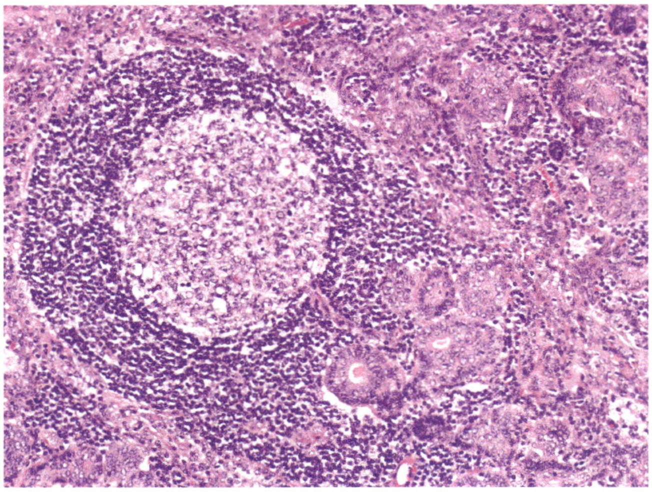

Fig. 15.13 (H&E, 200×) Lymphadenoma, non-sebaceous

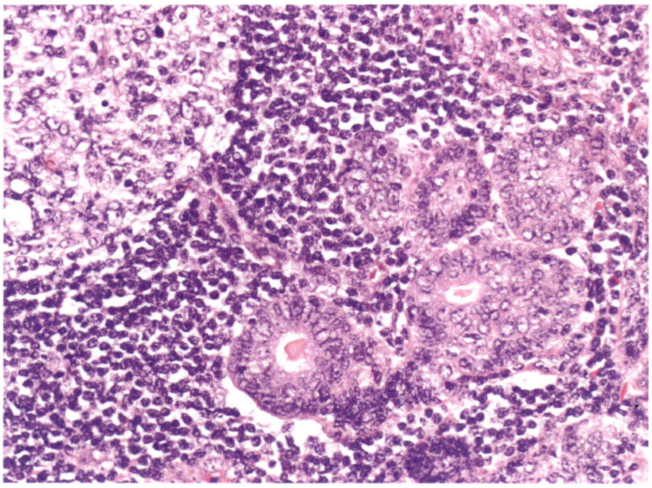

Fig. 15.14 (H&E, 400×) Lymphadenoma, non-sebaceous

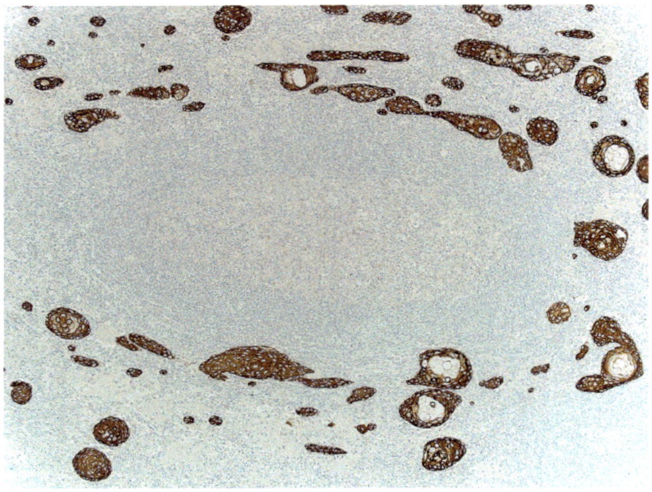

Fig. 15.15 (AE1/AE3, 100×) Lymphadenoma, diffuse immunoreactivity

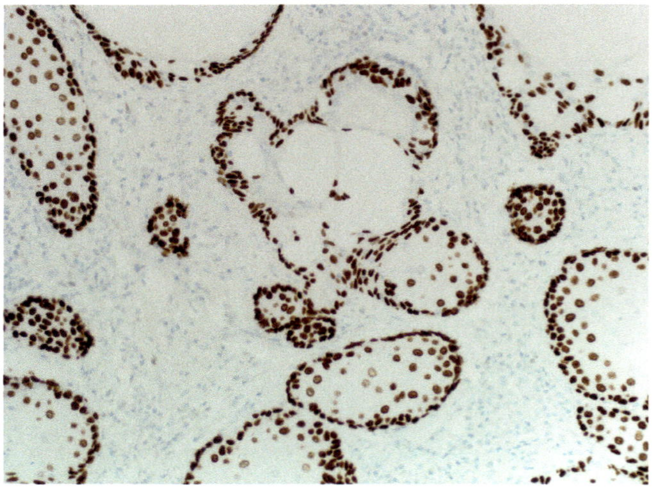

Fig. 15.16 (p63, 200×) Lymphadenoma, basal immunoreactivity

Suggested Reading

Abdool RA, Solomon LW, Papageorge MB. A clinic-pathologic correlation: sebaceous lymphadenoma. J Mass Dent Soc. 2008;57:36–7.

Castelino-Prabhu S, Li QK, Ali SZ. Non-sebaceous lymphadenoma of the parotid gland: cytopathologic findings and differential diagnosis. Diagn Cytopathol. 2010;38:137–40.

Croitoru CM, Mooney JE, Luna MA. Sebaceous lymphadenocarcinoma of salivary glands. Ann Diagn Pathol. 2003;7(4):236–9.

Dardick I, Thomas MJ. Lymphadenoma of parotid gland: two additional cases and a literature review. Oral Surg Oral Med Oral Pathol Oral Radiol Endod. 2008;105:491–4.

Gallego L, Junquera L, Fresno MF. Non-sebaceous lymphadenoma of the parotid gland: immunohistochemical study and DNA ploidy analysis. Oral Surg Oral Med Oral Pathol Oral Radiol Endod. 2009;107(4):555–8.

Liu G, He J, Zhang C, Fu S, He Y. Lymphadenoma of the salivary gland: report of 10 cases. Oncol Lett. 2014;7:1097–101.

Ma J, Chan JK, Chow CW, Orell SR. Lymphadnoma: a report of three cases of an uncommon salivary gland neoplasm. Histopathology. 2002;41:342–50.

Mori D, Akashi M, Shibaki M, Koike E, Miyazaki J. Nonsebaceous lympadenoma in the parotid gland: true neoplastic or reactive? A report of two cases. Int J Surg Pathol. 2013;21:509–13.

Seethala RR, Thompson LD, Gnepp DR, Barnes EL, Skalova A, Montone K, et al. Lymphadenoma of the salivary gland: clinicopathological and immunohistochemical analysis of 33 tumors. Mod Pathol. 2012;25(1):26–35.

Weiler C, Agaimy A, Zengel P, Zenk J, Kirchner T, Ihrler S. Non-sebaceous lymphadenoma of salivary glands: proposed development from intraparotid lymph nodes and risk of misdiagnosis. Virchows Arch. 2012;460:467–72.

16 Lymphoepithelial Carcinoma

Lymphoepithelial carcinoma affects children and adults and presents at a mean age of approximately 55 years. Women and men are involved with similar frequency. The majority of cases involve the parotid gland, presenting as single or multiple masses. Most cases of lymphoepithelial carcinoma behave as intermediate to high-grade malignancies. Lymphepithelial carcinoma may be circumscribed or infiltrative, comprised of multiple cell types (polygonal and spindled), and exhibit a variety of architectural patterns (solid, trabecular, and single cells) (Figs. 16.1–16.17).

J. J. García, *Atlas of Salivary Gland Pathology*, https://doi.org/10.1007/978-3-319-09021-4_16

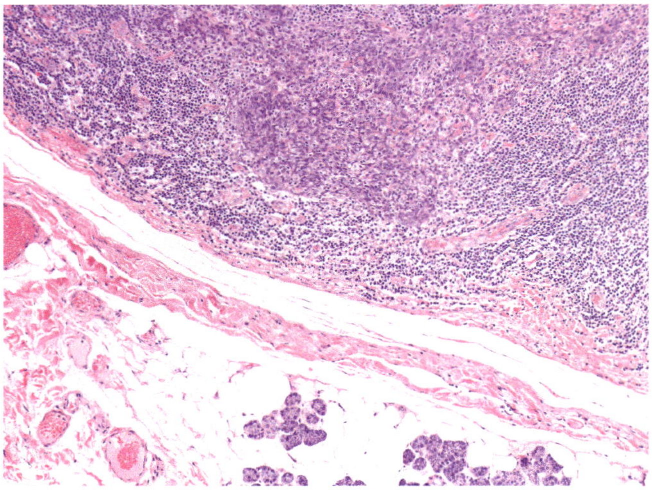

Fig. 16.1 (H&E, 100×) Lymphoepithelial carcinoma, circumscribed

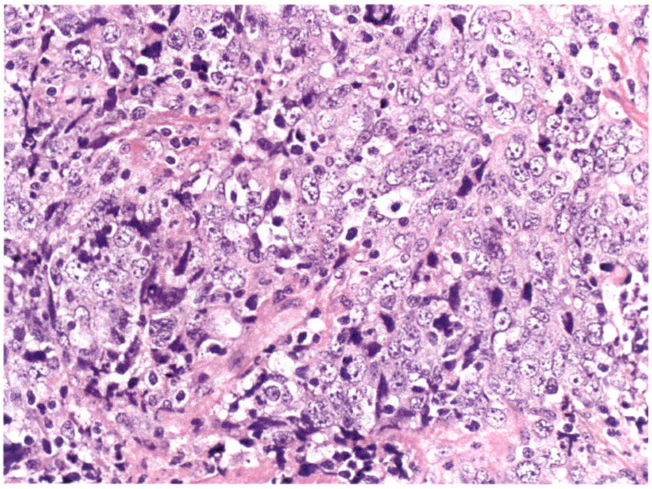

Fig. 16.2 (H&E, 400×) Lymphoepithelial carcinoma, biphasic

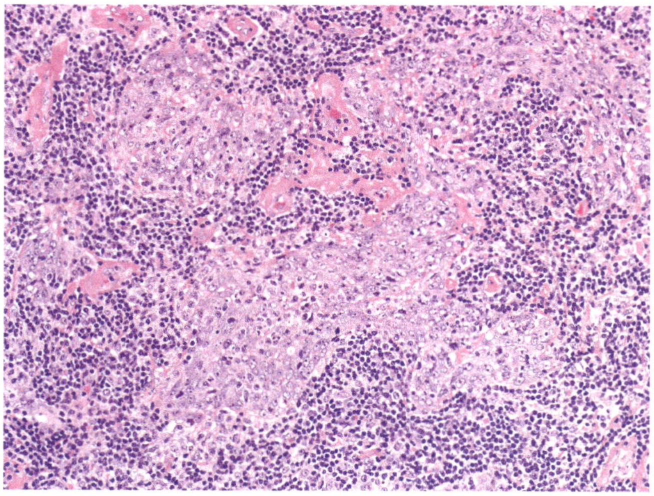

Fig. 16.3 (H&E, 200×) Lymphoepithelial carcinoma, tumor-associated lymphoid proliferation

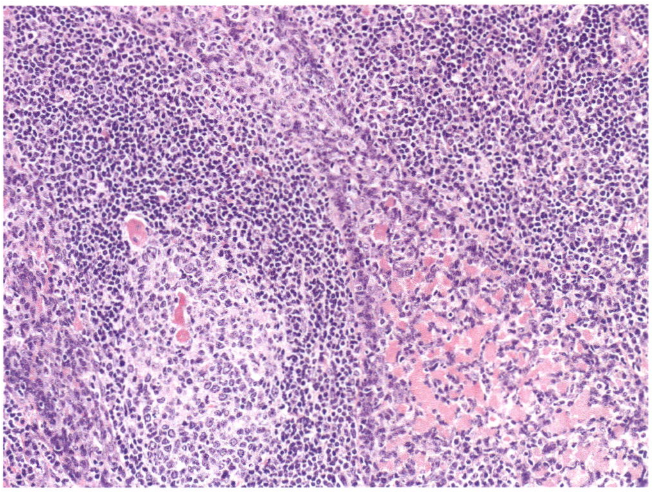

Fig. 16.4 (H&E, 200×) Lymphoepithelial carcinoma, tumor-associated lymphoid proliferation

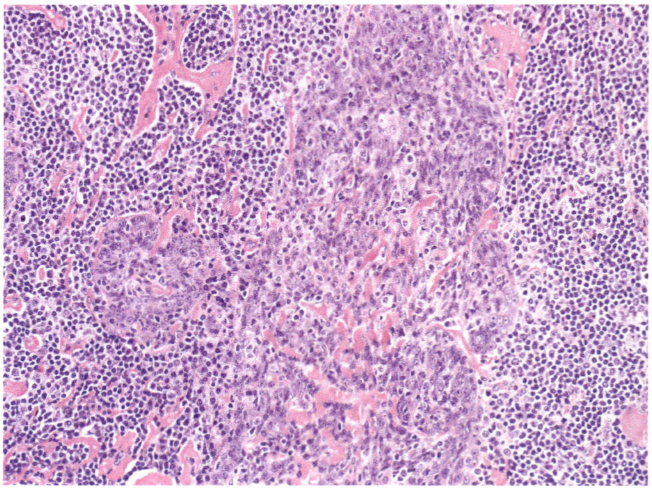

Fig. 16.5 (H&E, 200×) Lymphoepithelial carcinoma, tumor-associated lymphoid proliferation

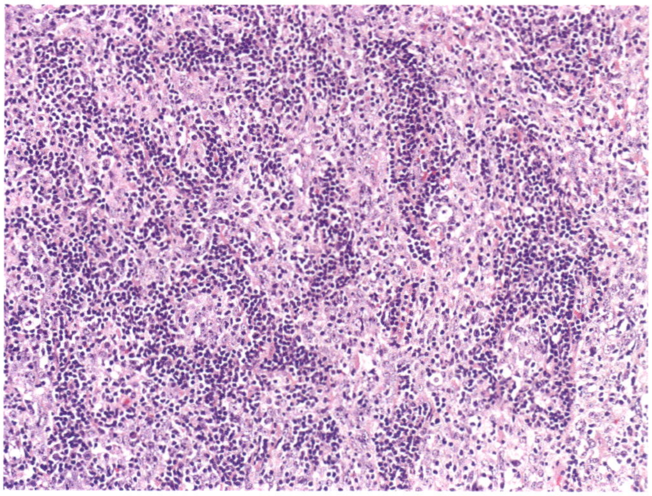

Fig. 16.6 (H&E, 200×) Lymphoepithelial carcinoma, tumor-associated lymphoid proliferation

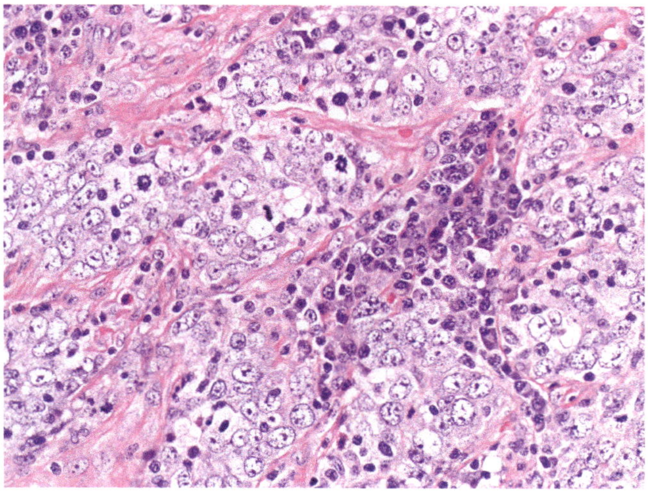

Fig. 16.7 (H&E, 400×) Lymphoepithelial carcinoma, cytomorphologic atypia

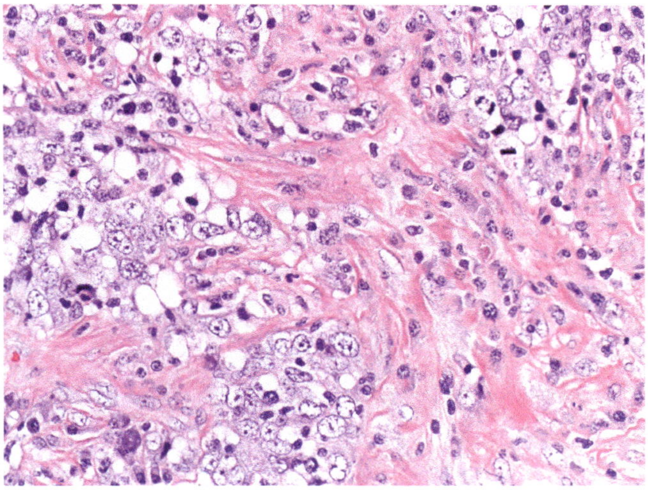

Fig. 16.8 (H&E, 400×) Lymphoepithelial carcinoma, cytomorphologic atypia

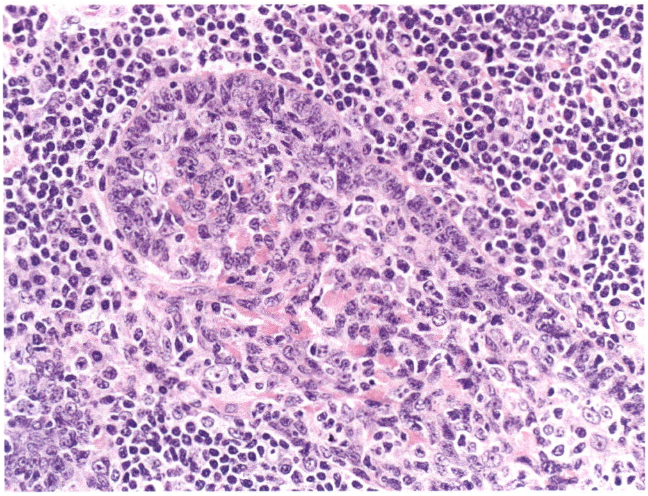

Fig. 16.9 (H&E, 400×) Lymphoepithelial carcinoma, cytomorphologic atypia

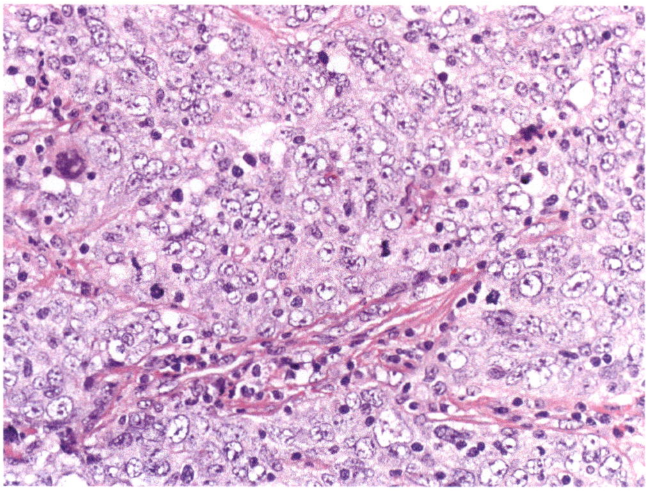

Fig. 16.10 (H&E, 400×) Lymphoepithelial carcinoma, mitotic activity

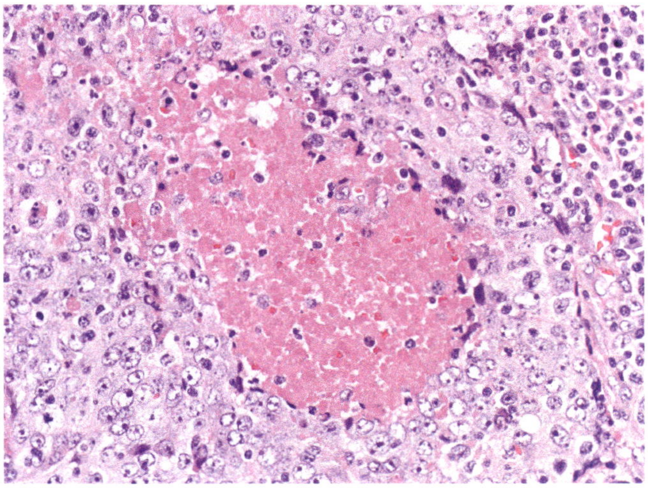

Fig. 16.11 (H&E, 400×) Lymphoepithelial carcinoma, necrosis

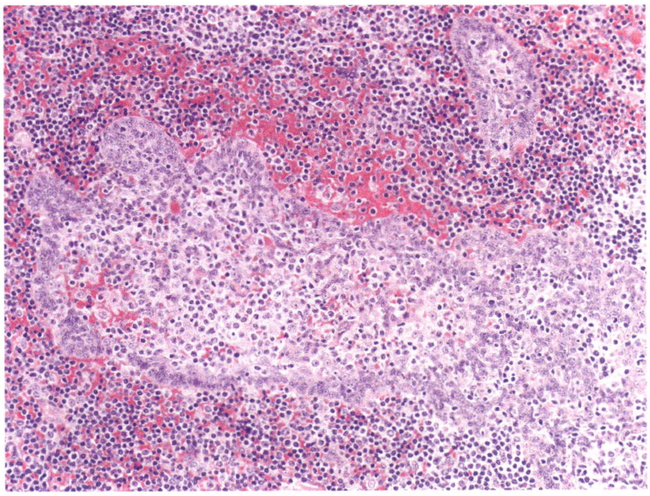

Fig. 16.12 (H&E, 200×) Lymphoepithelial carcinoma, hemorrhagic

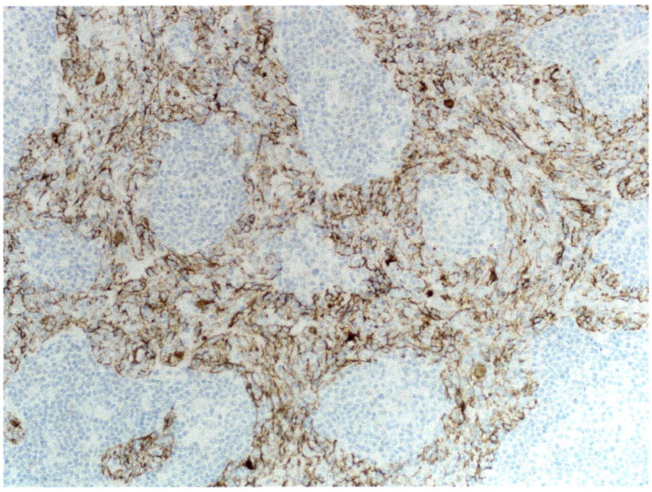

Fig. 16.13 (AE1/AE3, 200×) Lymphoepithelial carcinoma, diffuse immunoreactivity

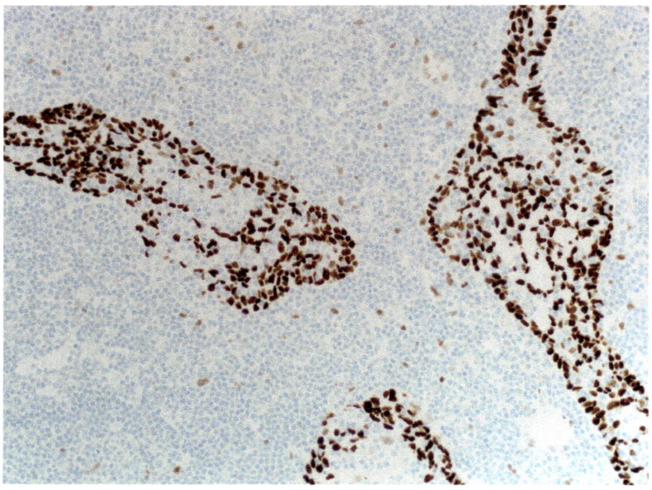

Fig. 16.14 (p63, 200×) Lymphoepithelial carcinoma, diffuse immunoreactivity

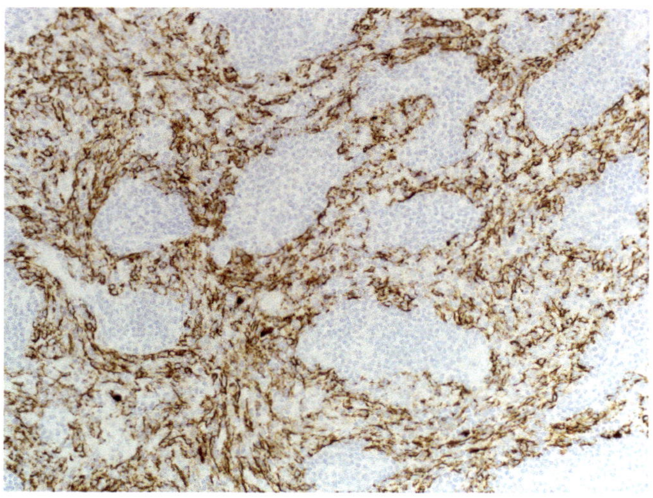

Fig. 16.15 (CK5/6, 200×) Lymphoepithelial carcinoma, diffuse immunoreactivity

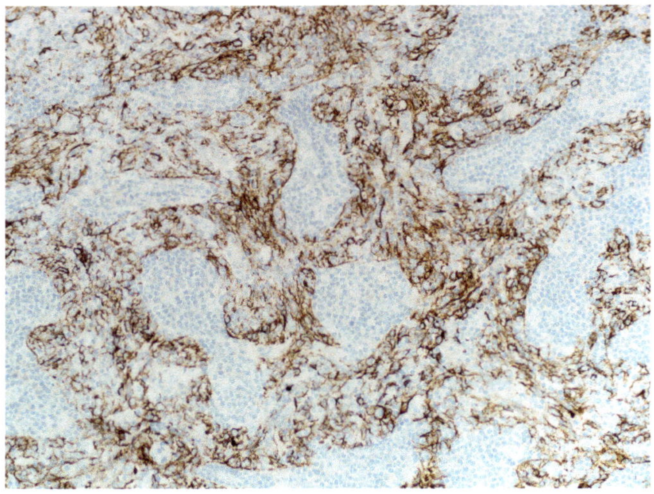

Fig. 16.16 (34βE12, 200×) Lymphoepithelial carcinoma, diffuse immunoreactivity

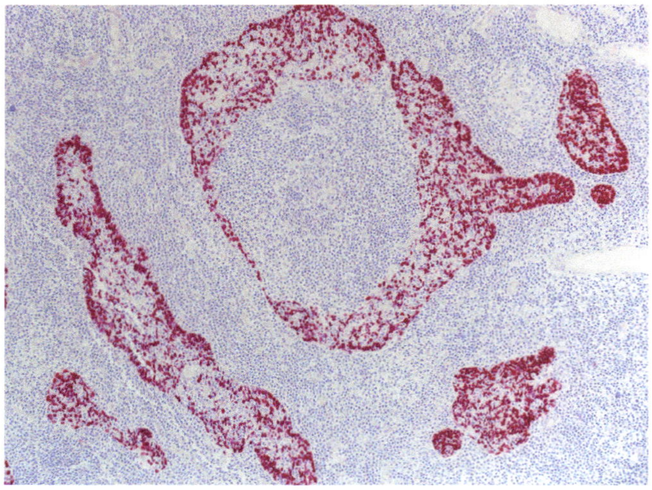

Fig. 16.17 (EBV in situ hybridization, 100×) Lymphoepithelial carcinoma, diffuse hybridization

Suggested Reading

Albeck H, Nielsen NH, Hansen HE, Bentzen J, Ockelmann HH, Bretlau P, et al. Epidemiology of nasopharyngeal and salivary gland carcinoma in Greenland. Arctic Med Res. 1992;51:189–95.

Ambrosio MR, Masrogiulio MG, Barone A, Rocca BJ, Gallo C, Lazzi S, et al. Lymphoepithelial-like carcinoma of the parotid gland: a case report and a brief review of the western literature. Diagn Pathol. 2013;8:115.

Bialas M, Sinczak A, Choinska-Stefanska A, Zygulska A. EBV-positive lymphoepithelial carcinoma of salivary gland in a woman of a non-endemic area--a case report. Pol J Pathol. 2002;53(4):235–8.

Friborg J, Hamilton-Therkildsen M, Homoe P, Kristensen C, Hui A, Liu FF, et al. A spectrum of basaloid morphology in a subset of EBV-associated "lymphoepithelial carcinomas" of major salivary glands. Head Neck Pathol. 2012;6:445–50.

Hamilton-Dutoit SJ, Therkildsen M, Neilsen NH, Jensen H, Hansen JP, Pallesen G. Undifferentiated carcinoma of the salivary gland in Greenlandic Eskimos: demonstration of Epstein-Barr virus DNA by in situ nucleic acid hybridization. Hum Pathol. 1991;22:811–5.

Hsiung CY, Huang CC, Wang CJ, Huang EY, Huang HY. Lymphoepithelioma-like carcinoma of salivary glands: treatment results and failure patterns. Br J Radiol. 2006;79:52–5.

Jen KY, Cheng J, Li J, Wu L, Li Y, Yu S, et al. Mutational events in LMP1 gene of Epstein-Barr virus in salivary gland lymphoepithelial carcinomas. Int J Cancer. 2003;105(5):654–60.

Jen KY, Higuchi M, Cheng J, Li J, Wu LY, Li YF, et al. Nucleotide sequences and functions of the Epstein-Barr virus latent membrane protein 1 genes isolated from salivary gland lymphoepithelial carcinomas. Virus Genes. 2005;30(2):223–35.

Kuo T, Hsueh C. Lymphoepithelioma-like salivary gland carcinoma in Taiwan: a clinicopathological study of nine cases demonstrating strong association with Epstein-Barr virus. Histopathology. 1997;31:75–82.

Leung SY, Chung LP, Yuen ST, Ho CM, Wong MP, Chan SY. Lymphoepithelial carcinoma of the salivary gland: in situ detection of Epstein-Barr virus. J Clin Pathol. 1995;48:1022–7.

Li F, Zhu G, Wang Y, Wang Y, Chent T, Ji Q. A clinical analysis of 37 cases with lymphoepithelial carcinoma of the major salivary gland treated by surgical resection and postoperative radiotherapy: a single institution study. Med Oncol. 2014;31:957.

Nagao T, Ishida Y, Sugano I, Tajima Y, Matsuzaki O, Hino T, et al. Epstein-Barr virus-associated undifferentiated carcinoma with lymphoid stroma of the salivary gland in Japanese patients: comparison with benign lymphoepithelial lesion. Cancer. 1996;78:695–703.

Saku T, Cheng J, Jen KY, Tokunaga M, Li J, Zhang W, et al. Epstein-Barr virus infected lymphoepithelial carcinomas of the salivary gland in the Russia-Asia area: a clinicopathologic study of 160 cases. Arkh Patol. 2003;65(2):35–9.

Sheen TS, Tsai CC, Ko JY, Chang YL, Hsu MM. Undifferentiated carcinoma of the major salivary glands. Cancer. 1997;80:357–63.

Tsai CC, Chen CL, Hsu HC. Expression of Epstein-Barr virus in carcinomas of major salivary glands: a strong association with lymphoepithelioma-like carcinoma. Hum Pathol. 1996;27: 258–62.

Wang CP, Chang YL, Ko JY, Lou PJ, Yeh CF, Sheen TS. Lymphoepithelial carcinoma versus large cell undifferentiated carcinoma of the major salivary glands. Cancer. 2004;101(9):2020–7.

Wenig BM. Lymphoepithlial-like carcinomas of the head and neck. Semin Diagn Pathol. 2015;32:74–86.

Wu DL, Shemen L, Brady T, Saw D. Malignant lymphoepithelial lesion of the parotid gland: a case report and review of the literature. Ear Nose Throat J. 2001;80(11):803–6.

17 Mucoepidermoid Carcinoma

Mucoepidermoid carcinoma affects children and adults and is the most common salivary gland malignancy. Women are involved slightly more than men. The majority of cases involve major salivary glands, presenting as single or multiple masses. Most cases of mucoepidermoid carcinoma behave as low to intermediate-grade malignancies. Mucoepidermoid carcinoma may be circumscribed or infiltrative, comprised of multiple cell types (mucous, epidermoid, intermediate, columnar, oncocytic, and clear), and exhibit a variety of architectural patterns (solid, cystic, papillary, and sclerosing) (Figs. 17.1–17.40).

J. J. García, *Atlas of Salivary Gland Pathology*, https://doi.org/10.1007/978-3-319-09021-4_17

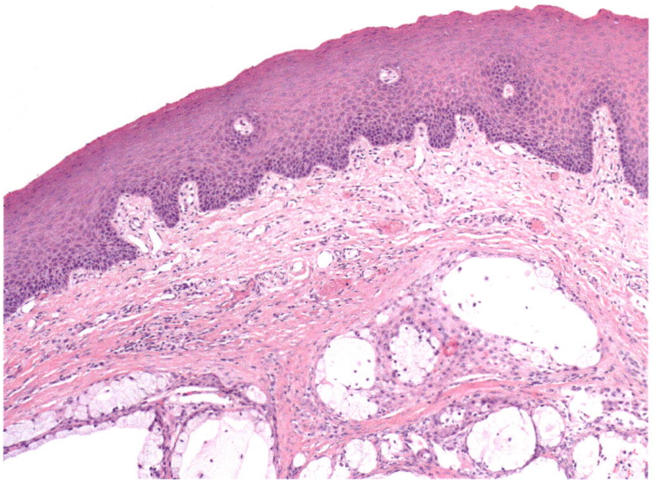

Fig. 17.1 (H&E, 100×) Mucoepidermoid carcinoma, circumscribed

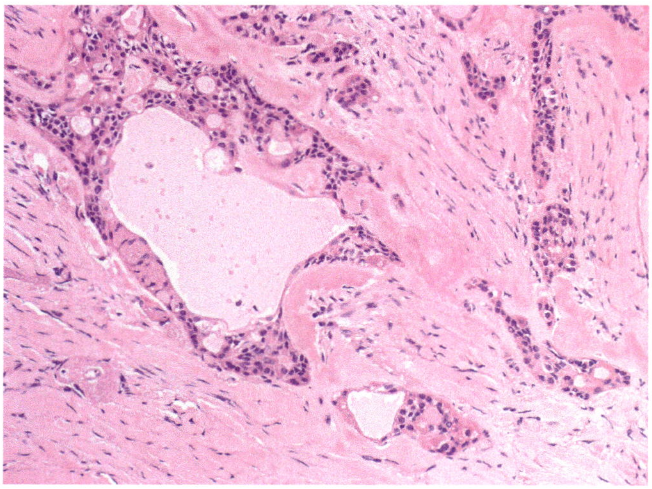

Fig. 17.2 (H&E, 200×) Mucoepidermoid carcinoma, infiltrative

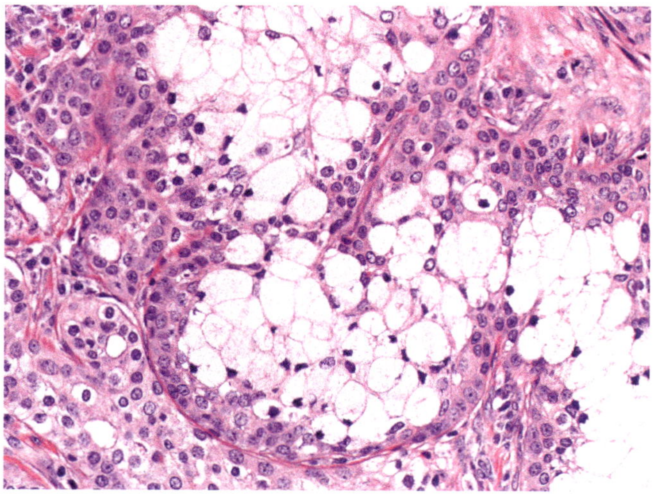

Fig. 17.3 (H&E, 400×) Mucoepidermoid carcinoma, triphasic or more

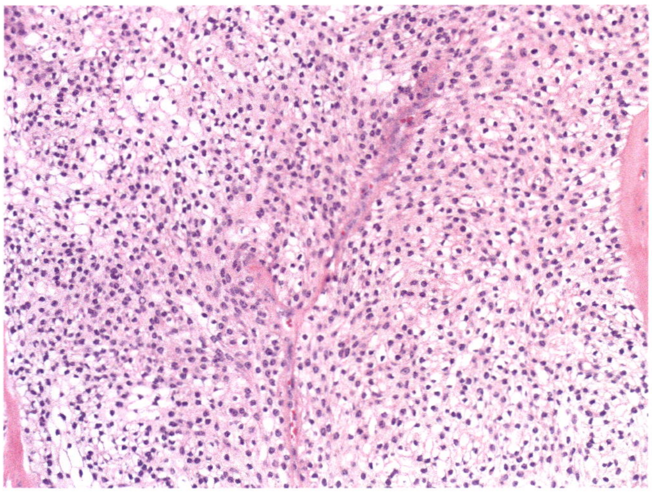

Fig. 17.4 (H&E, 200×) Mucoepidermoid carcinoma, solid

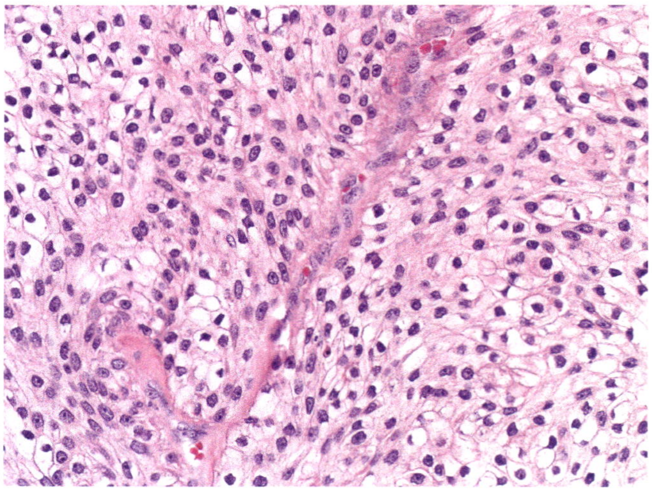

Fig. 17.5 (H&E, 400×) Mucoepidermoid carcinoma, solid

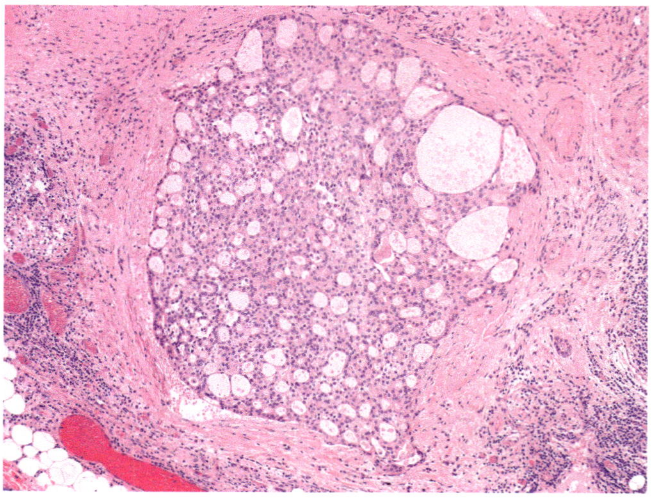

Fig. 17.6 (H&E, 100×) Mucoepidermoid carcinoma, microcystic

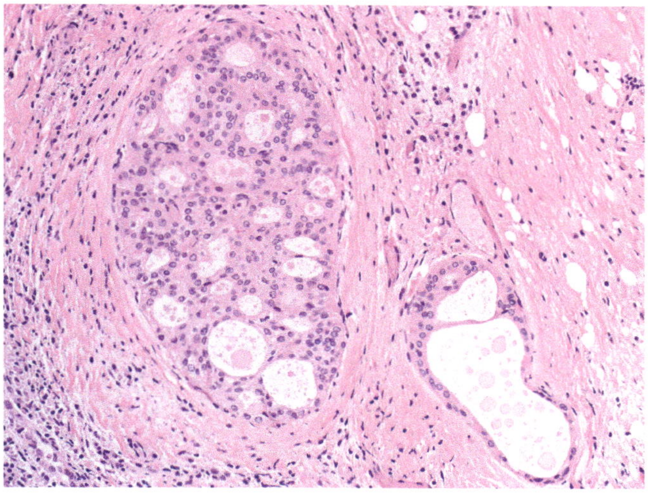

Fig. 17.7 (H&E, 200×) Mucoepidermoid carcinoma, microcystic

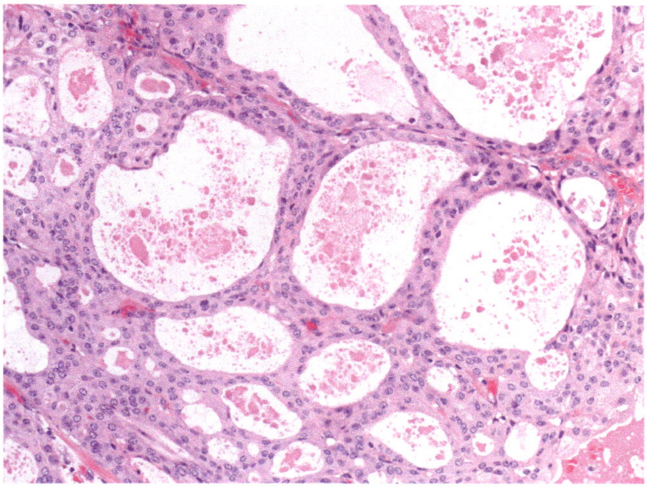

Fig. 17.8 (H&E, 200×) Mucoepidermoid carcinoma, microcystic

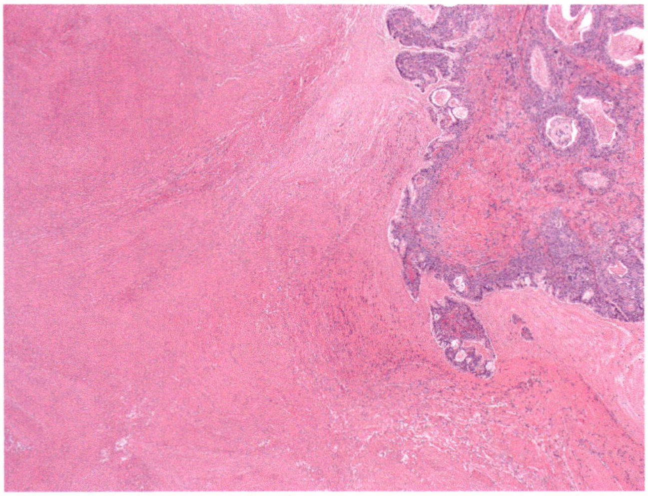

Fig. 17.9 (H&E, 40×) Mucoepidermoid carcinoma, cystic

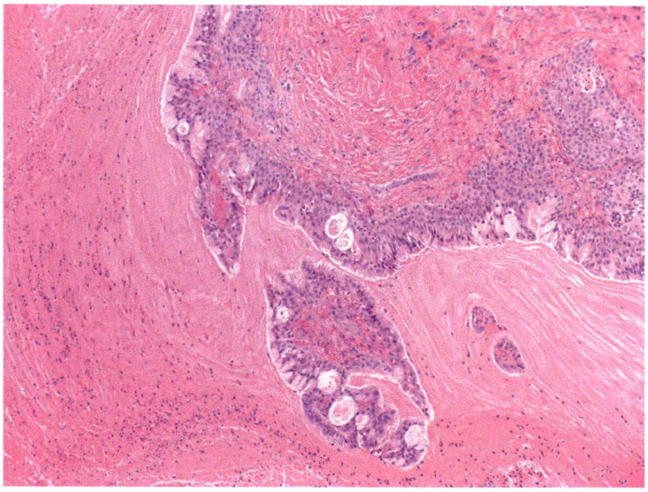

Fig. 17.10 (H&E, 100×) Mucoepidermoid carcinoma, cystic

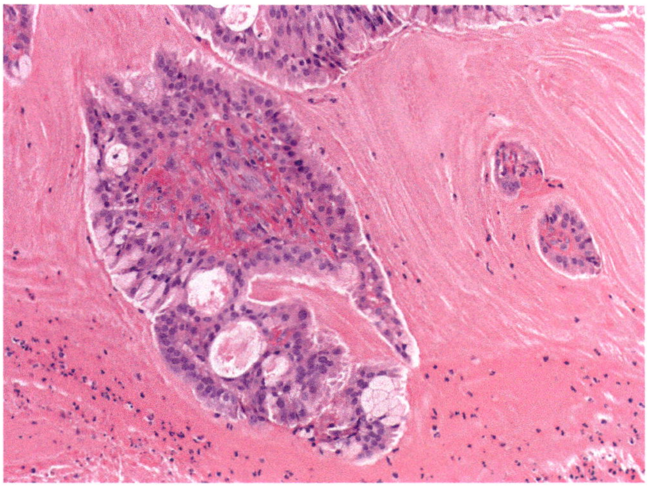

Fig. 17.11 (H&E, 200×) Mucoepidermoid carcinoma, cystic

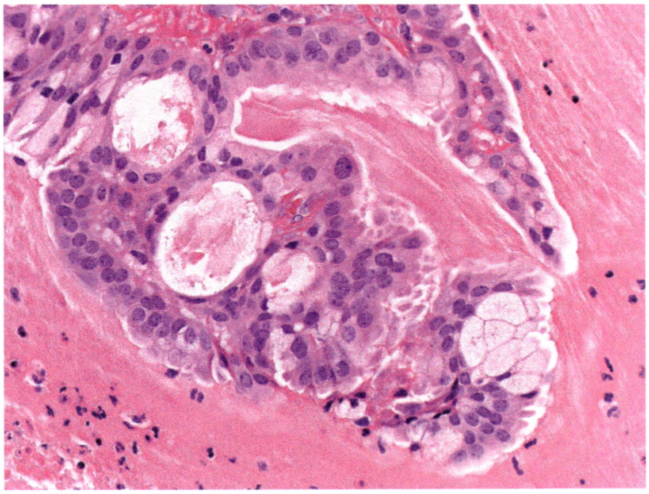

Fig. 17.12 (H&E, 400×) Mucoepidermoid carcinoma, cystic

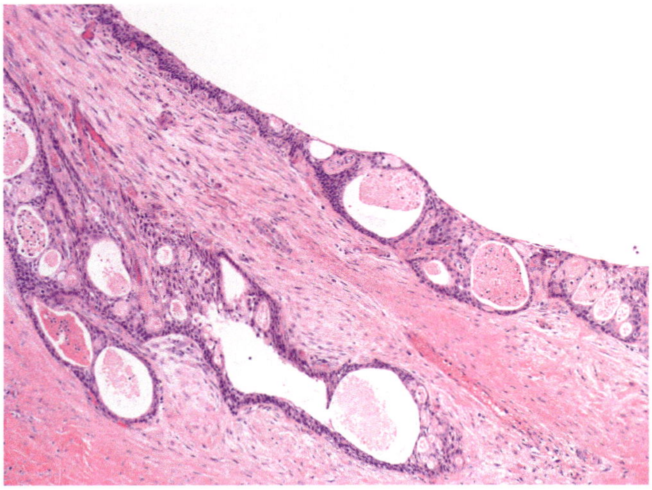

Fig. 17.13 (H&E, 100×) Mucoepidermoid carcinoma, cystic

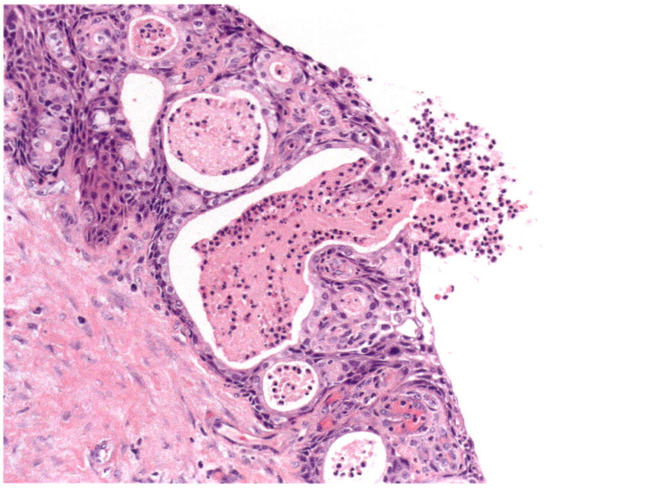

Fig. 17.14 (H&E, 100×) Mucoepidermoid carcinoma, cystic

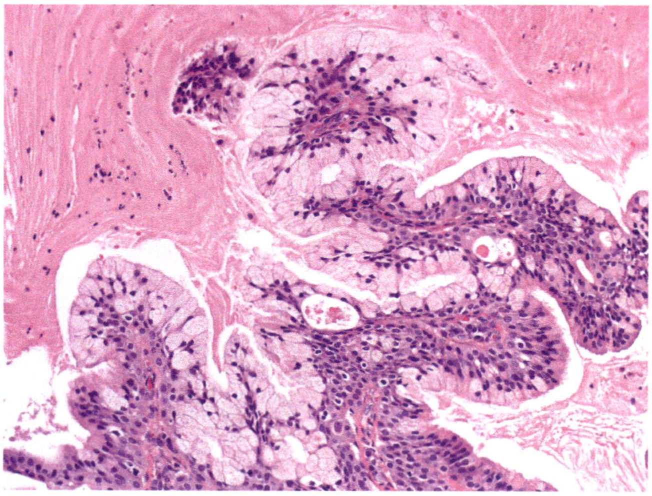

Fig. 17.15 (H&E, 200×) Mucoepidermoid carcinoma, cystic

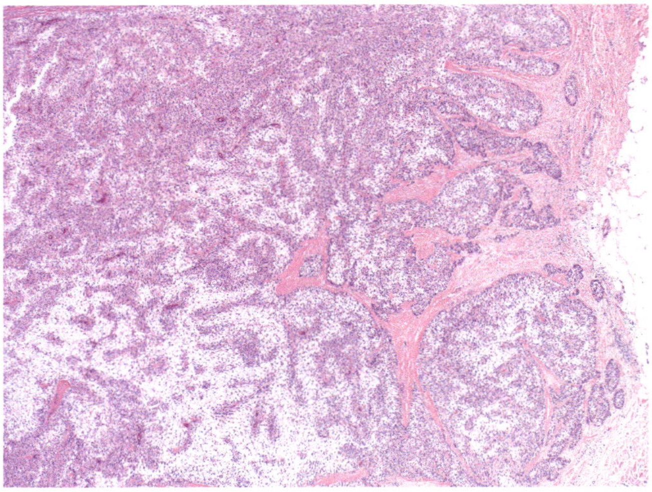

Fig. 17.16 (H&E, 40×) Mucoepidermoid carcinoma, clear

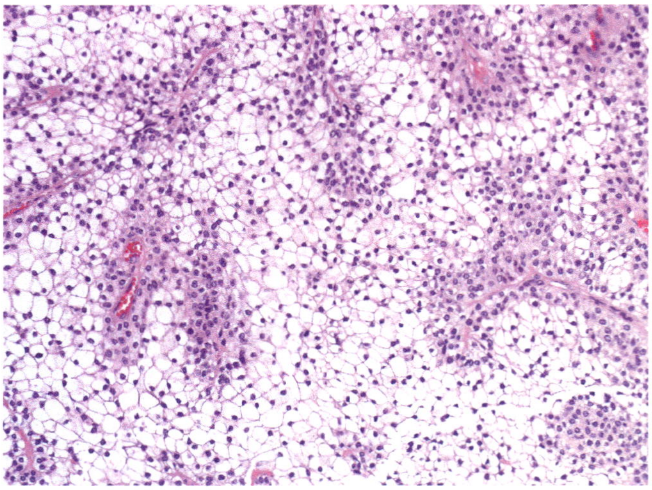

Fig. 17.17 (H&E, 200×) Mucoepidermoid carcinoma, clear

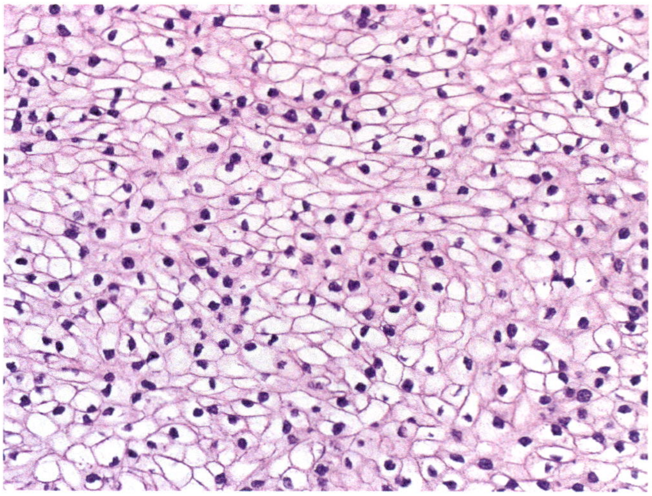

Fig. 17.18 (H&E, 400×) Mucoepidermoid carcinoma, clear

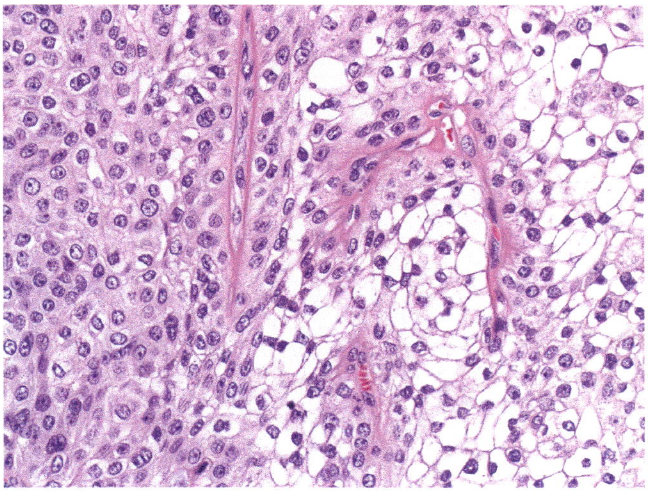

Fig. 17.19 (H&E, 400×) Mucoepidermoid carcinoma, clear

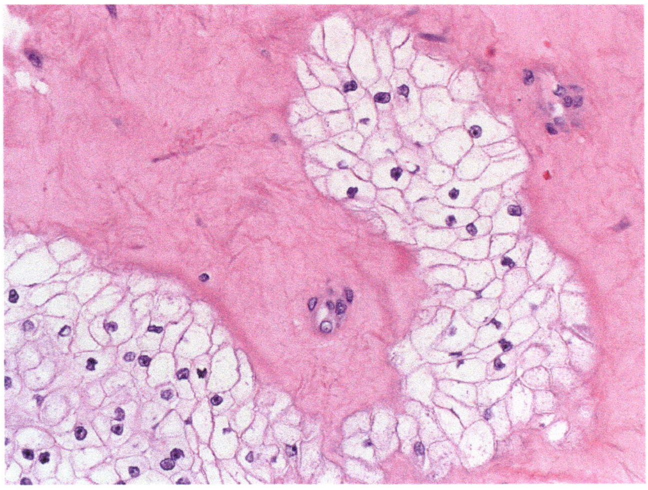

Fig. 17.20 (H&E, 400×) Mucoepidermoid carcinoma, clear

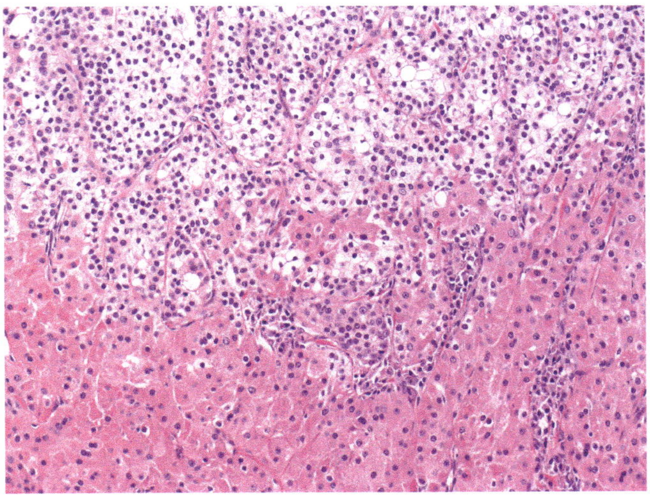

Fig. 17.21 (H&E, 200×) Mucoepidermoid carcinoma, oncocytic

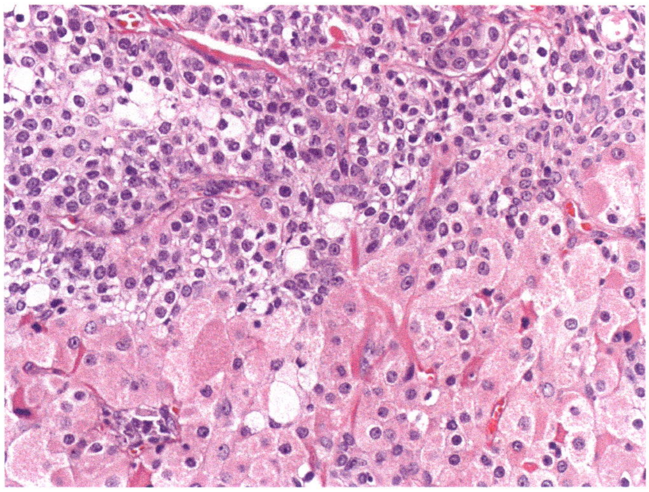

Fig. 17.22 (H&E, 400×) Mucoepidermoid carcinoma, oncocytic

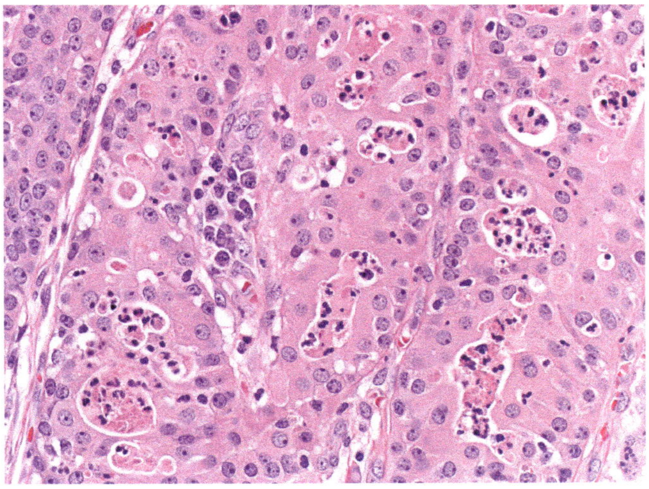

Fig. 17.23 (H&E, 400×) Mucoepidermoid carcinoma, oncocytic

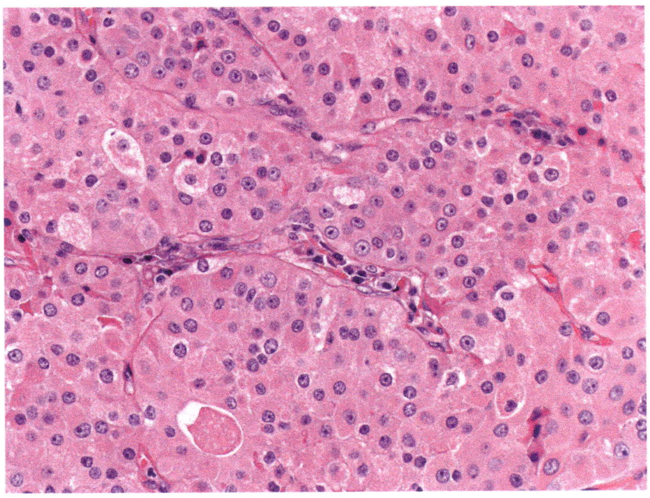

Fig. 17.24 (H&E, 400×) Mucoepidermoid carcinoma, oncocytic

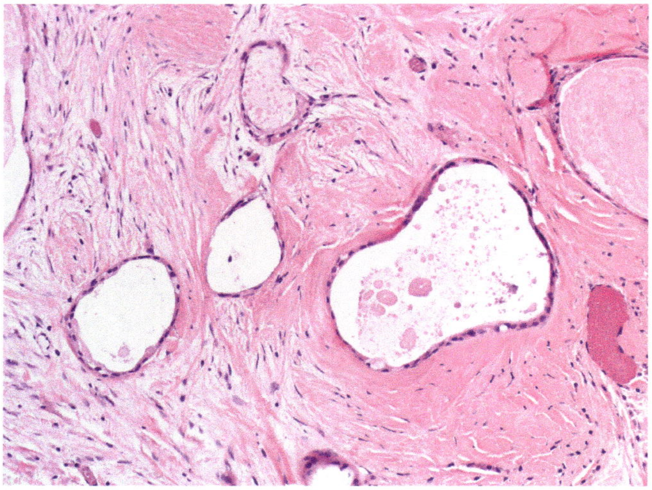

Fig. 17.25 (H&E, 200×) Mucoepidermoid carcinoma, sclerosing

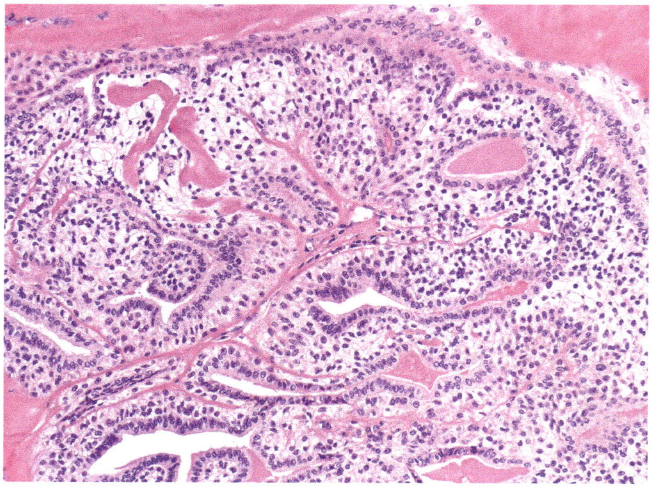

Fig. 17.26 (H&E, 200×) Mucoepidermoid carcinoma, columnar

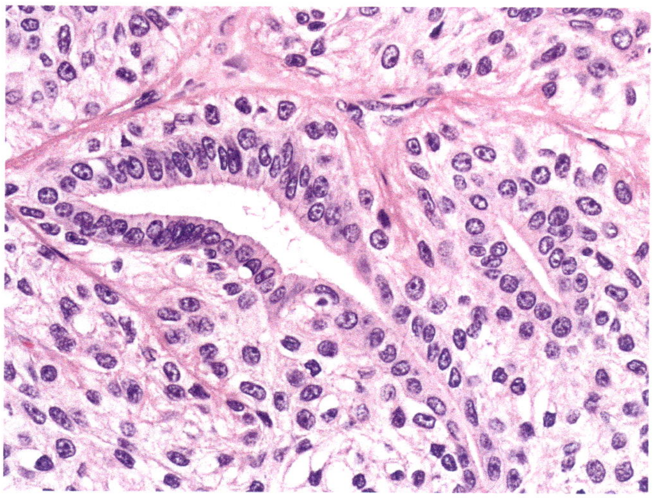

Fig. 17.27 (H&E, 400×) Mucoepidermoid carcinoma, columnar

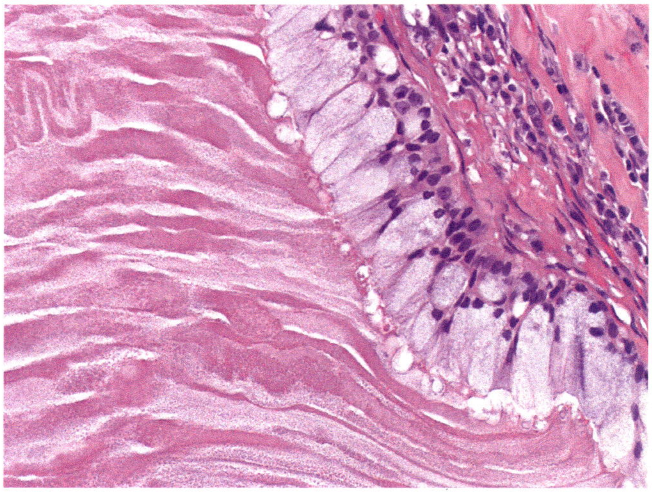

Fig. 17.28 (H&E, 400×) Mucoepidermoid carcinoma, mucin

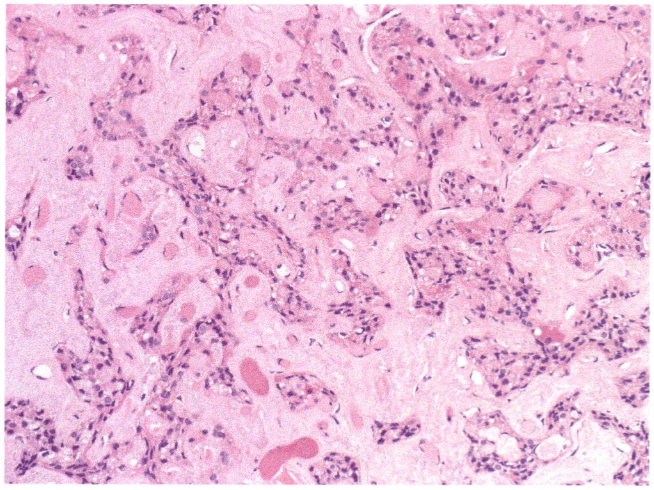

Fig. 17.29 (H&E, 200×) Mucoepidermoid carcinoma, myxoid

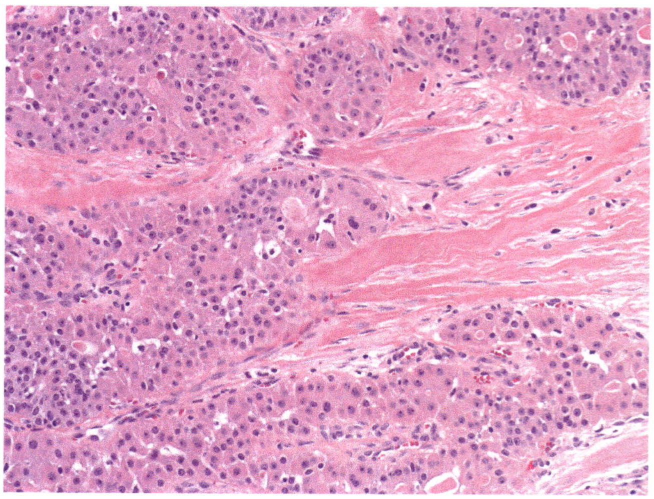

Fig. 17.30 (H&E, 200×) Mucoepidermoid carcinoma, hyalinized

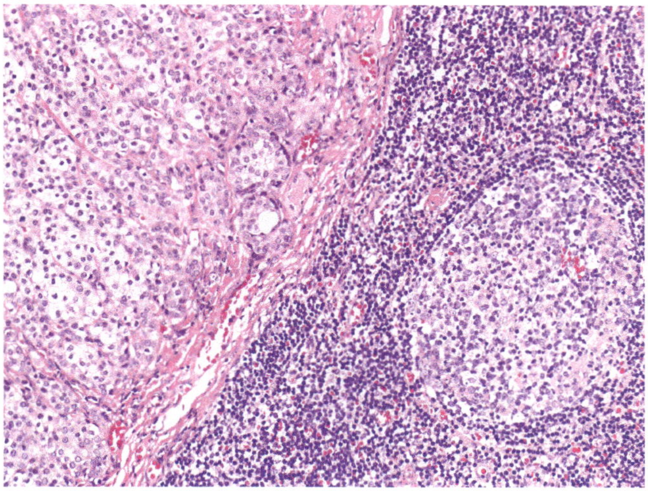

Fig. 17.31 (H&E, 200×) Mucoepidermoid carcinoma, tumor-associated lymphoid proliferation

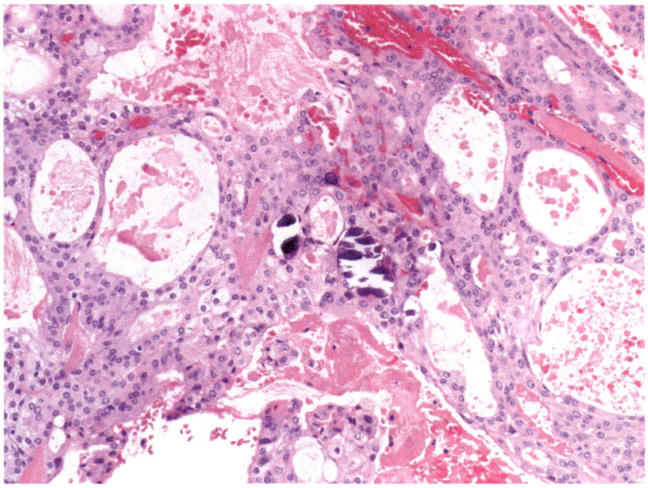

Fig. 17.32 (H&E, 200×) Mucoepidermoid carcinoma, microcalcifications

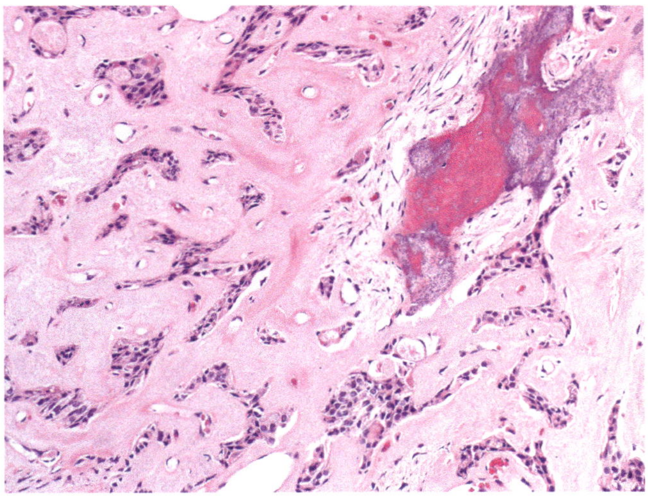

Fig. 17.33 (H&E, 200×) Mucoepidermoid carcinoma, osseous metaplasia

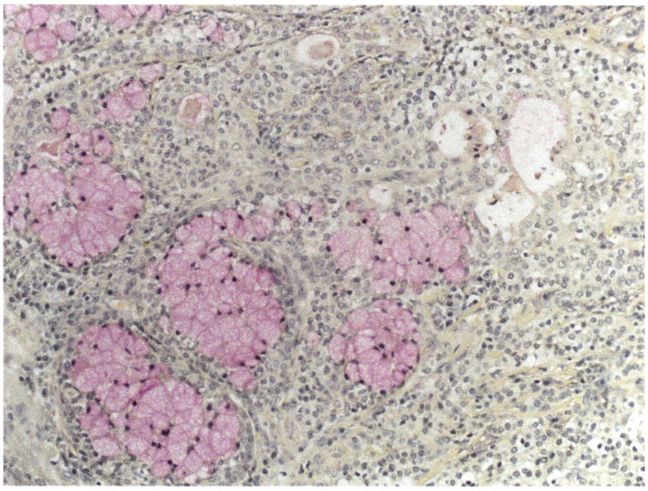

Fig. 17.34 (Mucicarmine, 200×) Mucoepidermoid carcinoma, intracytoplasmic reactivity

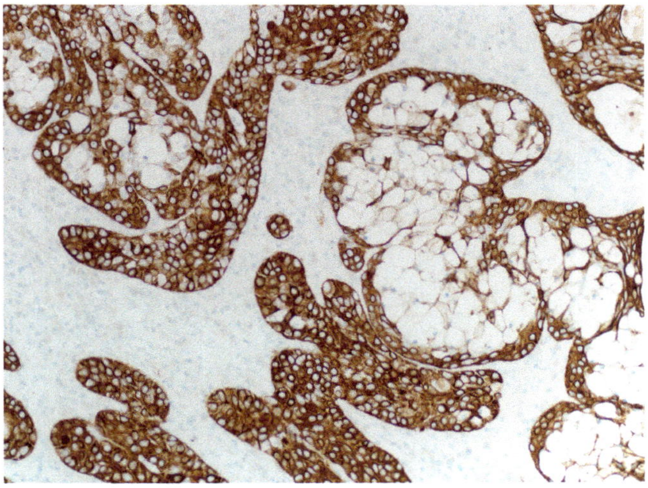

Fig. 17.35 (AE1/AE3, 200×) Mucoepidermoid carcinoma, diffuse immunoreactivity

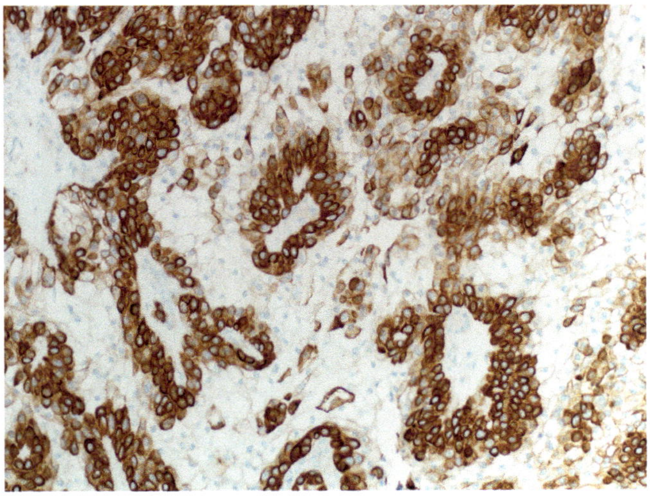

Fig. 17.36 (AE1/AE3, 200×) Mucoepidermoid carcinoma, focal immunoreactivity

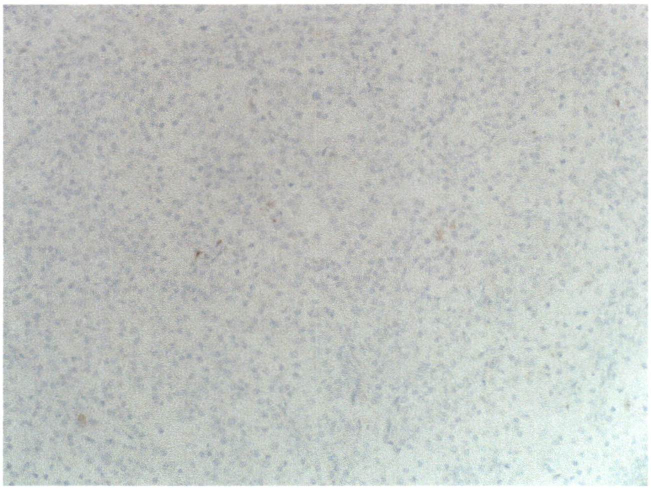

Fig. 17.37 (S-100, 200×) Mucoepidermoid carcinoma, negative immunoreactivity

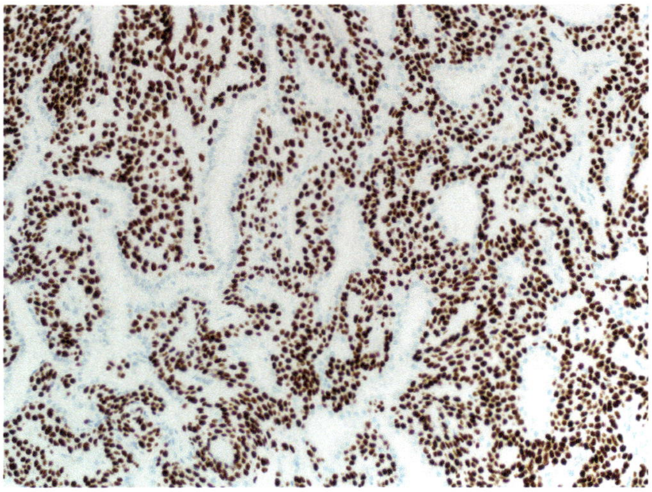

Fig. 17.39 (p63, 200×) Mucoepidermoid carcinoma, focal immunoreactivity

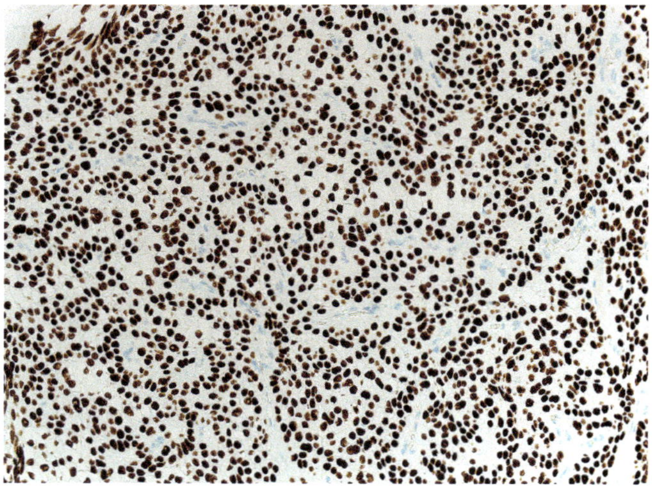

Fig. 17.38 (p63, 200×) Mucoepidermoid carcinoma, diffuse immunoreactivity

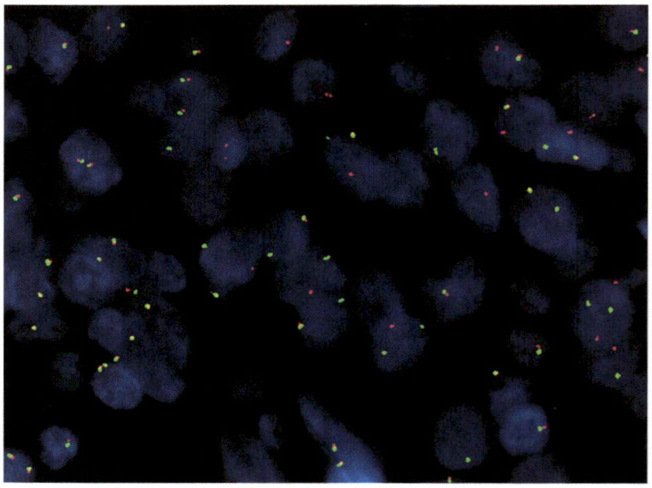

Fig. 17.40 (Fluorescent in situ hybridization, 600×) Mucoepidermoid carcinoma, *MAML2* rearrangement

Suggested Reading

Achcar Rde O, Nikiforova MN, Dacic S, Nicholson AG, Yousem SA. Mammalian mastermind like 2 11q21 gene rearrangement in bronchopulmonary mucoepidermoid carcinoma. Hum Pathol. 2009;40(6):854–60.

Aro K, Leivo I, Makitie AA. Management and outcome of patients with mucoepidermoid carcinoma of major salivary gland origin: a single institution's 30-year experience. Laryngoscope. 2008;118(2):258–62.

Auclair PL, Goode RK, Ellis GL. Mucoepidermoid carcinoma of intraoral salivary glands. Evaluation and application of grading criteria in 143 cases. Cancer. 1992;69:2021–30.

Bai S, Clubwala R, Adler E, Sarta C, Schiff B, Smith RV, et al. Salivary mucoepidermoid carcinoma: a multi-institutional review of 76 patients. Head Neck Pathol. 2013;7(2):105–12.

Bhaijee F, Pepper DJ, Pitman KT, Bell D. New developments in the molecular pathogenesis of head and neck tumors: a review of tumor-specific fusion oncogenes in mucoepidermoid carcinoma, adenoid cystic carcinoma, and NUT midline carcinoma. Ann Diagn Pathol. 2011;15(1):69–77.

Brandwein MS, Ivanov K, Wallace DI, Hille JJ, Wang B, Fahmy A, et al. Mucoepidermoid carcinoma: a clinicopathologic study of 80 patients with special reference to histological grading. Am J Surg Pathol. 2001;25(7):835–45.

Byrd SA, Spector ME, Carey TE, Bradford CR, McHugh JB. Predictors of recurrence and survival for head and neck mucoepidermoid carcinoma. Otoloaryngol Head Neck Surg. 2013;149:402–8.

Camelo-Piragua SI, Habib C, Kanumuri P, Lago CE, Mason HS, Otis CN. Mucoepidermoid carcinoma of the breast shares cytogenetic abnormality with mucoepidermoid carcinoma of the salivary gland: a case report with molecular analysis and review of the literature. Hum Pathol. 2009;40(6):887–92.

Fadare O, Hileeto D, Gruddin YL, Mariappan MR. Sclerosing mucoepidermoid carcinoma of the parotid gland. Arch Pathol Lab Med. 2004;128(9):1046–9.

Fehr A, Roser K, Heidorn K, Hallas C, Loning T, Bullerdiek J. A new type of MAML2 fusion in mucoepidermoid carcinoma. Genes Chromosomes Cancer. 2008;47(3):203–6.

Foschini MP, Marucci G, Eusebi V. Low-grade mucoepidermoid carcinoma of salivary glands: characteristic immunohistochemical profile and evidence of striated duct differentiation. Virchows Arch. 2002;440(5):536–42.

Garcia JJ, Hunt JL, Weinreb I, McHugh JB, Barnes EL, Cieply K, et al. Fluorescence in situ hybridization for detection of MAML2 rearrangements in oncocytic mucoepidermoid carcinoma: utility as a diagnostic test. Hum Pathol. 2011;42:2001–9.

Goode RK, Auclair PL, Ellis GL. Mucoepidermoid carcinoma of the major salivary glands: clinical and histopathologic analysis of 234 cases with evaluation of grading criteria. Cancer. 1998;82:1217–24.

Guzzo M, Andreola S, Sirizzotti G, Cantu G. Mucoepidermoid carcinoma of the salivary glands: clinicopathologic review of 108 patients treated at the National Cancer Institute of Milan. Ann Surg Oncol. 2002;9(7):688–95.

Han SW, Kim HP, Jeon YK, Oh DY, Lee SH, Kim DW, et al. Mucoepidermoid carcinoma of lung: potential target of EGFR-directed treatment. Lung Cancer. 2008;61(1):30–4.

Jarvis SJ, Giangrande V, Brennan PA. Mucoepidermoid carcinoma of the tonsil: a very rare presentation. Acta Otorhinolaryngol Ital. 2013;33(4):286–8.

Katabi N, Ghossein R, Ali S, Dogan S, Klimstra D, Ganly I. Prognostic features in mucoepidermoid carcinoma of major salivary glands with emphasis on tumor histologic grading. Histopathology. 2014;65:793–804.

Li Y, Li LJ, Huang J, Han B, Pan J. Central malignant salivary gland tumors of the jaw: retrospective clinical analysis of 22 cases. J Oral Maxillofac Surg. 2008;66:2247–53.

Martins C, Cavaco B, Tonon G, Kaye FJ, Soares J, Fonseca I. A study of MECT1-MAML2 in mucoepidermoid carcinoma and Warthin's tumor of salivary glands. J Mol Diagn. 2004;6(3):205–10.

McHugh CH, Roberts DB, El-Naggar AK, Hanna EY, Garden AS, Kies MS, et al. Prognostic factors in mucoepidermoid carcinoma of the salivary glands. Cancer. 2012;118:3928–36.

Mendelson AA, al-Macki K, Chauvin P, Kost KM. Sclerosing mucoepidermoid carcinoma of the salivary gland: case report and literature review. Ear Nose Throat J. 2010;890:600–3.

Nakayama T, Miyabe S, Okabe M, Sakuma H, Ijichi K, Hasegawa Y, et al. Clinicopathological significance of the CRTC3-MAML2 fusion transcript in mucoepidermoid carcinoma. Mod Pathol. 2009;22(12):1575–81.

Nance MA, Seethala RR, Wang Y, Chiosea SI, Myers EN, Johnson JT, et al. Treatment and survival outcomes based on histologic grading in patients with head and neck mucoepidermoid carcinoma. Cancer. 2008;113(8):2082–9.

O'Neill ID. t(11;19) translocation and CRTC1-MAML2 fusion oncogene in mucoepidermoid carcinoma. Oral Oncol. 2009;45(1):2–9.

Pires FR, de Almeida OP, de Araujo VC, Kowalski LP. Prognostic factors in head and neck muoepidermoid carcinoma. Arch Otolaryngol Head Neck Surg. 2004;130:174–80.

Raut D, Khedkar S. Primary intraosseous mucoepidermoid carcinoma of the maxilla: a case report and review of literature. Dentomaxillofac Radiol. 2009;38(3):163–8.

Ritwik P, Cordell KG, Brannon RB. Minor salivary gland mucoepidermoid carcinoma in children and adolescents: a case series and review of the literature. J Med Case Rep. 2012;6:182.

Roden AC, Erickson-Johnson MR, Yi ES, Garcia JJ. Analysis of MAML2 rearrangement in mucoepidermoid carcinoma of the thymus. Hum Pathol. 2013;44(12):2799–805.

Roden AC, Garcia JJ, Wehrs RN, Colby TV, Khoor A, Leslie KO, et al. Histopathologic, immunophenotypic and cytogenetic features of pulmonary mucoepidermoid carcinoma. Mod Pathol. 2014;27(11):1479–88.

Seethala RR, Dacic S, Cieply K, Kelly LM, Nikiforova MN. A reappraisal of the MECT1/MAML2 translocation in salivary mucoepidermoid carcinomas. Am J Surg Pathol. 2010;34:1106–21.

Tasaki T, Matsuyama A, Tabata T, Suzuki H, Yamada S, Sasaguri Y, et al. Sclerosing mucoepidermoid carcinoma with eosinophilia of the salivary gland: case report and review of the literature. Pathol Int. 2013;63:125–31.

Tonon G, Modi S, Wu L, Kubo A, Coxon AB, Komiya T, et al. t(11;19)(q21;p13) translocation in mucoepidermoid carcinoma creates a novel fusion product that disrupts a notch signaling pathway. Nat Genet. 2003;33(2):208–13.

Tsubochi H, Suzuki T, Suzuki S, Ohashi Y, Ishibashi S, Moriya T, et al. Immunohistochemical study of basaloid squamous cell carcinoma, adenoid cystic and mucoepidermoid carcinoma in the upper aerodigestive tract. Anticancer Res. 2000;20(2B):1205–11.

Veras EF, Sturgis E, Luna MA. Sclerosing mucoepidermoid carcinoma of the salivary glands. Ann Diagn Pathol. 2007;11(6):407–12.

18 Myoepithelioma

Myoepithelioma is the benign counterpart of myoepithelial carcinoma. Myoepithelioma affects children and adults and presents at a mean age of approximately 45 years. Women and men are involved with similar frequency. The majority of cases involve major salivary glands, presenting as single or multiple masses. Myoepithelioma may be circumscribed or multi-nodular, comprised almost exclusively of one cell type (myoepithelial), and exhibit a variety of architectural patterns (solid, trabecular, and cystic) (Figs. 18.1–18.23).

J. J. García, *Atlas of Salivary Gland Pathology*, https://doi.org/10.1007/978-3-319-09021-4_18

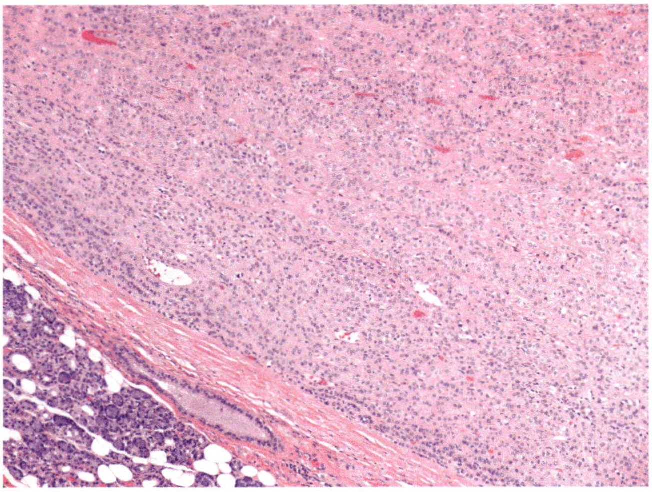

Fig. 18.1 (H&E, 100×) Myoepithelioma, circumscribed

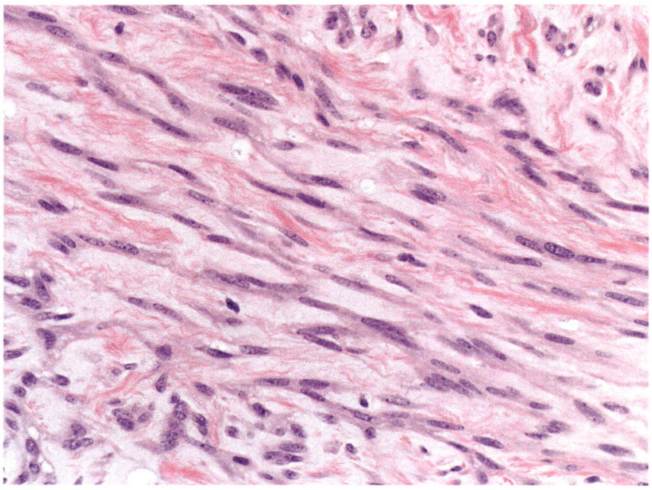

Fig. 18.2 (H&E, 400×) Myoepithelioma, monophasic

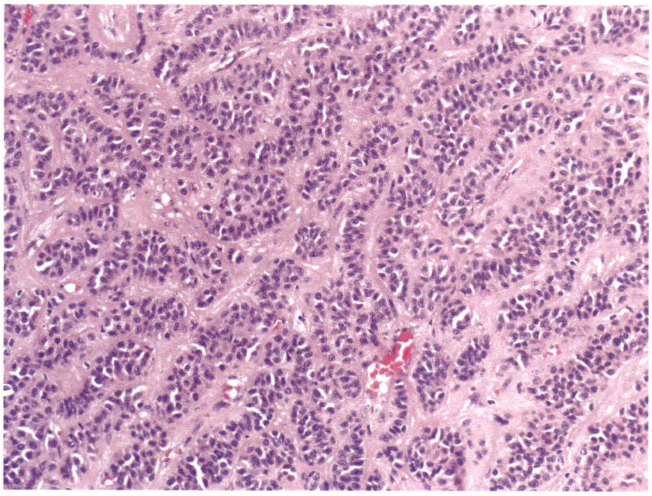

Fig. 18.3 (H&E, 200×) Myoepithelioma, trabecular

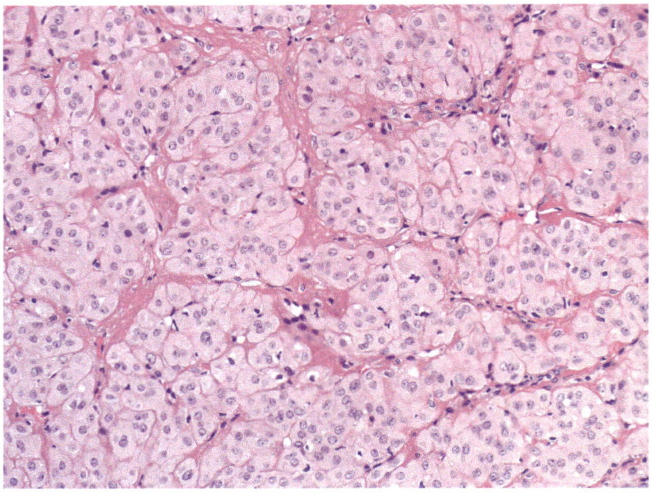

Fig. 18.4 (H&E, 200×) Myoepithelioma, epithelioid

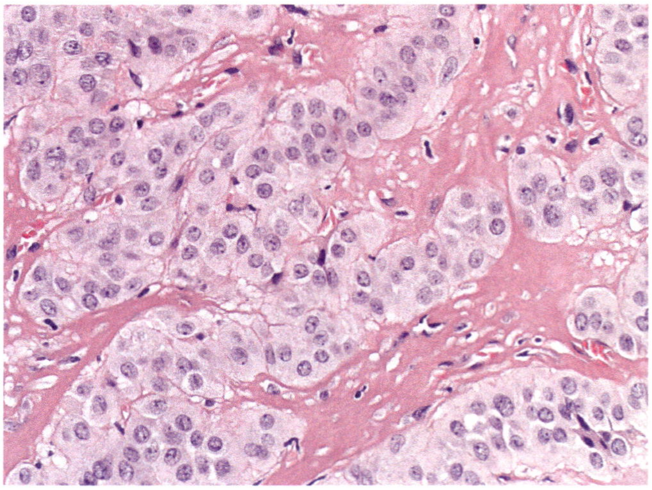

Fig. 18.5 (H&E, 400×) Myoepithelioma, epithelioid

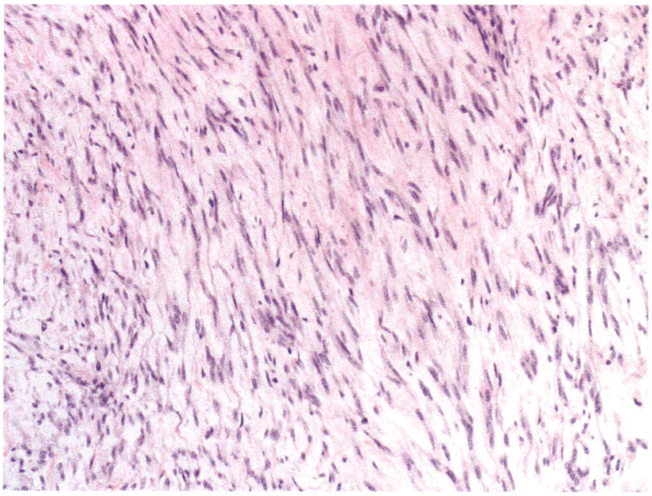

Fig. 18.6 (H&E, 200×) Myoepithelioma, spindled

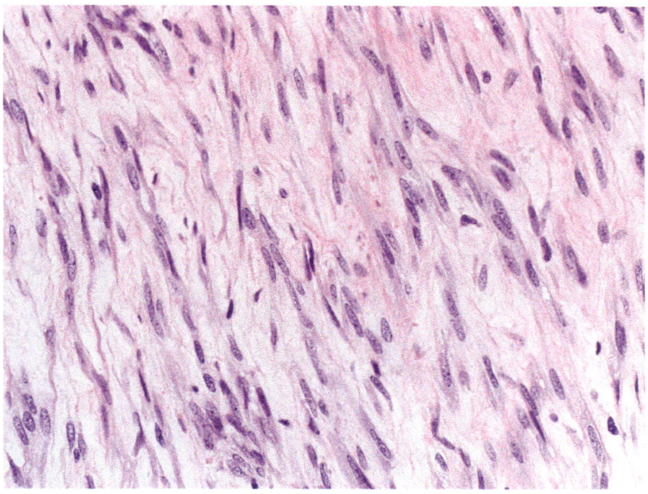

Fig. 18.7 (H&E, 400×) Myoepithelioma, spindled

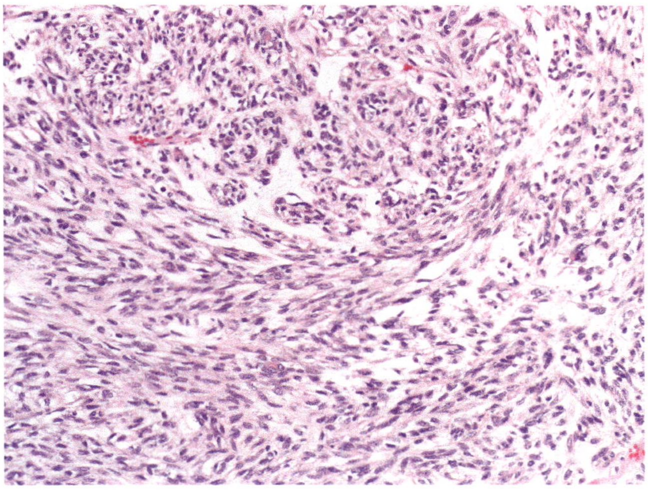

Fig. 18.8 (H&E, 200×) Myoepithelioma, spindled

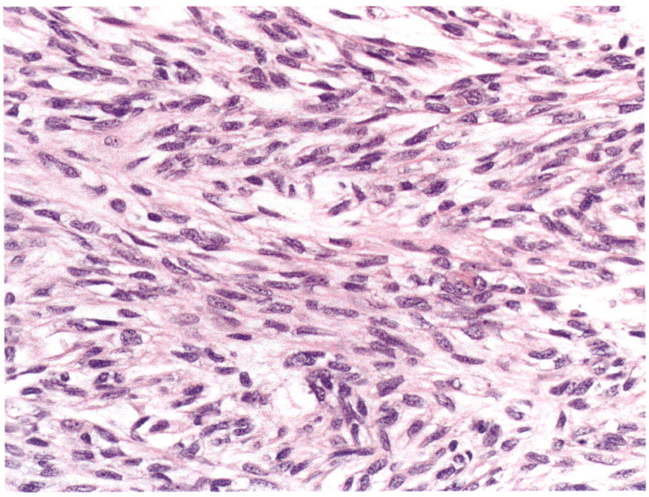

Fig. 18.9 (H&E, 400×) Myoepithelioma, spindled

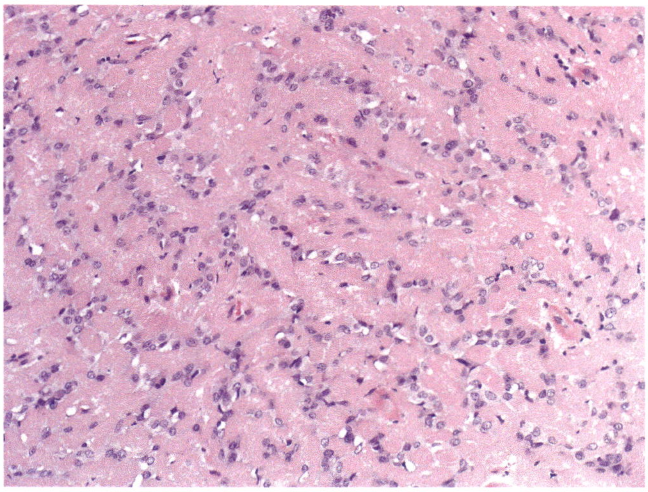

Fig. 18.10 (H&E, 200×) Myoepithelioma, plasmacytoid

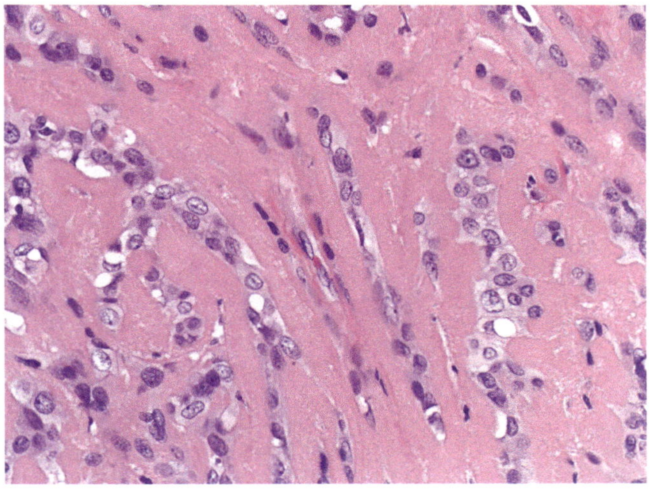

Fig. 18.11 (H&E, 400×) Myoepithelioma, plasmacytoid

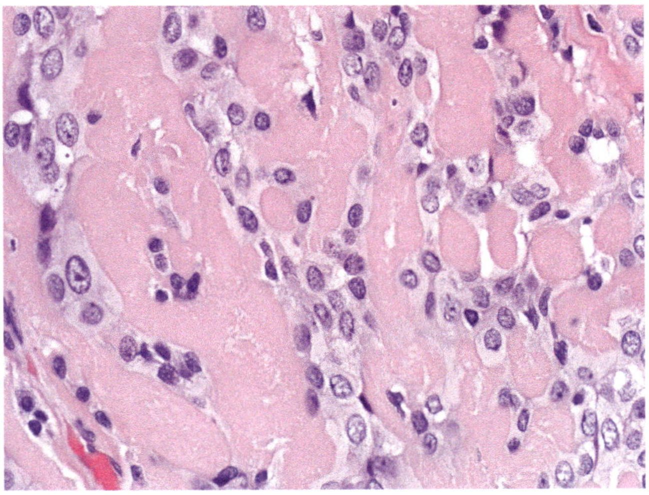

Fig. 18.12 (H&E, 600×) Myoepithelioma, plasmacytoid

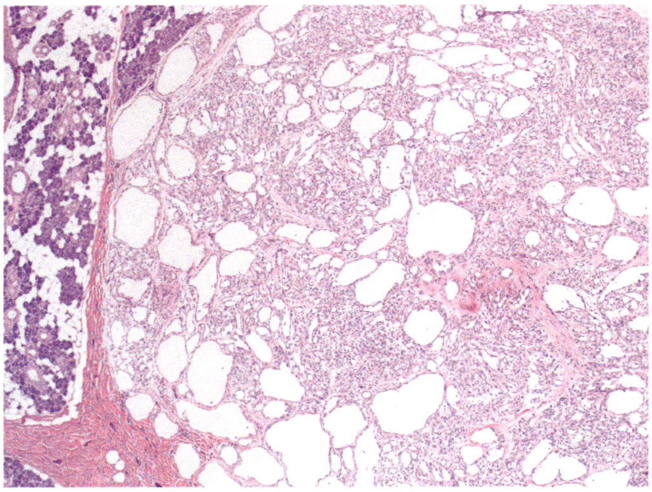

Fig. 18.13 (H&E, 40×) Myoepithelioma, cystic

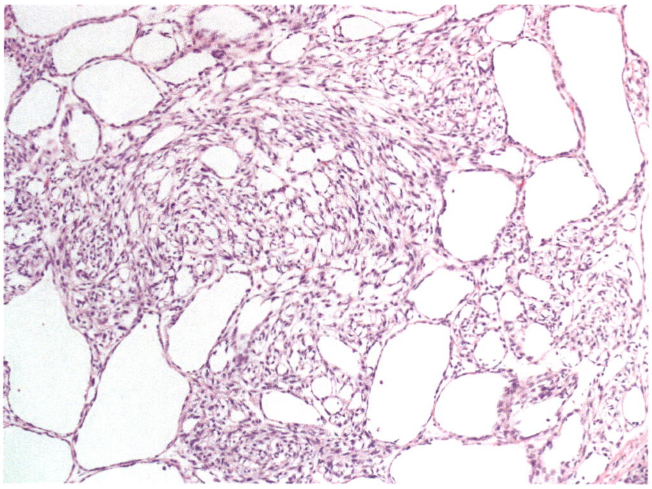

Fig. 18.14 (H&E, 100×) Myoepithelioma, cystic

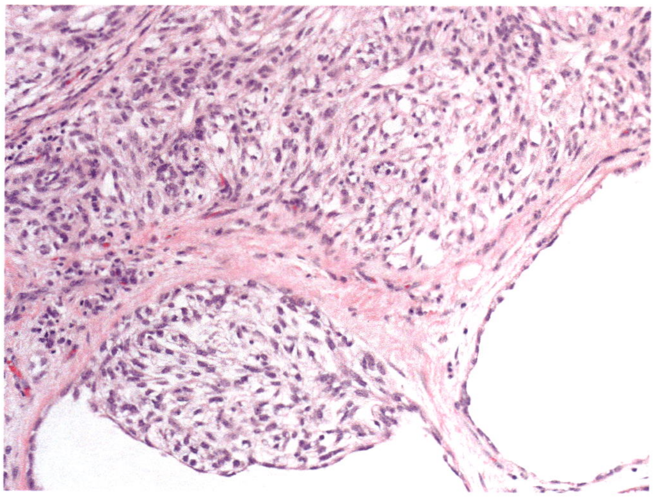

Fig. 18.15 (H&E, 200×) Myoepithelioma, cystic

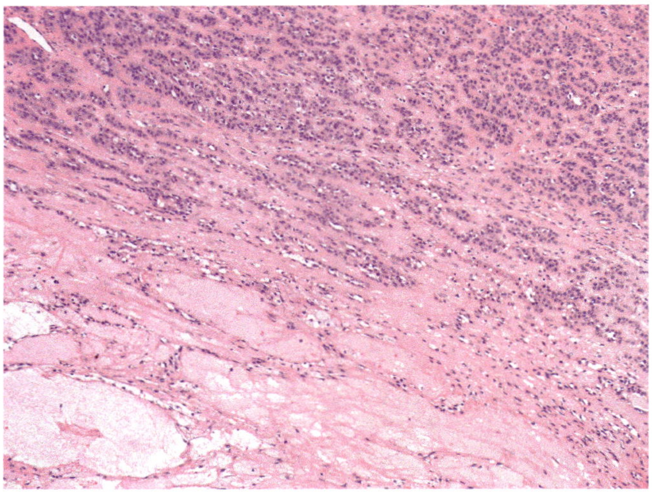

Fig. 18.16 (H&E, 100×) Myoepithelioma, myxoid

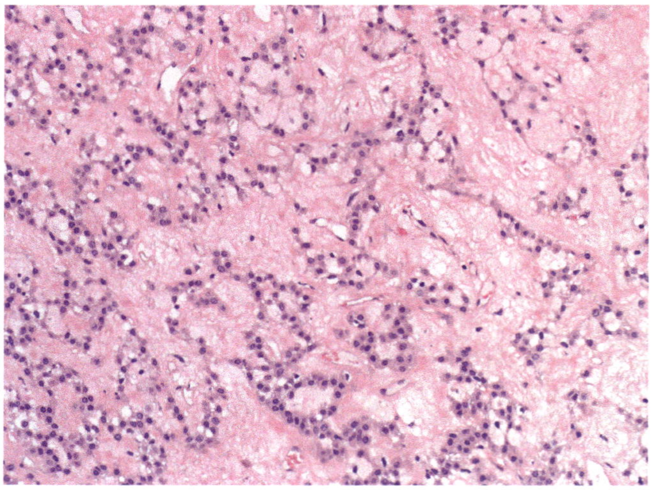

Fig. 18.17 (H&E, 200×) Myoepithelioma, myxoid

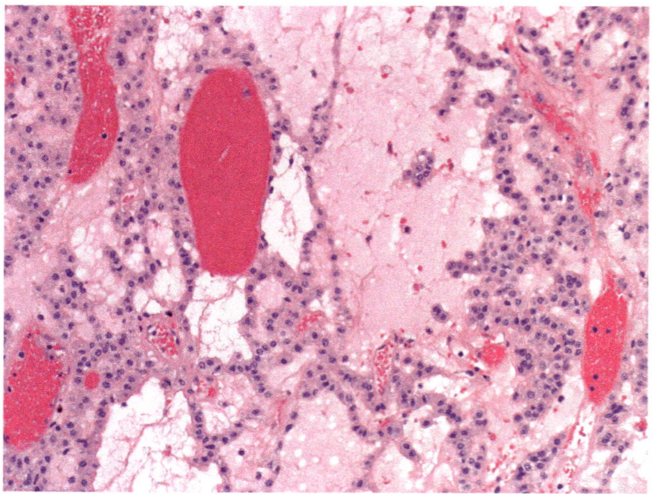

Fig. 18.18 (H&E, 200×) Myoepithelioma, myxoid

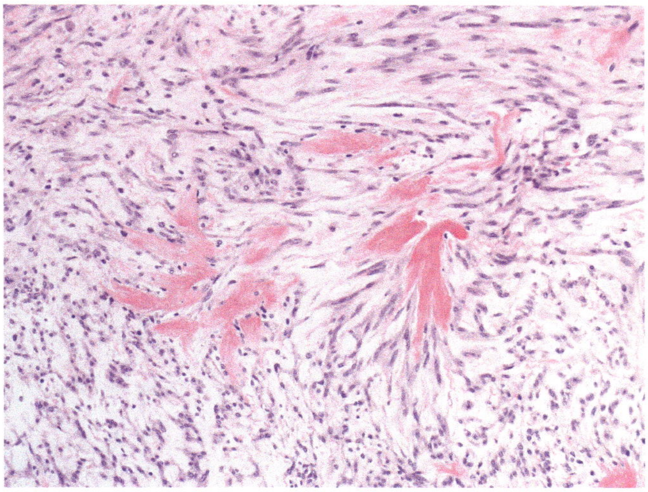

Fig. 18.19 (H&E, 200×) Myoepithelioma, hyalinized

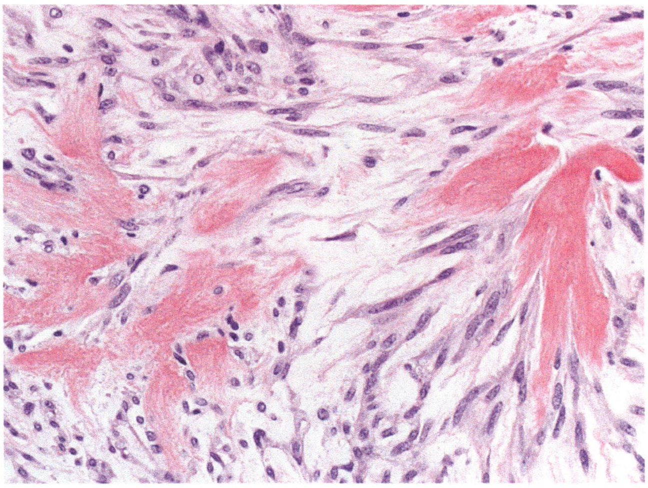

Fig. 18.20 (H&E, 400×) Myoepithelioma, hyalinized

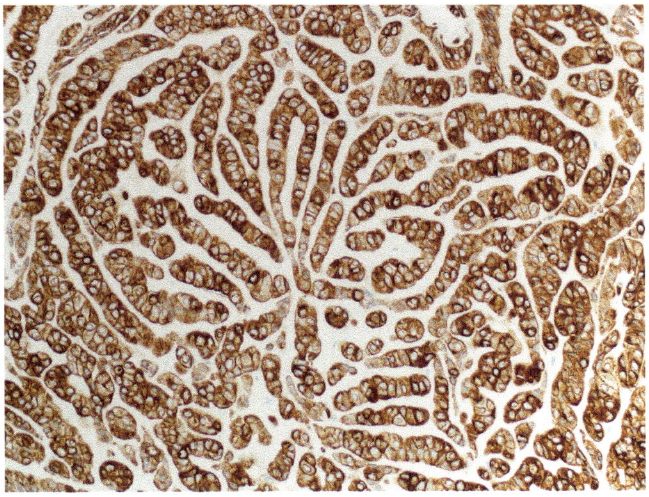

Fig. 18.21 (AE1/AE3, 200×) Myoepithelioma, diffuse immunoreactivity

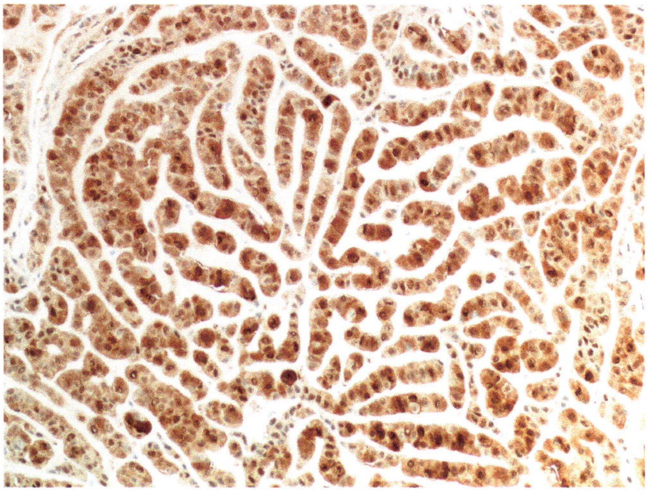

Fig. 18.22 (S-100, 200×) Myoepithelioma, diffuse immunoreactivity

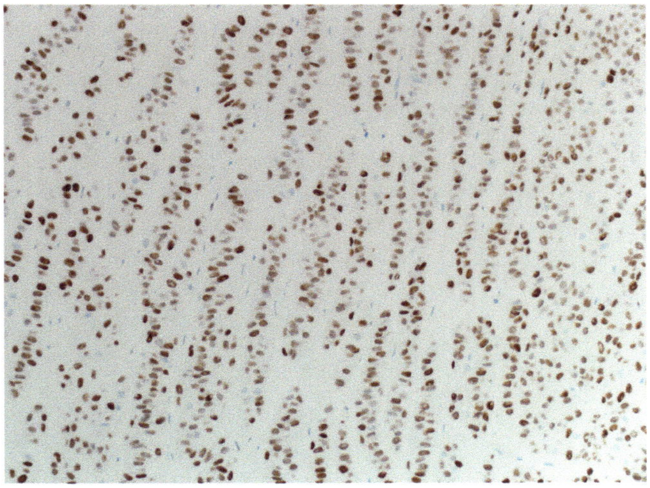

Fig. 18.23 (p63, 200×) Myoepithelioma, diffuse immunoreactivity

Suggested Reading

Alos L, Cardesa A, Bombi JA, Mallofre C, Cuchi A, Traserra J. Myoepithelial tumors of salivary glands: a clinicopathologic, immunohistochemical, ultrastructural, and flow-cytometric study. Semin Diagn Pathol. 1996;13:138–47.

Barnes L, Appel BN, Perez H, El-Attar AM. Myoepithelioma of the head and neck: case report and review. J Surg Oncol. 1985;28:21–8.

Dardick I, Cavell S, Boivin M, Hoppe D, Parks WR, Stinson J, et al. Salivary gland myoepithelioma variants. Histological, ultrastructural, and immunocytological features. Virchows Arch A Pathol Anat Histopathol. 1989a;416(1):25–42.

Dardick I, Thomas MJ, van Nostrand AW. Myoepithelioma—new concepts of histology and classification: a light and electron microscopic study. Ultrastruct Pathol. 1989b;13(2–3):187–224.

Dardick I, Ostrynski VL, Ekem JK, Leung R, Burford-Mason AP. Immunohistochemical and ultrastructural correlates of muscle-actin expression in pleomorphic adenomas and myoepitheliomas based on comparison of formalin and methanol fixation. Virchows Arch A Pathol Anat Histopathol. 1992;421:95–104.

Di Palma S, Guzzo M. Malignant myoepithelioma of salivary glands: clinicopathological features of ten cases. Virchows Arch A Pathol Anat Histopathol. 1993;423(5):389–96.

DiPalma S, Alasio L, Pilotti S. Fine needle aspiration (FNA) appearances of malignant myoepithelioma of the parotid gland. Cytopathology. 1996;7(5):357–65.

Ellis GL, Auclair PL. Tumors of the salivary glands. In: AFIP atlas of tumor pathology, 4th series. Silver Spring: ARP Press; 2008. p. 495–7.

Gnepp DR. Mucinous myoepithelioma, a recently described new myoepithelioma variant. Head Neck Pathol. 2013;7(Suppl 1): S85–9.

Hungermann D, Roeser K, Buerger H, Jakel T, Loning T, Herbst H. Relative paucity of gross genetic alterations in myoepitheliomas and myoepithelial carcinomas of salivary glands. J Pathol. 2002;198(4):487–94.

Laikui L, Hongwei L, Hongbing J, Zhixiu H. Epithelial salivary gland tumors of children and adolescents in West China population: a clinicopathologic study of 79 cases. J Oral Pathol Med. 2008;37:201–5.

Leifer C, Miller AS, Putong PB, Harwick RD. Myoepithelioma of the parotid gland. Arch Pathol. 1974;98:312–9.

Nagao T, Sugano I, Ishida Y, Tajima Y, Matsuzaki O, Konno A, et al. Salivary gland malignant myoepithelioma: a clinicopathologic and immunohistochemical study of ten cases. Cancer. 1998;83(7):1292–9.

Sciubba JJ, Brannon RB. Myoepithelioma of salivary glands: report of 23 cases. Cancer. 1982;49(3):562–72.

Simpson RH, Jones H, Beasley P. Benign myoepithelioma of the salivary glands: a true entity? Histopathology. 1995;27:1–9.

Turgut S, Cekic A, Ergul G, Aksoy F, Seckin S, Ozdem C. Myoepithelioma of the parotid gland: a report of two cases. Ear Nose Throat J. 2001;80:155–8.

Yaman H, Gerek M, Tosun F, Deveci S, Kilic E, Arslan HH. Myoepithelioma of the parotid gland in a child: a case report. J Pediatr Surg. 2010;45:E5–7.

19 Myoepithelial Carcinoma

Myoepithelial carcinoma is the malignant counterpart of myoepithelioma. Myoepithelial carcinoma affects children and adults. Women and men are involved with similar frequency. The majority of cases involve major salivary glands, presenting as single or multiple masses. Most cases of myoepithelial carcinoma behave as intermediate to high-grade malignancies. Myoepithelial carcinoma may be circumscribed or infiltrative, comprised almost exclusively of one cell type (myoepithelial), and exhibit a variety of architectural patterns (solid, trabecular, and cystic) (Figs. 19.1–19.22).

J. J. García, *Atlas of Salivary Gland Pathology*, https://doi.org/10.1007/978-3-319-09021-4_19

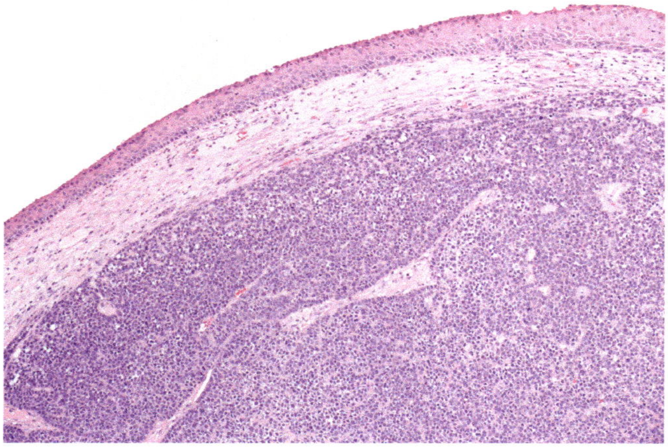

Fig. 19.1 (H&E, 100×) Myoepithelial carcinoma, circumscribed

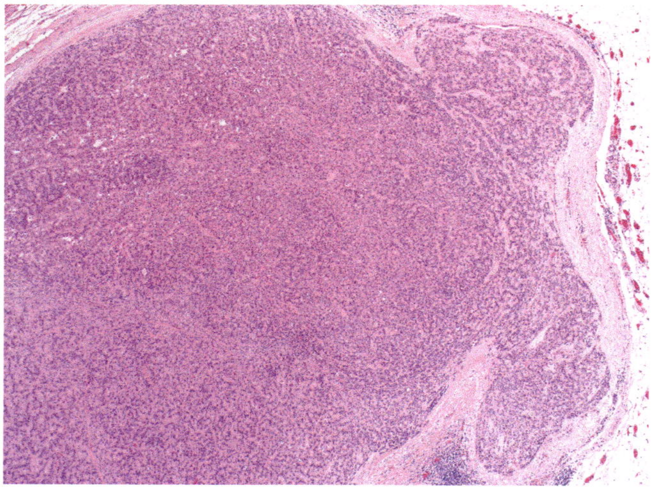

Fig. 19.2 (H&E, 40×) Myoepithelial carcinoma, encapsulated

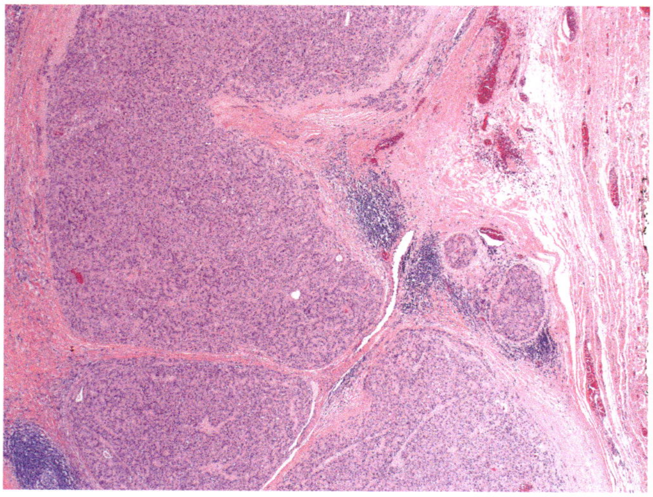

Fig. 19.3 (H&E, 40×) Myoepithelial carcinoma, infiltrative

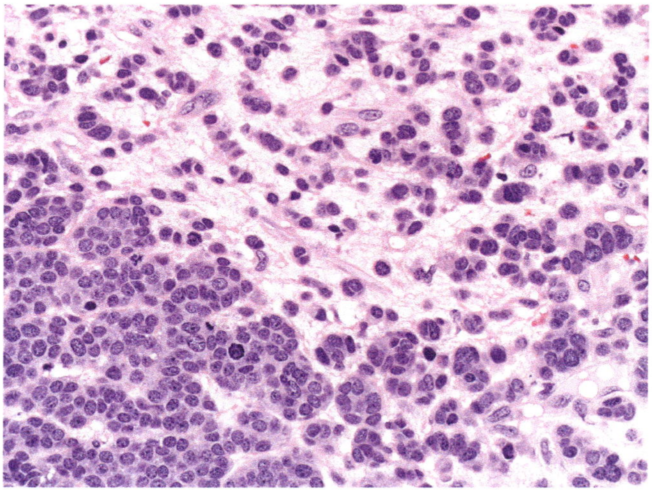

Fig. 19.4 (H&E, 400×) Myoepithelial carcinoma, monophasic

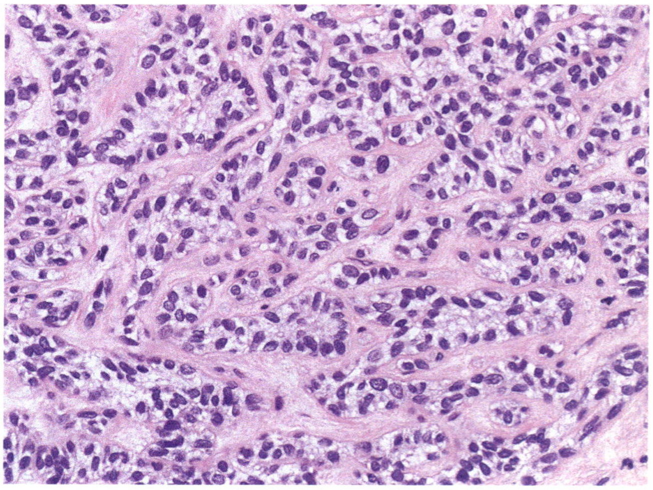

Fig. 19.5 (H&E, 400×) Myoepithelial carcinoma, cords

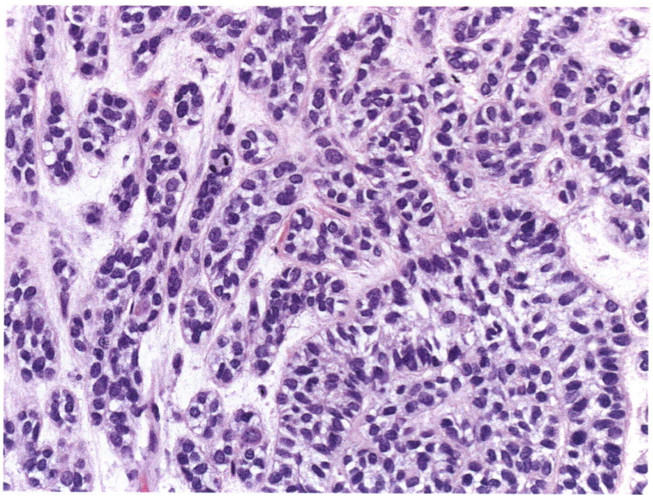

Fig. 19.6 (H&E, 400×) Myoepithelial carcinoma, cords

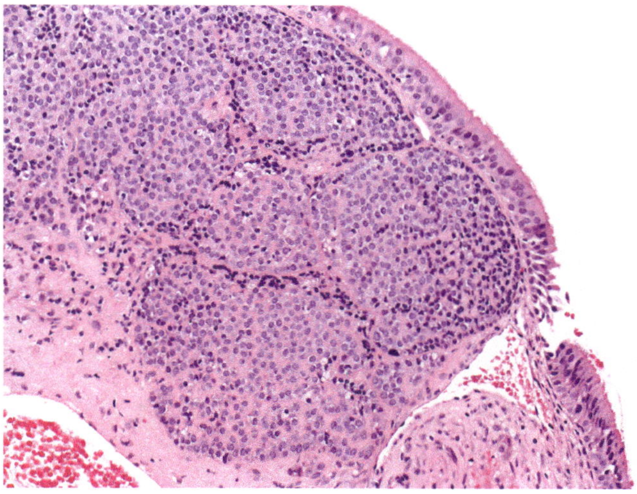

Fig. 19.7 (H&E, 200×) Myoepithelial carcinoma, nests

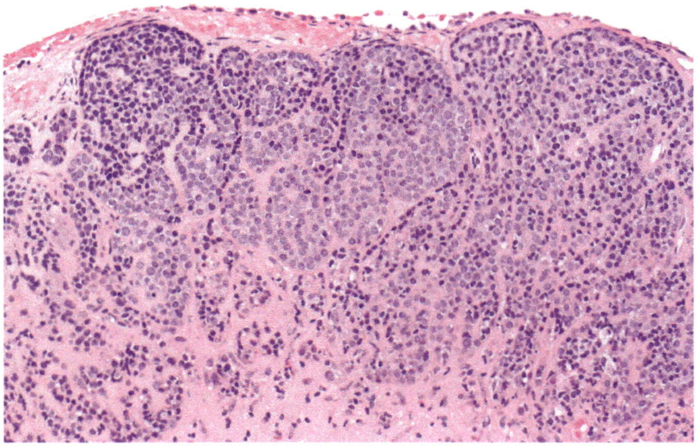

Fig. 19.8 (H&E, 200×) Myoepithelial carcinoma, nests

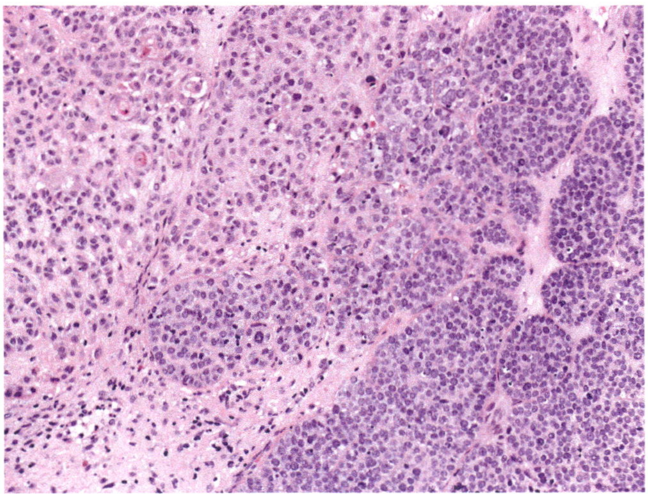

Fig. 19.9 (H&E, 200×) Myoepithelial carcinoma, nests

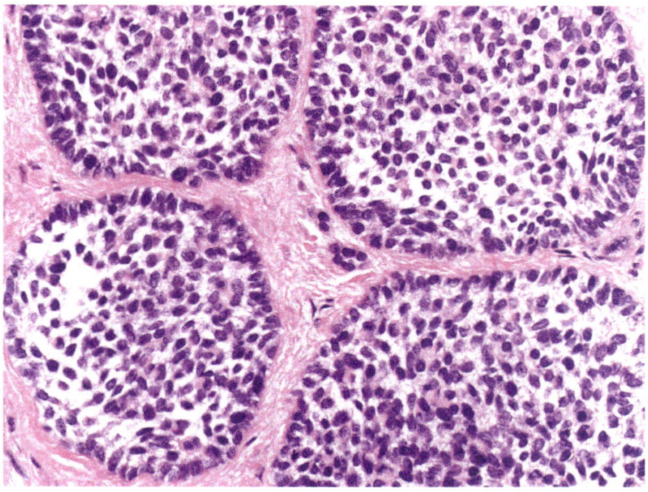

Fig. 19.10 (H&E, 400×) Myoepithelial carcinoma, nests

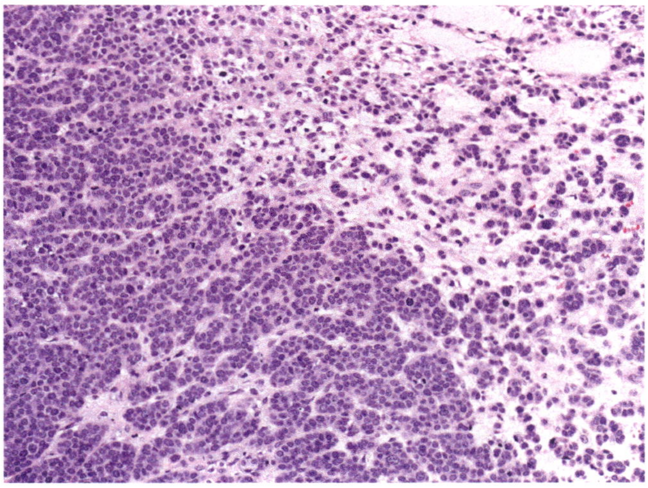

Fig. 19.11 (H&E, 200×) Myoepithelial carcinoma, cords and nests

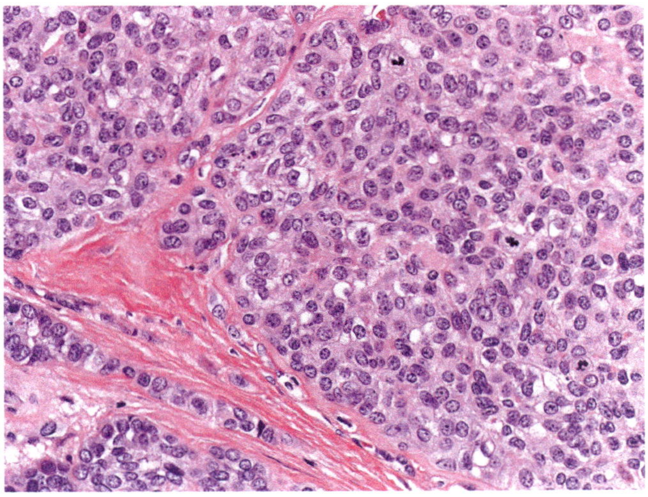

Fig. 19.12 (H&E, 400×) Myoepithelial carcinoma, solid

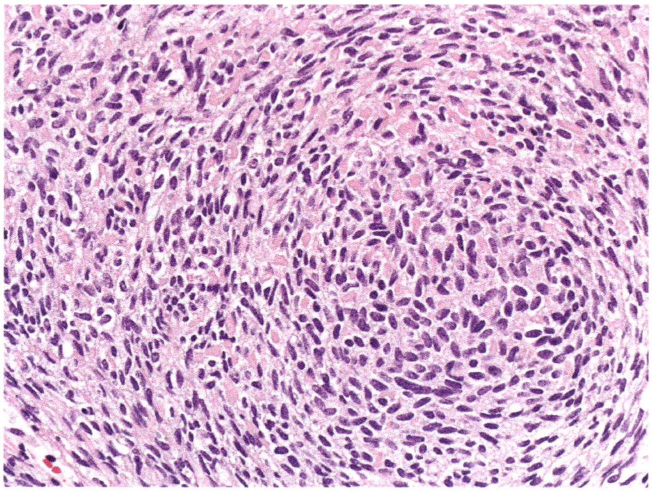

Fig. 19.13 (H&E, 400×) Myoepithelial carcinoma, solid

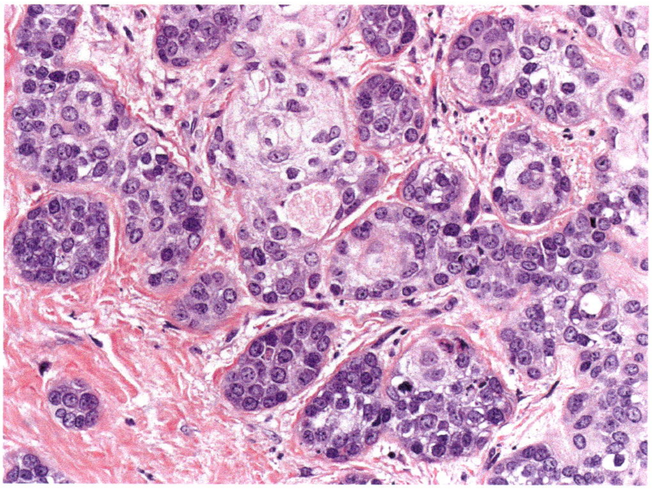

Fig. 19.14 (H&E, 400×) Myoepithelial carcinoma, cytomorphologic atypia

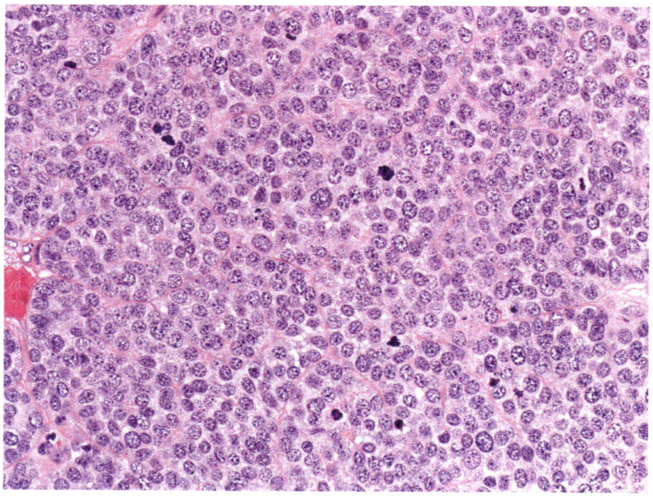

Fig. 19.15 (H&E, 400×) Myoepithelial carcinoma, mitotic activity

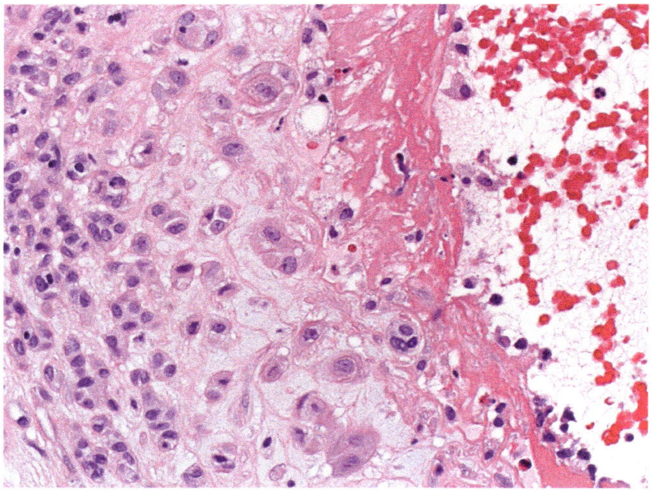

Fig. 19.16 (H&E, 400×) Myoepithelial carcinoma, vascular

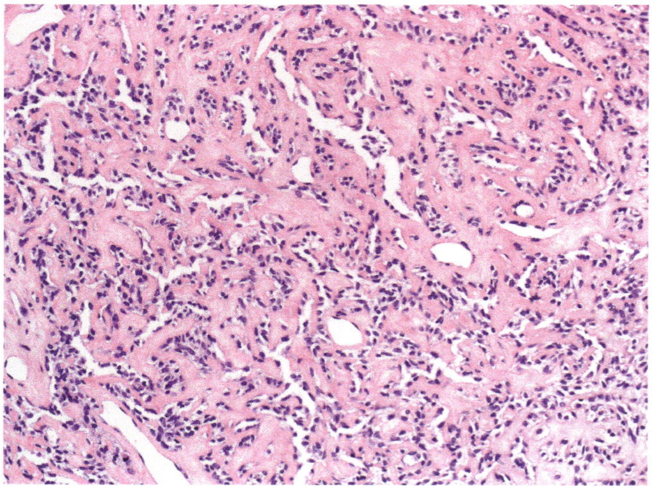

Fig. 19.17 (H&E, 200×) Myoepithelial carcinoma, pseudo-vascular

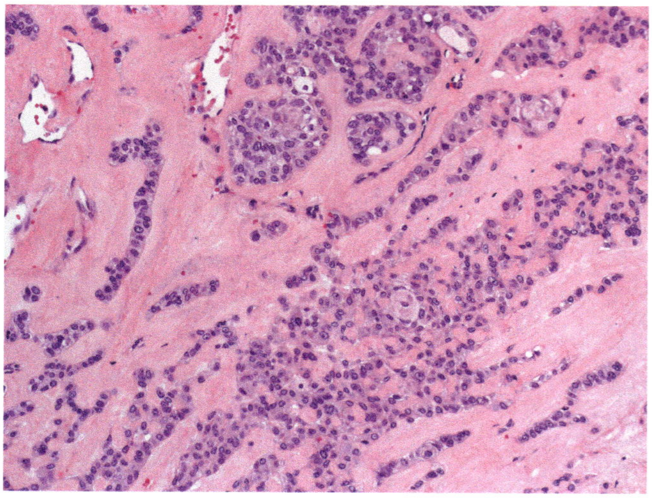

Fig. 19.18 (H&E, 200×) Myoepithelial carcinoma, hyalinized

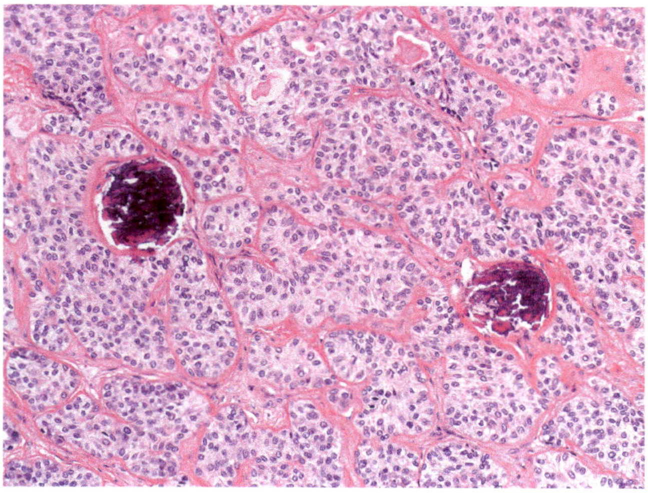

Fig. 19.19 (H&E, 200×) Myoepithelial carcinoma, microcalcifications

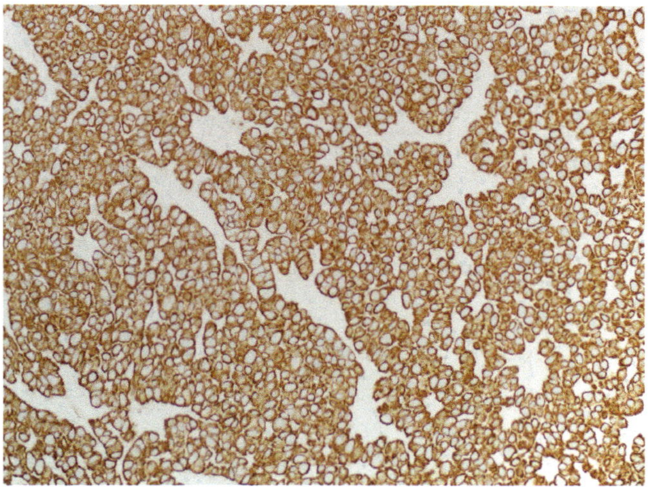

Fig. 19.20 (AE1/AE3, 200×) Myoepithelial carcinoma, diffuse immunoreactivity

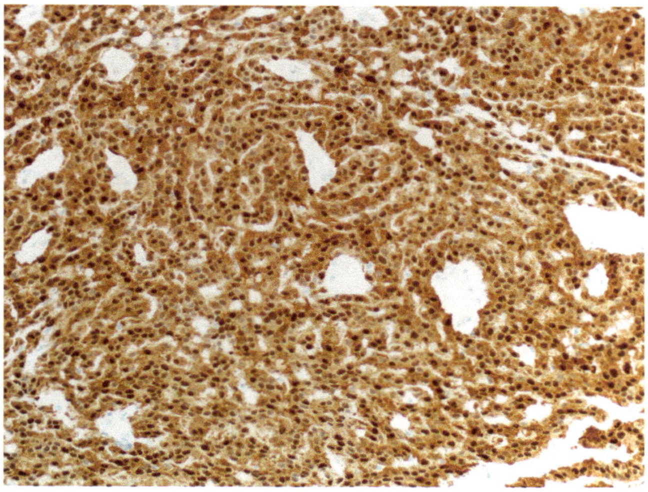

Fig. 19.21 (S-100, 200×) Myoepithelial carcinoma, diffuse immunoreactivity

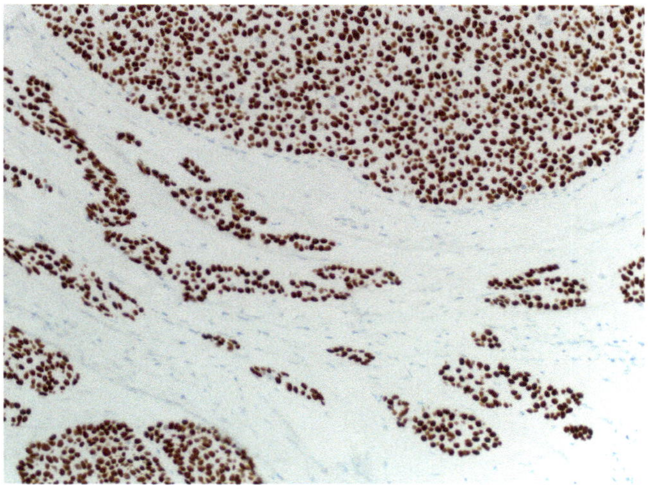

Fig. 19.22 (p63, 200×) Myoepithelial carcinoma, diffuse immunoreactivity

Suggested Reading

Bastaki JM, Purgina BM, Dacic S, Seethala RR. Secretory myoepithelial carcinoma: a histologic and molecular survey and a proposed nomenclature for mucin producing signet ring tumors. Head Neck Pathol. 2014;8:250–60.

Chhieng DC, Paulino AF. Cytology of myoepithelial carcinoma of the salivary gland. Cancer. 2002;96(1):32–6.

Di Palma S, Guzzo M. Malignant myoepithelioma of salivary glands: clinicopathological features of ten cases. Virchows Arch A Pathol Anat Histopathol. 1993;423:389–96.

Gnepp DR. Malignant mixed tumors of the salivary glands: a review. Pathol Annu. 1993;28:279–328.

Kong M, Drill EN, Morris L, West L, Klimstra D, Gonen M, et al. Prognostic factors in myoepithelial carcinoma of salivary glands: a clinicopathologic study of 48 cases. Am J Surg Pathol. 2015;39:931–8.

Savera AT, Sloman A, Huvos AG, Klimstra DS. Myoepithelial carcinoma of the salivary glands: a clinicopathologic study of 25 patients. Am J Surg Pathol. 2000;24(6):761–74.

Skalova A, Weinreb I, Hyrcza M, Simpson RH, Laco J, Agaimy A, et al. Clear cell myoepithelial carcinoma of salivary glands showing EWSR1 rearrangement: molecular analysis of 94 salivary gland carcinomas with prominent clear cell component. Am J Surg Pathol. 2015;39:338–48.

Su YX, Roberts DB, Hanna EY, El-Naggar A, Saylam G, Frank SJ, et al. Risk factors and prognosis for myoepithelial carcinoma of the major salivary glands. Ann Surg Oncol. 2015;22:3701–7.

Yu G, Ma D, Sun K, Li T, Zhang Y. Myoepithelial carcinoma of the salivary glands: behavior and management. Chin Med J. 2003;116(2):163–5.

20 Oncocytoma

Oncocytoma is the benign counterpart of oncocytic carcinoma. Oncocytoma affects predominantly adults and presents at a mean age of approximately 65 years. Women and men are involved with similar frequency. The majority of cases involve the parotid gland, presenting as single or multiple masses. Oncocytoma may be circumscribed or multi-nodular, comprised of multiple cell types (oncocyte, basal), and exhibit a variety of architectural patterns (solid, organoid, trabecular, cystic, and duct-like) (Figs. 20.1–20.26).

J. J. García, *Atlas of Salivary Gland Pathology*, https://doi.org/10.1007/978-3-319-09021-4_20

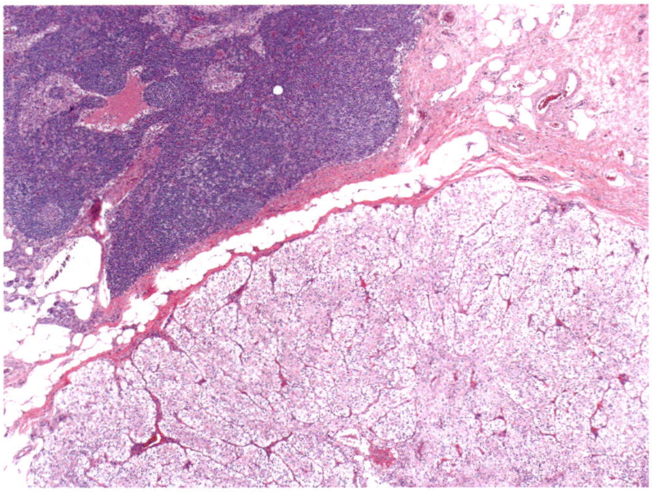

Fig. 20.1 (H&E, 40×) Oncocytoma, circumscribed

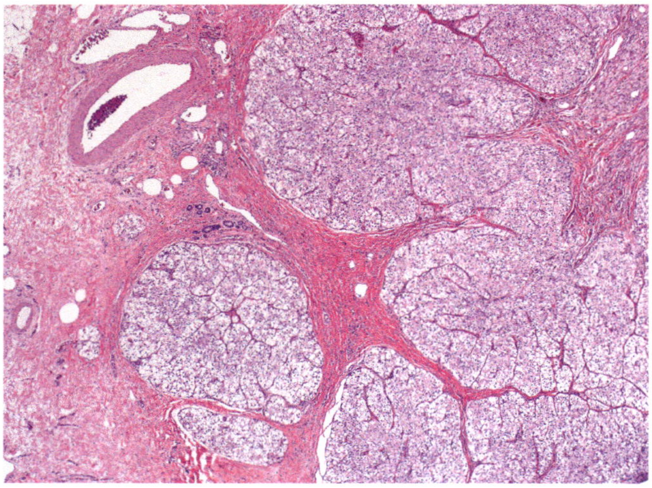

Fig. 20.2 (H&E, 40×) Oncocytoma, nodular

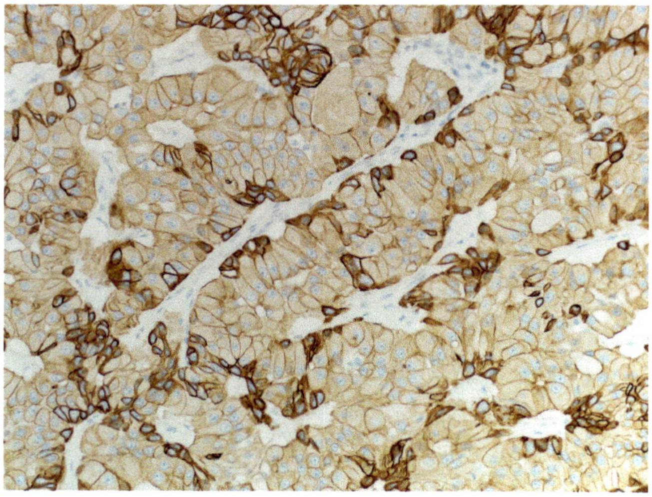

Fig. 20.3 (AE1/AE3, 200x) Oncocytoma, biphasic

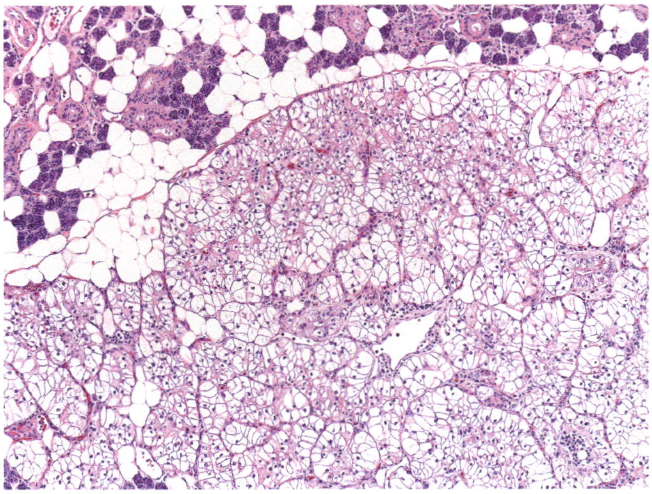

Fig. 20.4 (H&E, 100×) Oncocytoma, clear and eosinophilic

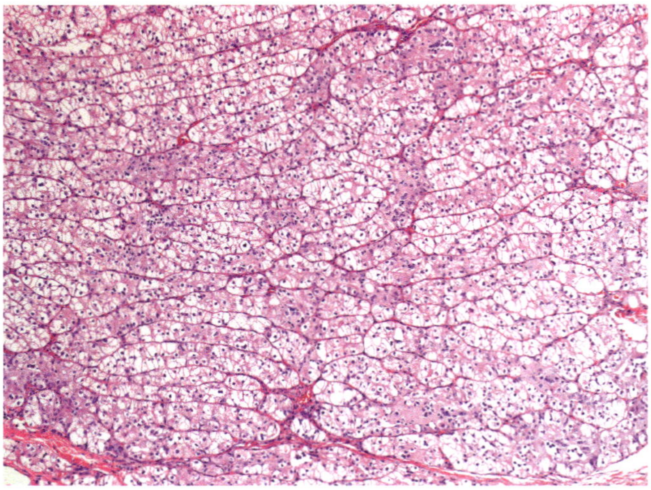

Fig. 20.5 (H&E, 100×) Oncocytoma, clear and eosinophilic

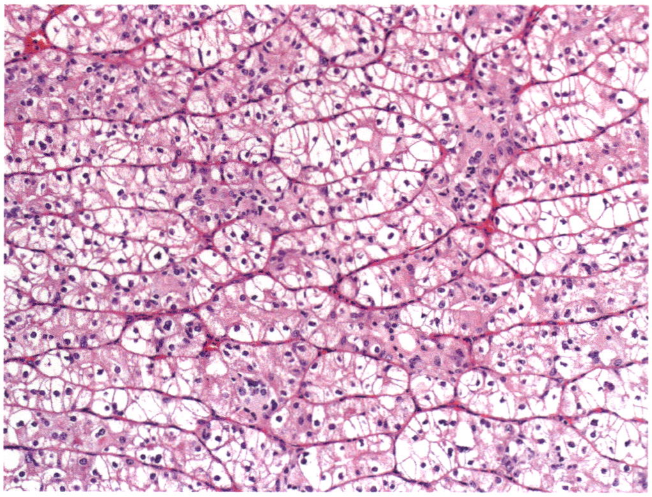

Fig. 20.6 (H&E, 200×) Oncocytoma, clear and eosinophilic

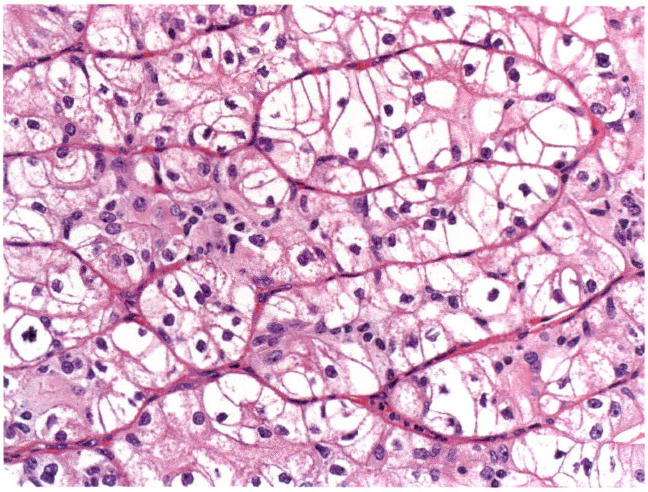

Fig. 20.7 (H&E, 400×) Oncocytoma, clear and eosinophilic

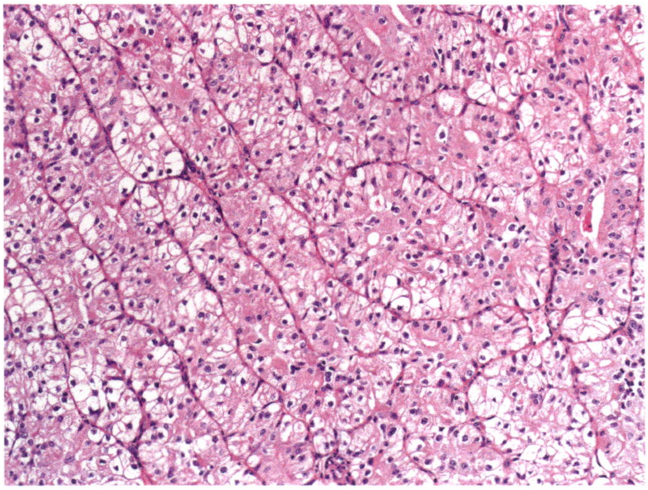

Fig. 20.8 (H&E, 200×) Oncocytoma, clear and eosinophilic

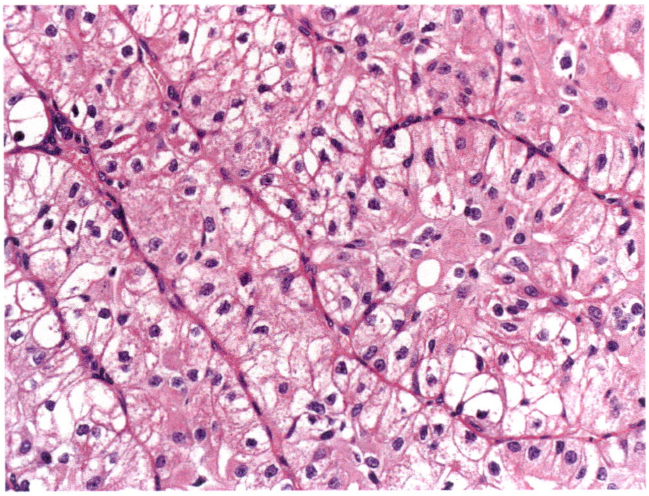

Fig. 20.9 (H&E, 400×) Oncocytoma, clear and eosinophilic

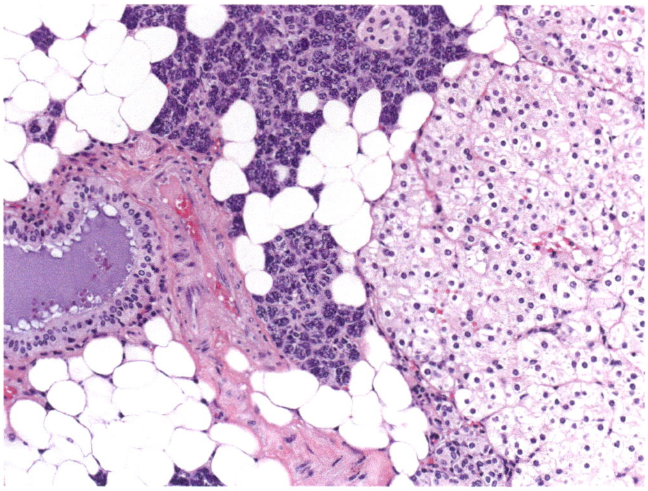

Fig. 20.10 (H&E, 200×) Oncocytoma, adjacent serous acini

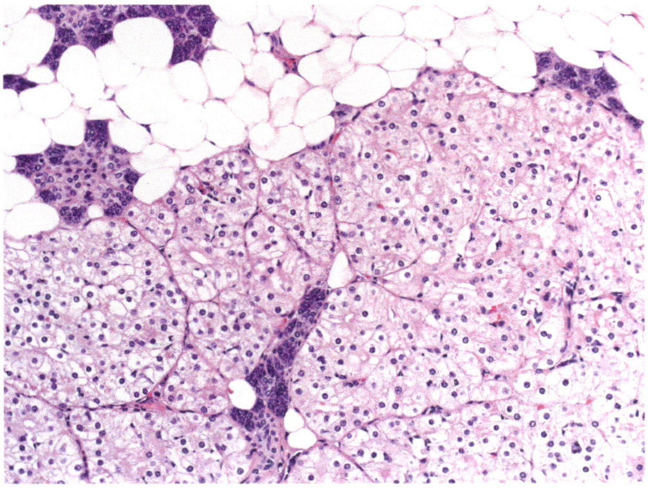

Fig. 20.11 (H&E, 200×) Oncocytoma, entrapped serous acini

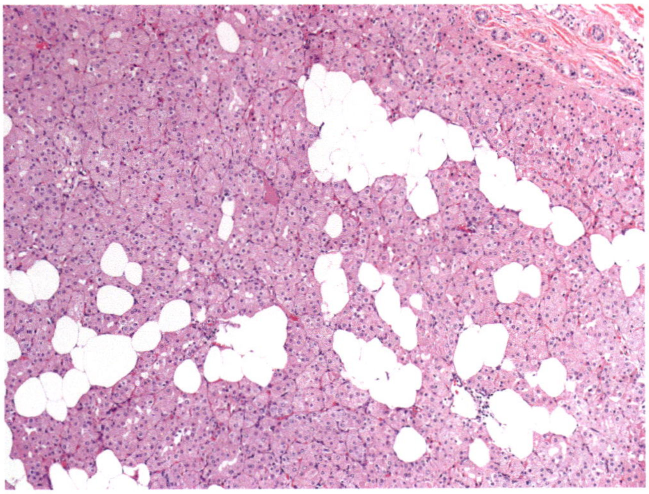

Fig. 20.12 (H&E, 100×) Oncocytoma, adipocytic metaplasia

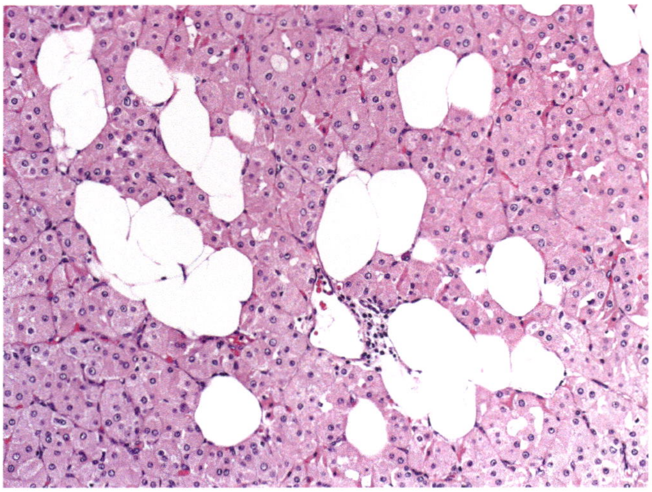

Fig. 20.13 (H&E, 200×) Oncocytoma, adipocytic metaplasia

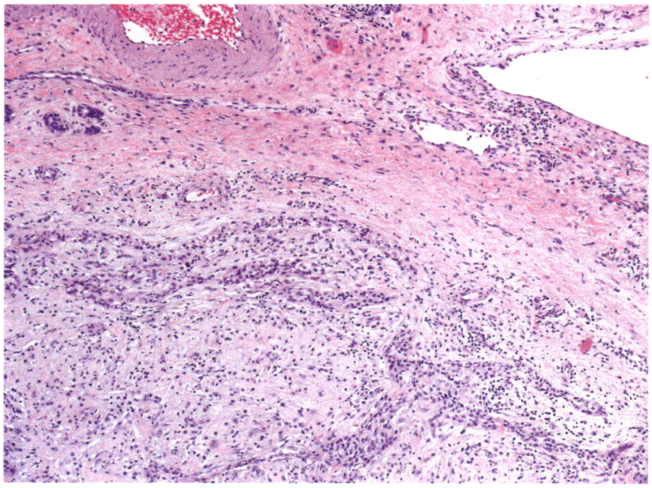

Fig. 20.14 (H&E, 100×) Oncocytoma, squamous metaplasia (biopsy-related)

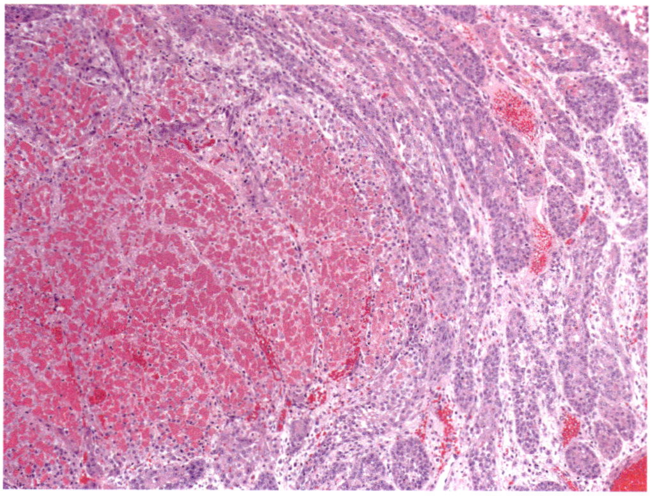

Fig. 20.15 (H&E, 100×) Oncocytoma, squamous metaplasia and necrosis (biopsy-related)

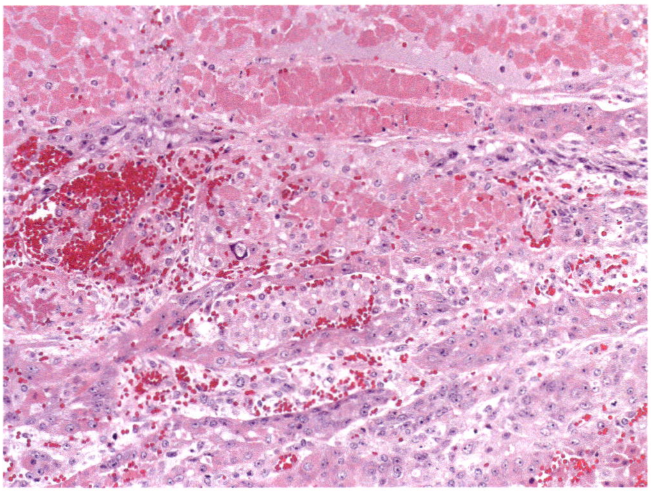

Fig. 20.16 (H&E, 200×) Oncocytoma, squamous metaplasia and necrosis (biopsy-related)

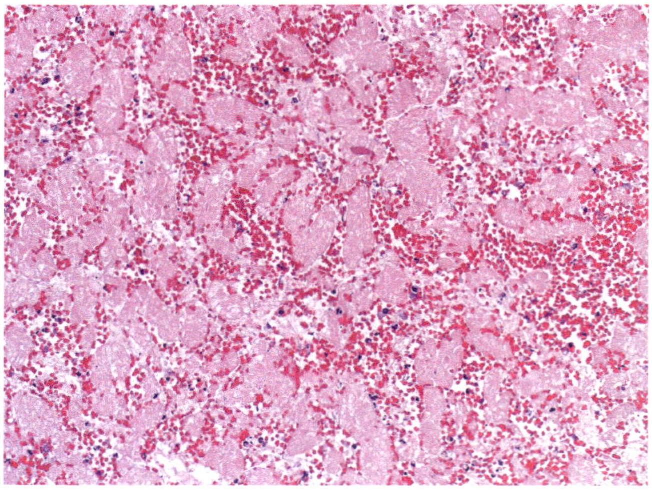

Fig. 20.17 (H&E, 200×) Oncocytoma, necrosis (biopsy-related)

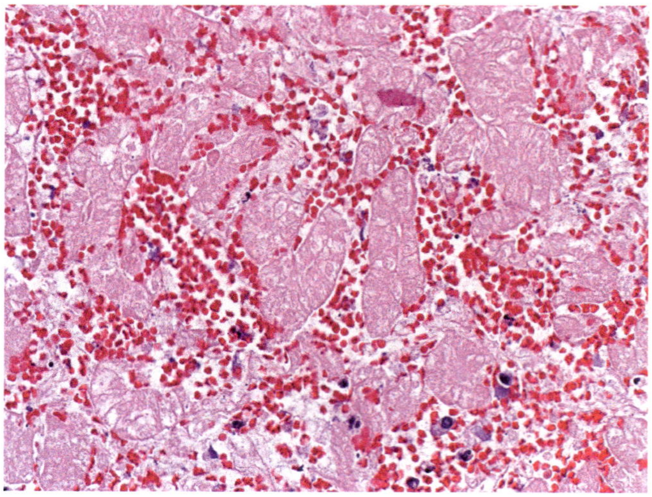

Fig. 20.18 (H&E, 400×) Oncocytoma, necrosis (biopsy-related)

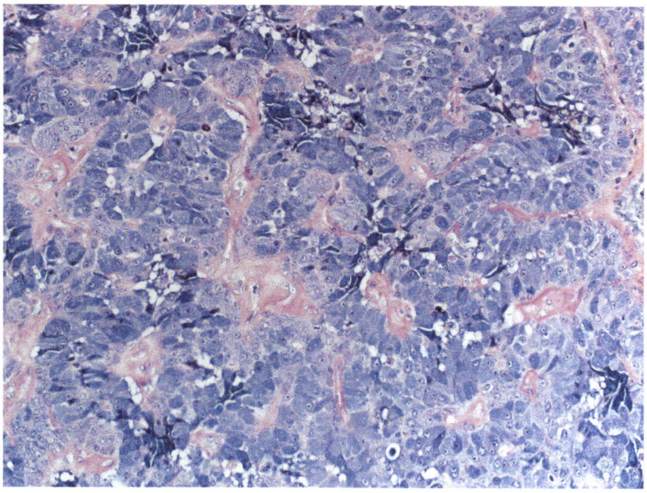

Fig. 20.19 (PTAH, 200×) Oncocytoma, intracytoplasmic reactivity

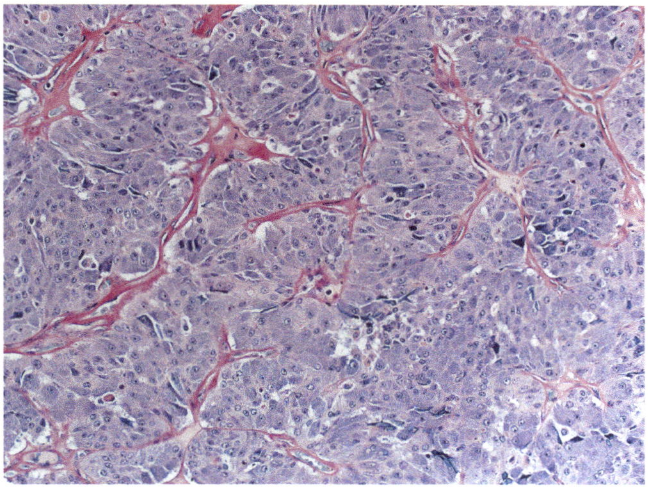

Fig. 20.20 (PTAH, 200×) Oncocytoma, negative reactivity

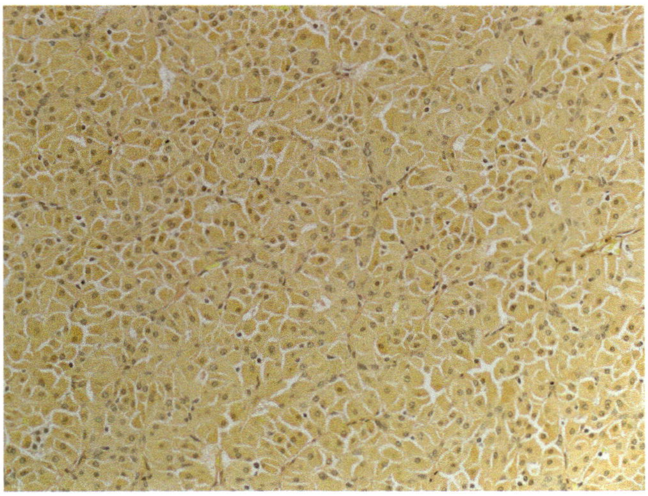

Fig. 20.21 (Mucicarmine, 200×) Oncocytoma, negative reactivity

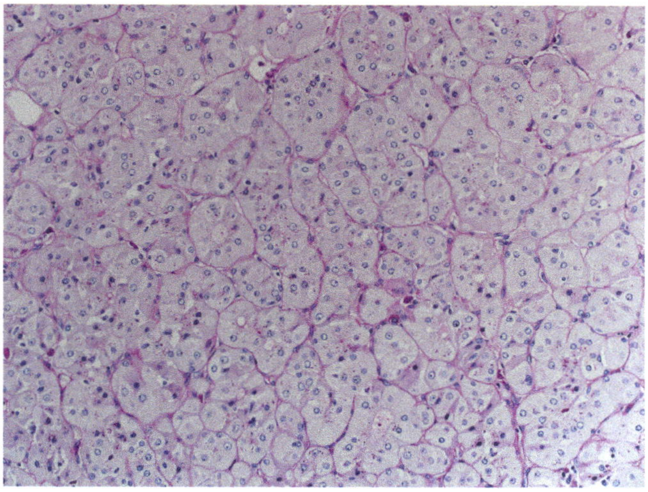

Fig. 20.22 (PAS-D, 200×) Oncocytoma, cytoplasmic granules

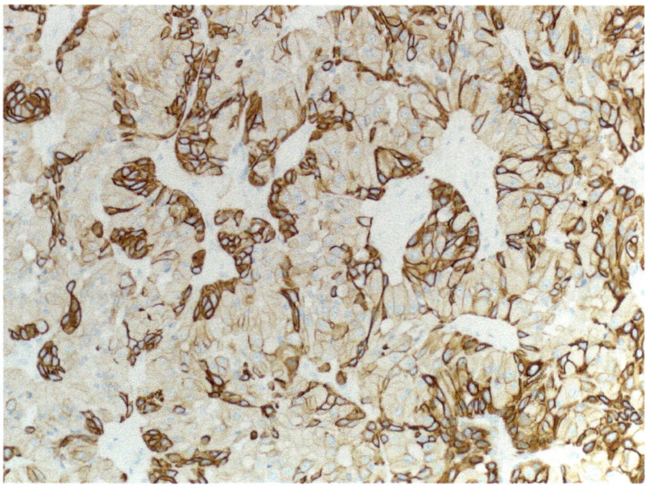

Fig. 20.23 (AE1/AE3, 200×) Oncocytoma, diffuse immunoreactivity

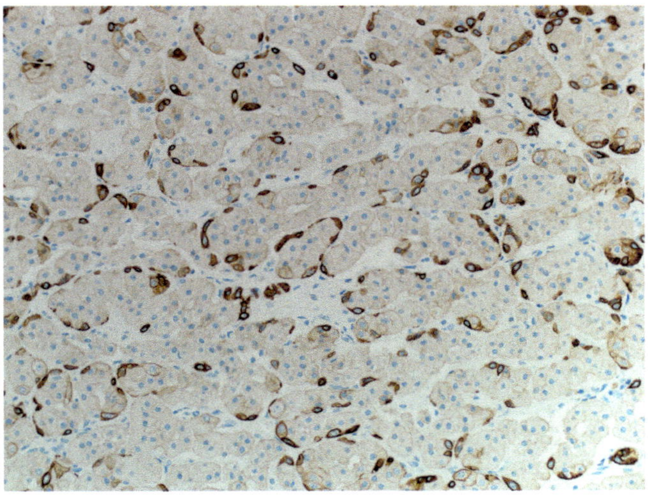

Fig. 20.24 (AE1/AE3, 200×) Oncocytoma, basal immunoreactivity

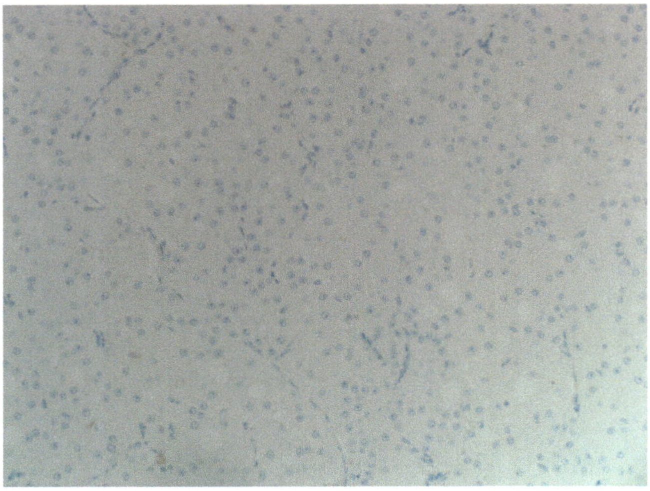

Fig. 20.25 (S-100, 200×) Oncocytoma, negative immunoreactivity

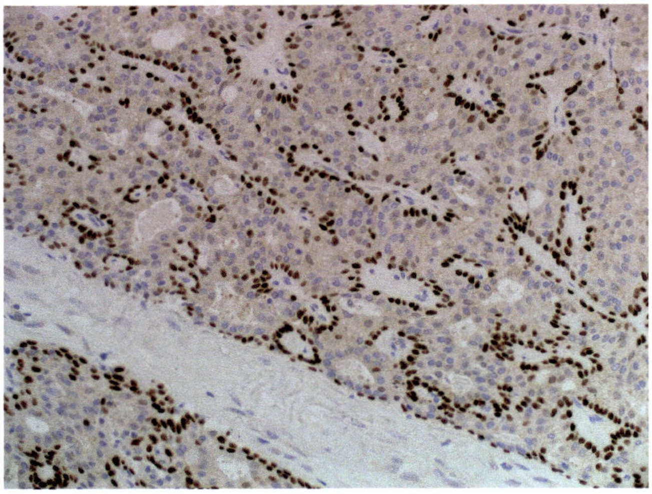

Fig. 20.26 (p63, 200×) Oncocytoma, basal immunoreactivity

Suggested Reading

Barnes L, editor. Surgical pathology of the head and neck. 3rd ed. New York: CRC Press Inc; 2008.

Blanck C, Eneroth CM, Jakobsson PA. Oncocytoma of the parotid gland: neoplasm or nodular hyperplasia? Cancer. 1970;25: 919–25.

Capone RB, Ha PK, Westra WH, Pilkington TM, Sciubba JJ, Koch WM, et al. Oncocytic neoplasms of the parotid gland: a 16-year institutional review. Otolaryngol Head Neck Surg. 2002;126(6): 657–62.

Deutsch E, Eilon A, Zelig S, Ariel I. Synchronous bilateral oncocytoma of the parotid glands. A case report. ORL J Otorhinolaryngol Relat Spec. 1984;46:66–8.

Garcia JJ, Hunt JL, Weinreb I, McHugh JB, Barnes EL, Cieply K, et al. Fluorescence in situ hybridization for detection of MAML2 rearrangements in oncocytic mucoepidermoid carcinoma: utility as a diagnostic test. Hum Pathol. 2011;42:2001–9.

Ghandur-Mnaymneh L. Multinodular oncocytoma of the parotid gland: a benign; lesion simulating malignancy. Hum Pathol. 1984;15:485–6.

McHugh JB, Hoschar AP, Dvorakova M, Parwani AV, Barnes EL, Seethala RR. p63 immunohistochemistry differentiates salivary gland oncocytoma and oncocytic carcinoma from metastatic renal cell carcinoma. Head Neck Pathol. 2007;1(2):123–31.

Ozolek JA, Bastacky SI, Myers EN, Hunt JL. Immunophenotypic comparison of salivary gland oncocytoma and metastatic renal cell carcinoma. Laryngoscope. 2005;115(6):1097–100.

Sorensen M, Baunsgaard P, Frederiksen P, Haahr PA. Multifocal adenomatous oncocytic hyperplasia of the parotid gland (unusual clear cell variant in two female siblings). Pathol Res Pract. 1986;181:254–9.

Thompson LD, Wenig BM, Ellis GL. Oncocytomas of the submandibular gland: a series of 22 cases and a review of the literature. Cancer. 1996;78:2281–7.

Verma K, Kapila K. Salivary gland tumors with a prominent oncocytic component. Cytologic findings and differential diagnosis of oncocytomas and Warthin's tumor on fine needle aspirates. Acta Cytol. 2003;47(2):221–6.

Weiler C, Reu S, Zengel P, Kirchner T, Ihrler S. Obligate basal cell component in salivary oncocytoma facilitates distinction from acinic cell carcinoma. Pathol Res Pract. 2009;205:838–42.

Zhou CX, Gao Y. Oncocytoma of the salivary glands: a clinicopathologic and immunohistochemical study. Oral Oncol. 2009;45(12):e232–8.

21 Oncocytic Carcinoma

Oncocytic carcinoma is the malignant counterpart of oncocytoma. Oncocytic carcinoma affects children and adults. Women and men are involved with similar frequency. The majority of cases involve the parotid gland, presenting as single or multiple masses. Oncocytic carcinoma may be circumscribed or infiltrative, comprised of multiple cell types (oncocyte, basal), and exhibit a variety of architectural patterns (solid, organoid, trabecular, cystic, and duct-like) (Figs. 21.1–21.12).

J. J. García, *Atlas of Salivary Gland Pathology*, https://doi.org/10.1007/978-3-319-09021-4_21

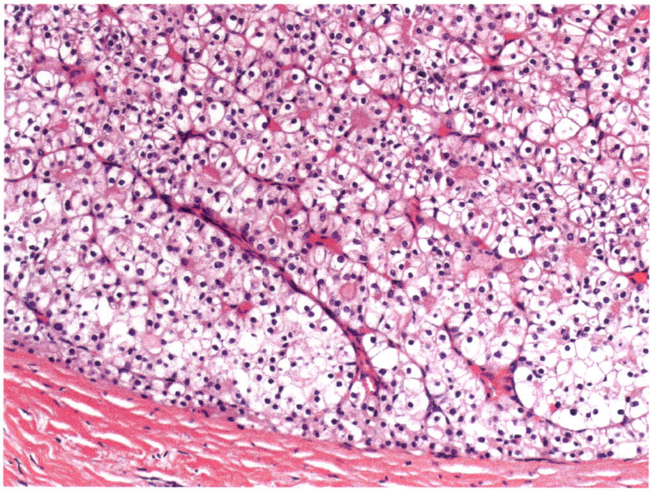

Fig. 21.1 (H&E, 200×) Oncocytic carcinoma, circumscribed

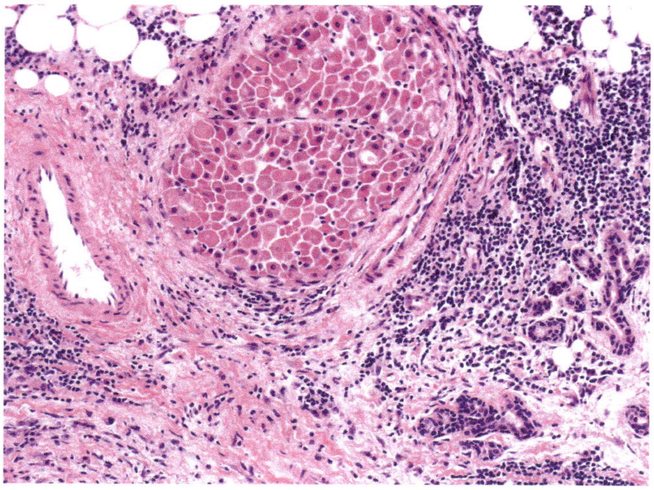

Fig. 21.2 (H&E, 200×) Oncocytic carcinoma, infiltrative

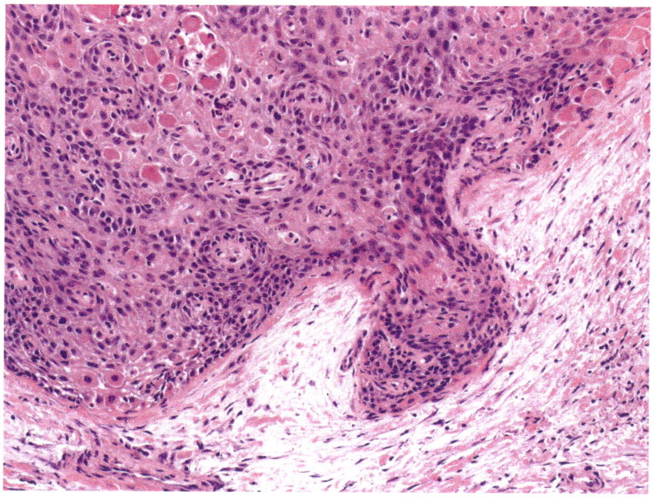

Fig. 21.3 (H&E, 200×) Oncocytic carcinoma, infiltrative

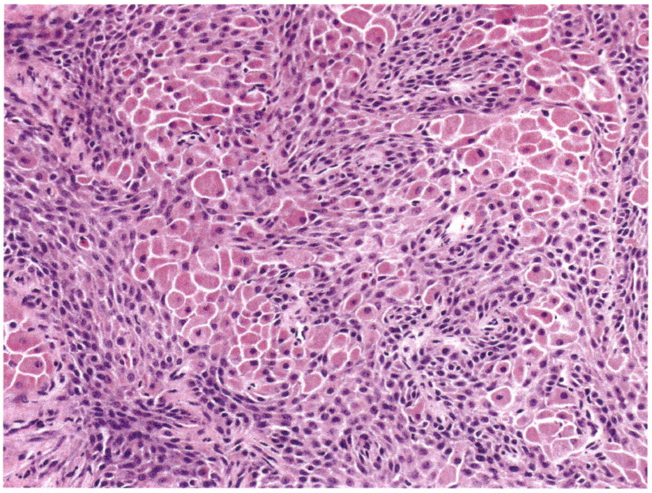

Fig. 21.4 (H&E, 200×) Oncocytic carcinoma, biphasic

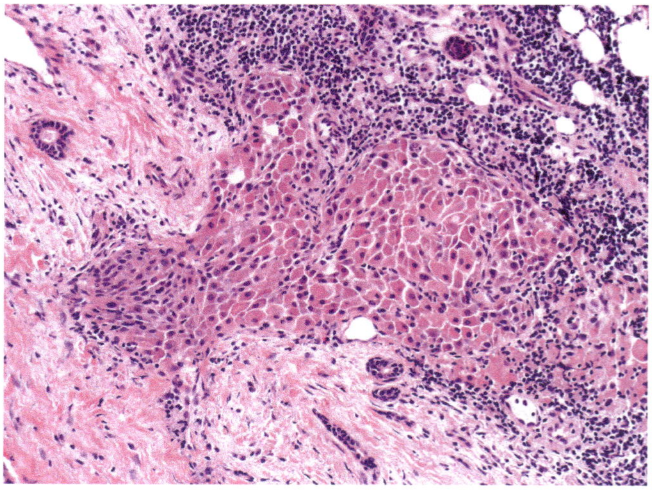

Fig. 21.5 (H&E, 200×) Oncocytic carcinoma, eosinophilic

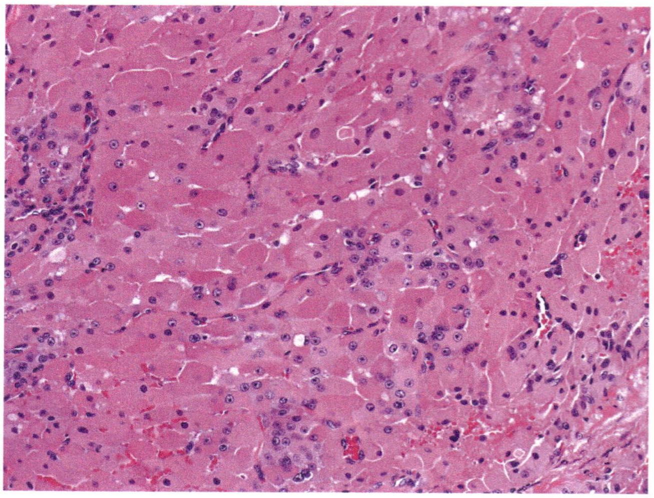

Fig. 21.6 (H&E, 200×) Oncocytic carcinoma, eosinophilic

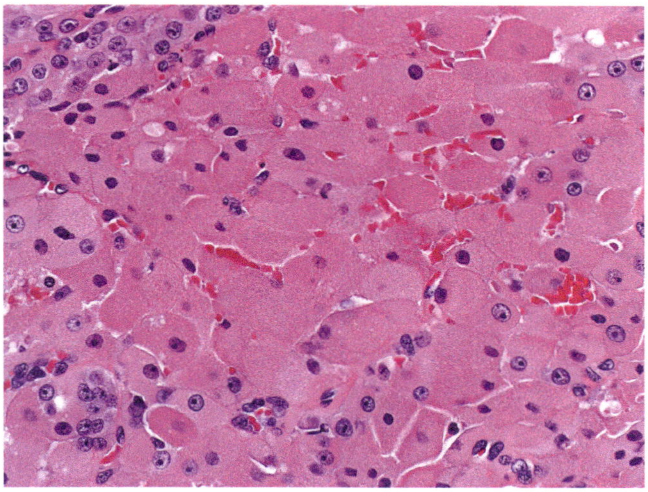

Fig. 21.7 (H&E, 400×) Oncocytic carcinoma, eosinophilic

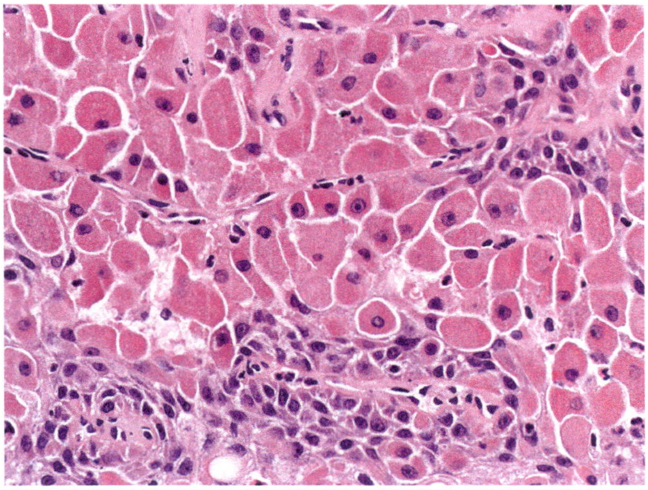

Fig. 21.8 (H&E, 400×) Oncocytic carcinoma, eosinophilic

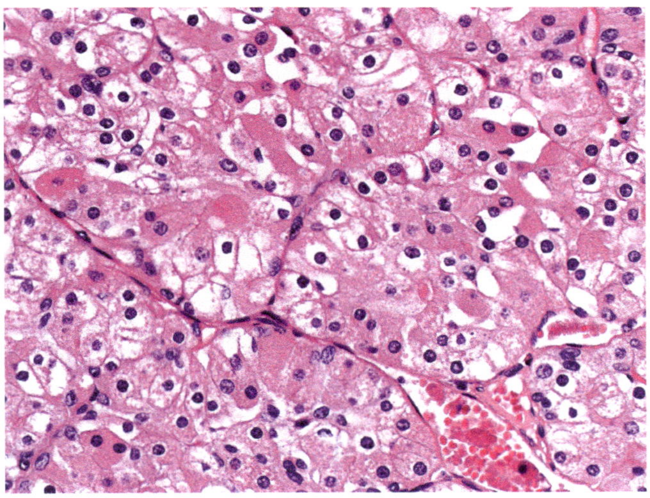

Fig. 21.9 (H&E, 400×) Oncocytic carcinoma, eosinophilic and clear

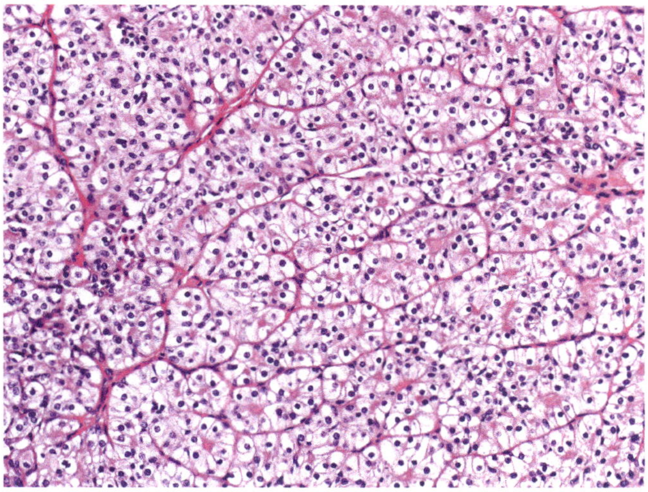

Fig. 21.10 (H&E, 200×) Oncocytic carcinoma, clear

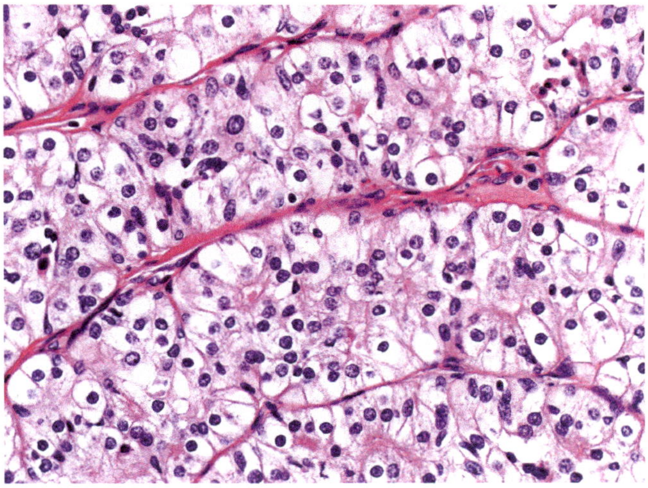

Fig. 21.11 (H&E, 400×) Oncocytic carcinoma, clear

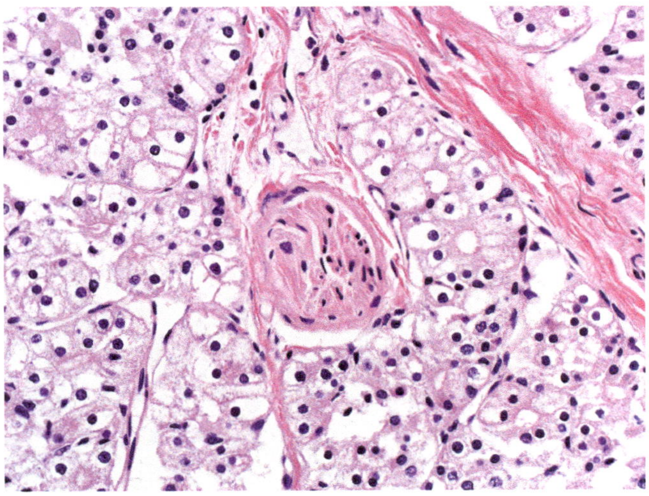

Fig. 21.12 (H&E, 400×) Oncocytic carcinoma, perineural invasion

Suggested Reading

Capone RB, Ha PK, Westra WH, Pilkington TM, Sciubba JJ, Koch WM, et al. Oncocytic neoplasms of the parotid gland: a 16-year institutional review. Otolaryngol Head Neck Surg. 2002;126(6):657–62.

Ferreiro JA, Stylopoulos N. Oncocytic differentiation in salivary gland tumors. J Laryngol Otol. 1995;109:569–71.

McHugh JB, Hoschar AP, Dvorakova M, Parwani AV, Barnes EL, Seethala RR. p63 immunohistochemistry differentiates salivary gland oncocytoma and oncocytic carcinoma from metastatic renal cell carcinoma. Head Neck Pathol. 2007;1(2):123–31.

Muramatsu T, Hashimoto S, Lee MW, Chung CK, Matsuzaki K, Inoue T, et al. Oncocytic carcinoma arising in submandibular gland with immunohistochemical observations and review of the literature. Oral Oncol. 2003;39(2):199–203.

Nakada M, Nishizaki K, Akagi H, Masuda Y, Yoshino T. Oncocytic carcinoma of the submandibular gland: a case report and literature review. J Oral Pathol Med. 1998;27(5):225–8.

Sugimoto T, Wakizono S, Uemura T, Tsuneyoshi M, Enjoji M. Malignant oncocytoma of the parotid gland: a case report with an immunohistochemical and ultrastructural study. J Laryngol Otol. 1993;107:69–74.

Weinreb I, Seethala RR, Perez-Ordonez B, Chetty R, Hoschar AP, Hunt JL. Oncocytic mucoepidermoid carcinoma: clinicopathologic description in a series of 12 cases. Am J Surg Pathol. 2009;33:409–16.

22 Pleomorphic Adenoma

Pleomorphic adenoma is the benign counterpart of carcinoma ex pleomorphic adenoma. Pleomorphic adenoma affects children and adults and presents at a mean age of approximately 45 years. Women are involved more than men. The majority of cases involve the parotid gland, presenting as single or multiple masses. Pleomorphic adenoma may be encapsulated, circumscribed, or multi-nodular, comprised of multiple cell types (ductal, myoepithelial, and mesenchymal), and exhibit a variety of architectural patterns (solid, trabecular, and cystic) (Figs. 22.1–22.36).

J. J. García, *Atlas of Salivary Gland Pathology*, https://doi.org/10.1007/978-3-319-09021-4_22

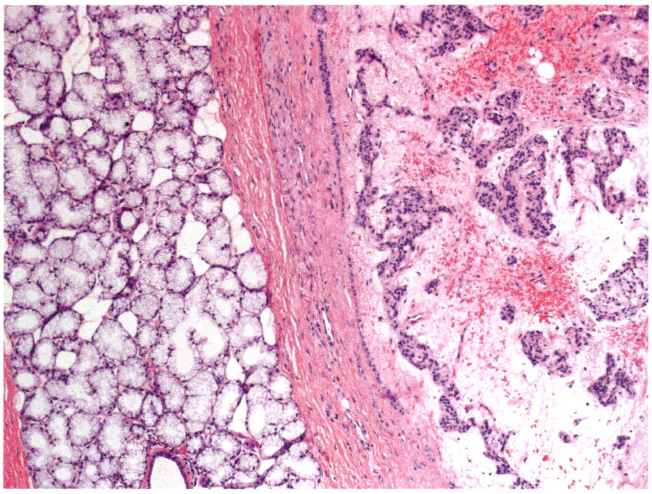

Fig. 22.1 (H&E, 100×) Pleomorphic adenoma, encapsulated

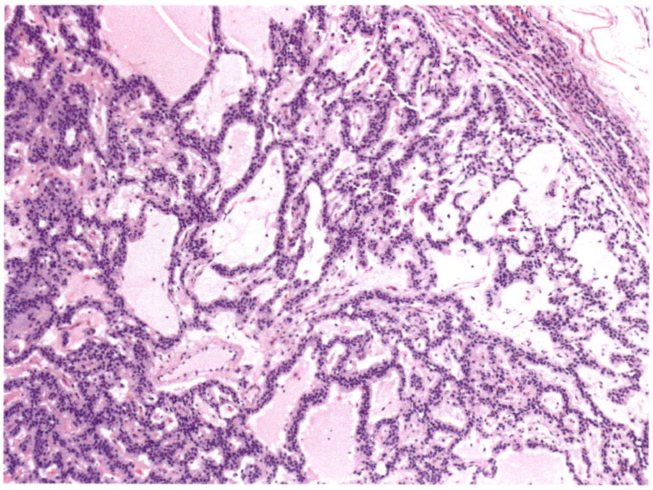

Fig. 22.2 (H&E, 100×) Pleomorphic adenoma, circumscribed

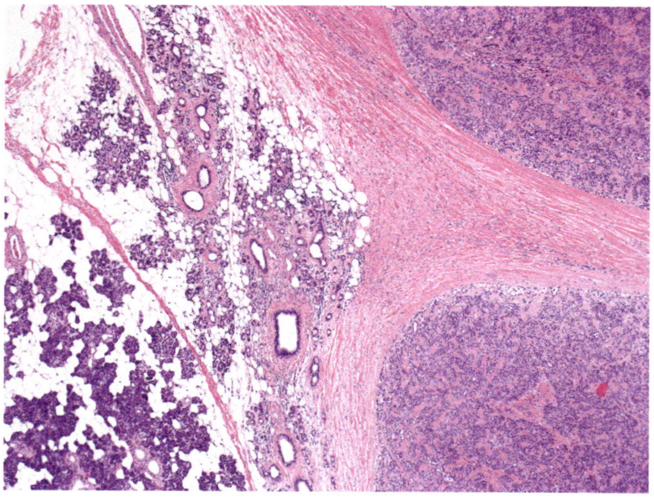

Fig. 22.3 (H&E, 40×) Pleomorphic adenoma, nodular

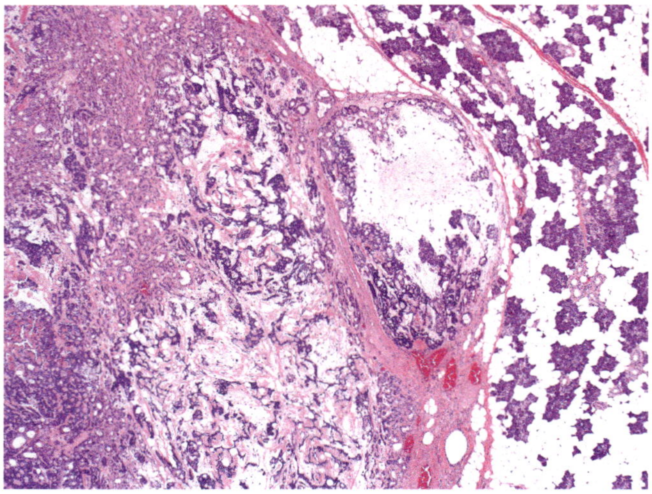

Fig. 22.4 (H&E, 40×) Pleomorphic adenoma, triphasic or more

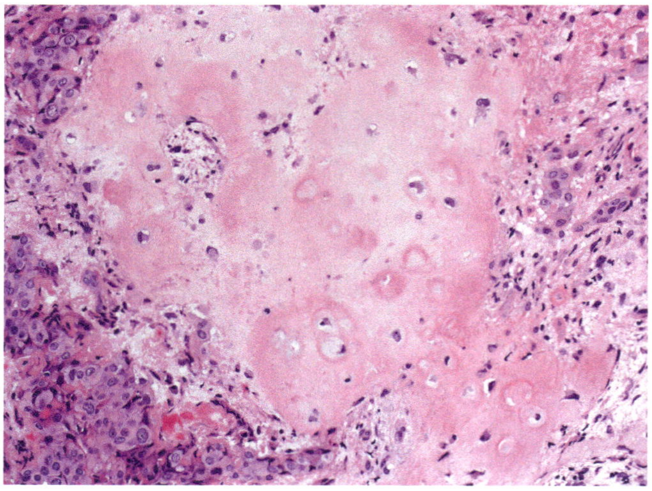

Fig. 22.5 (H&E, 200×) Pleomorphic adenoma, triphasic or more

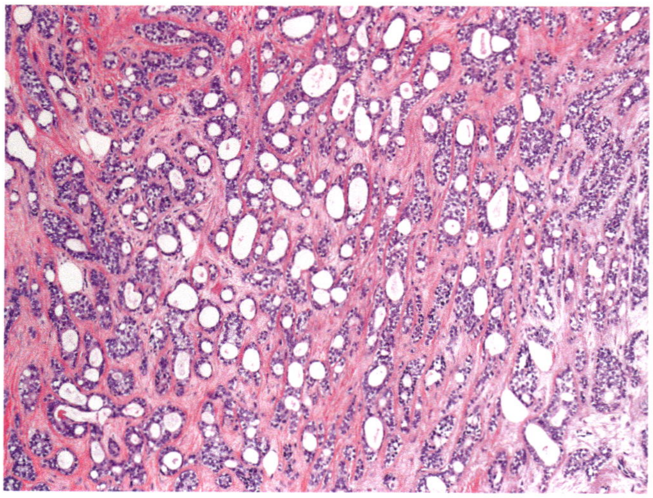

Fig. 22.6 (H&E, 100×) Pleomorphic adenoma, ducts

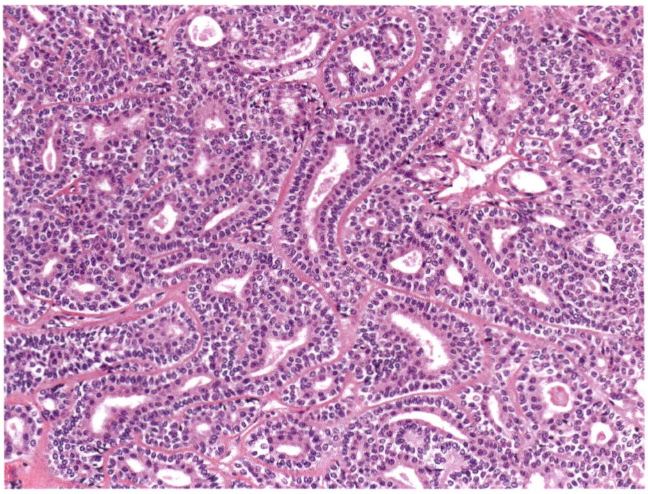

Fig. 22.7 (H&E, 200×) Pleomorphic adenoma, ducts

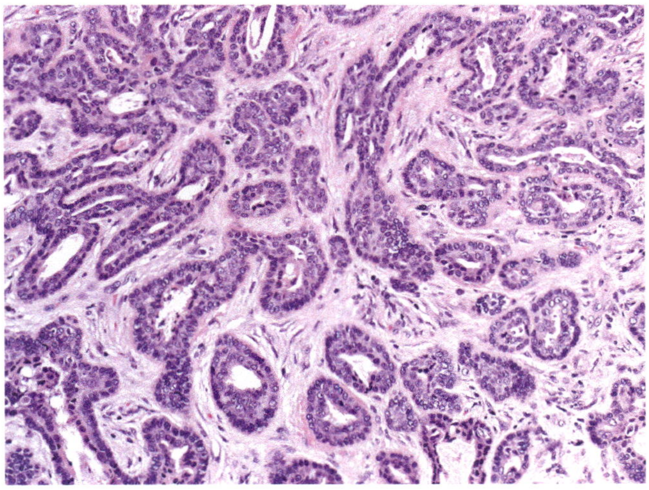

Fig. 22.8 (H&E, 200×) Pleomorphic adenoma, ducts

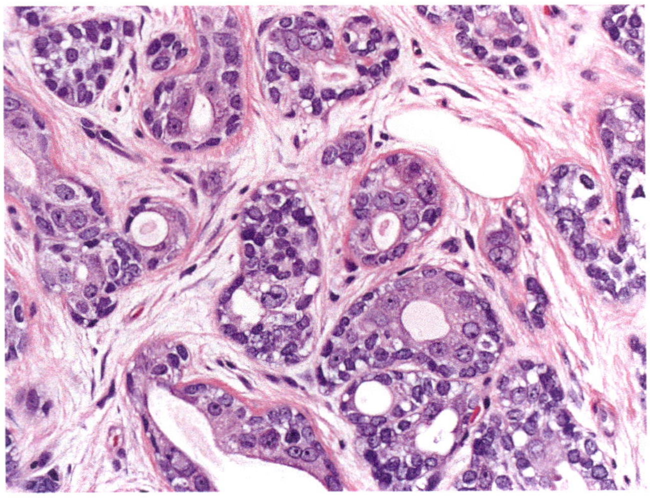

Fig. 22.9 (H&E, 400×) Pleomorphic adenoma, ducts

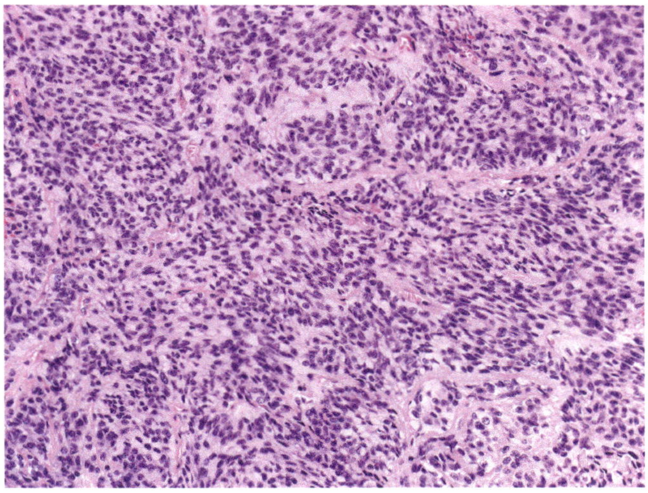

Fig. 22.10 (H&E, 200×) Pleomorphic adenoma, myoepithelial cells, spindled

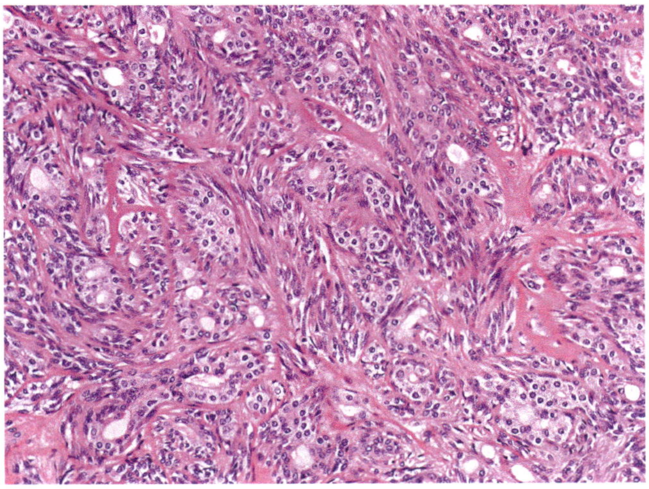

Fig. 22.11 (H&E, 200×) Pleomorphic adenoma, myoepithelial cells, spindled

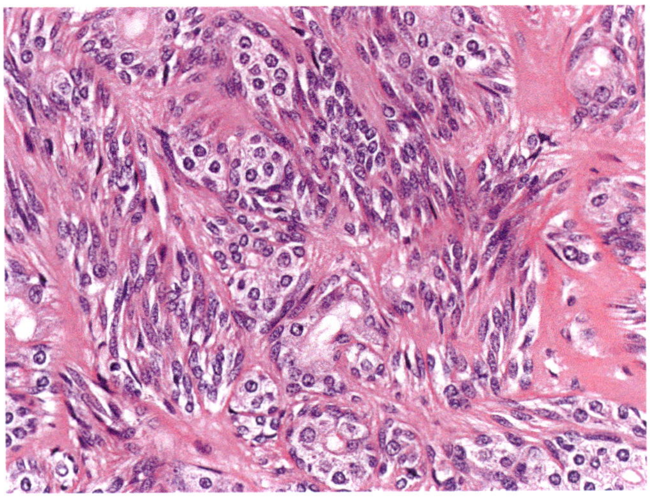

Fig. 22.12 (H&E, 400×) Pleomorphic adenoma, myoepithelial cells, spindled

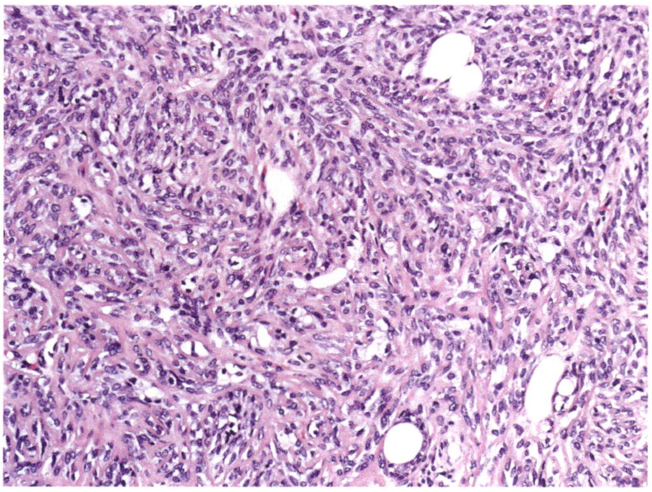

Fig. 22.13 (H&E, 200×) Pleomorphic adenoma, myoepithelial cells, spindled

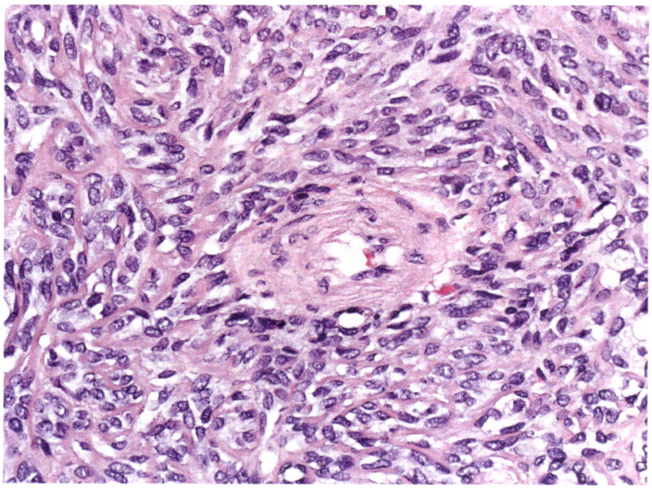

Fig. 22.14 (H&E, 400×) Pleomorphic adenoma, myoepithelial cells, spindled

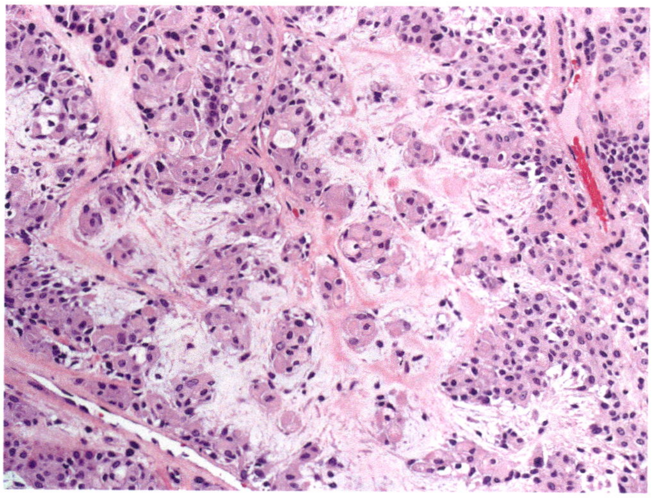

Fig. 22.15 (H&E, 200×) Pleomorphic adenoma, myoepithelial cells, plasmacytoid

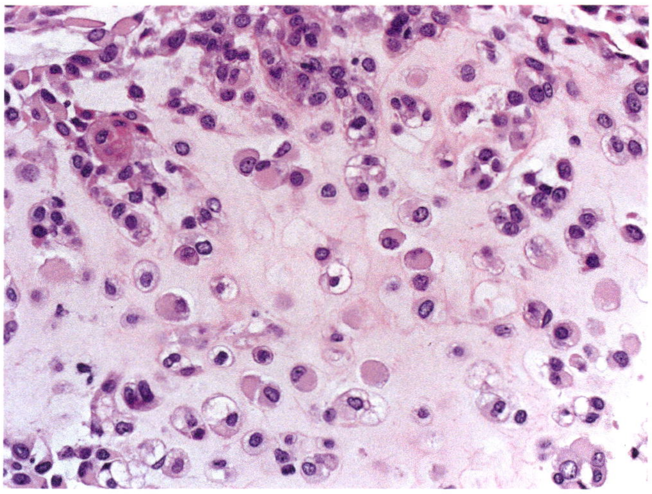

Fig. 22.16 (H&E, 400×) Pleomorphic adenoma, myoepithelial cells, plasmacytoid

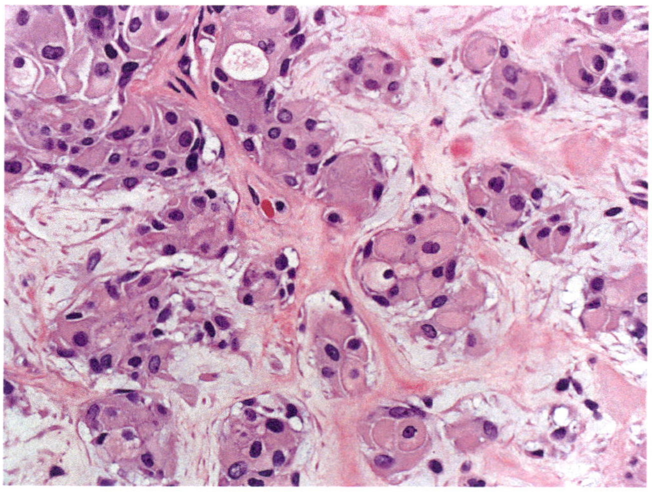

Fig. 22.17 (H&E, 400×) Pleomorphic adenoma, myoepithelial cells, plasmacytoid

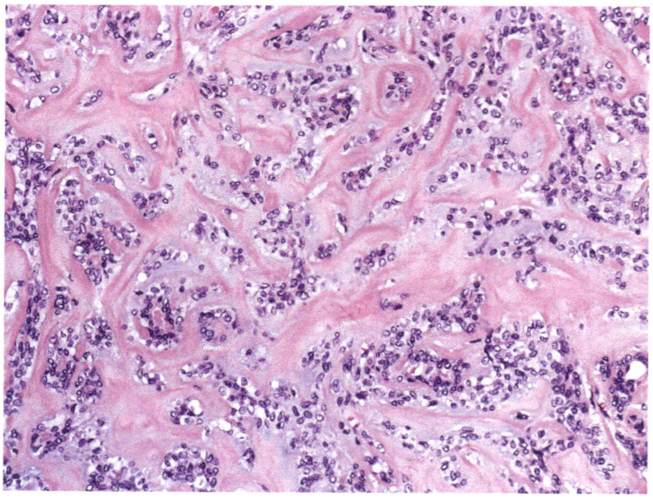

Fig. 22.18 (H&E, 200×) Pleomorphic adenoma, myoepithelial cells, clear

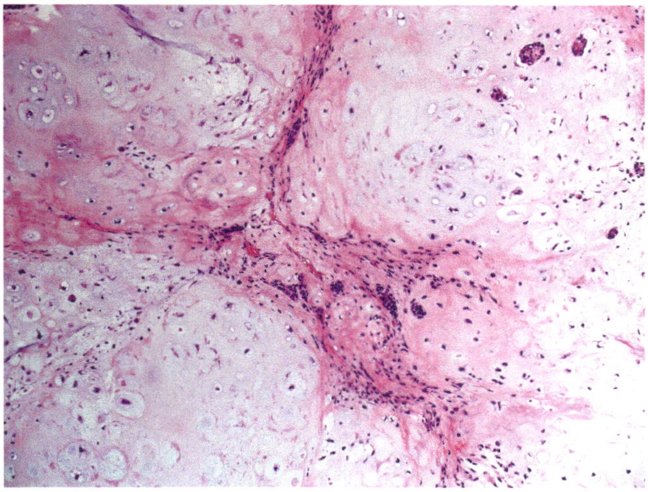

Fig. 22.19 (H&E, 100×) Pleomorphic adenoma, chondroid differentiation

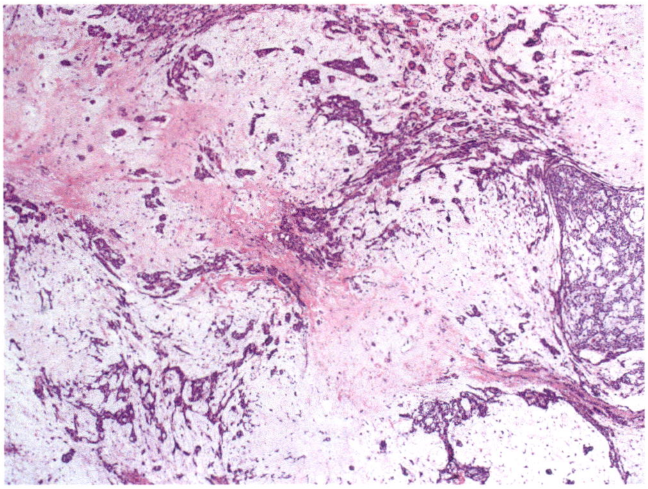

Fig. 22.20 (H&E, 40×) Pleomorphic adenoma, myxoid

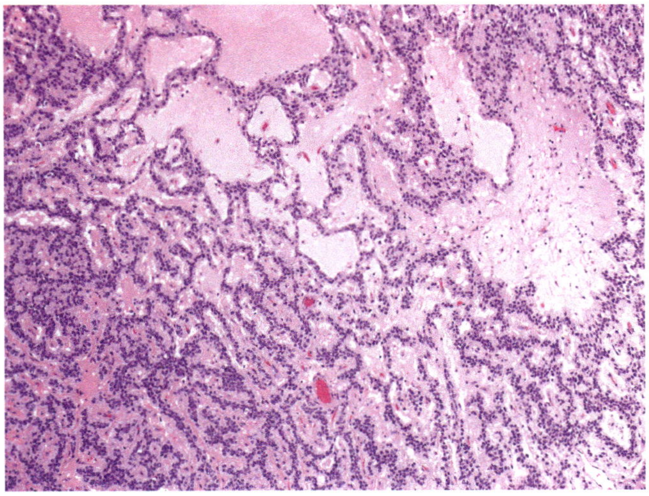

Fig. 22.21 (H&E, 100×) Pleomorphic adenoma, myxoid

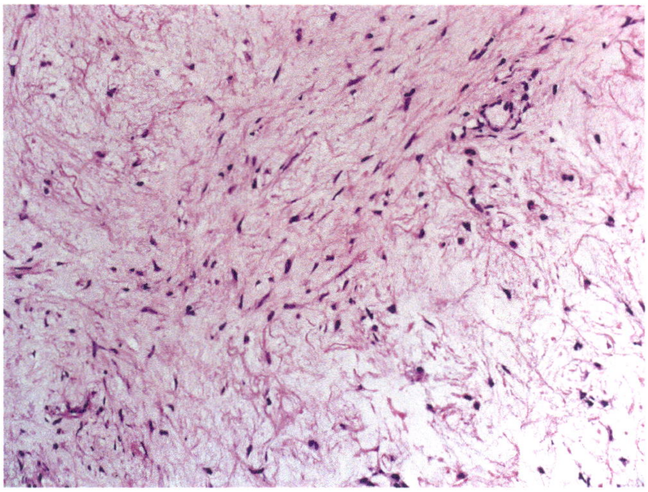

Fig. 22.22 (H&E, 200×) Pleomorphic adenoma, myxoid

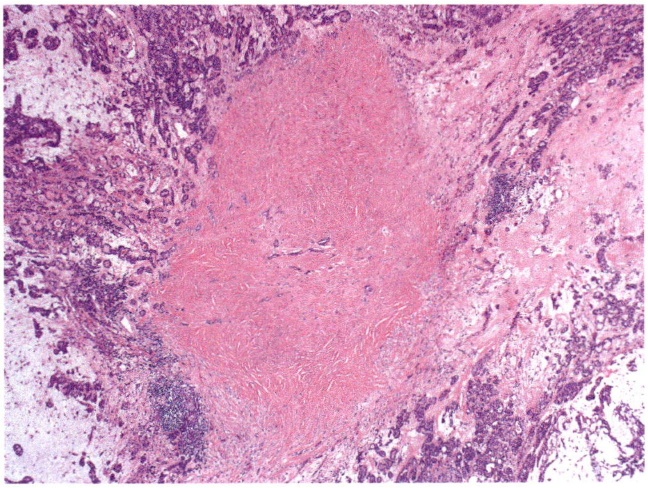

Fig. 22.23 (H&E, 40×) Pleomorphic adenoma, hyalinized

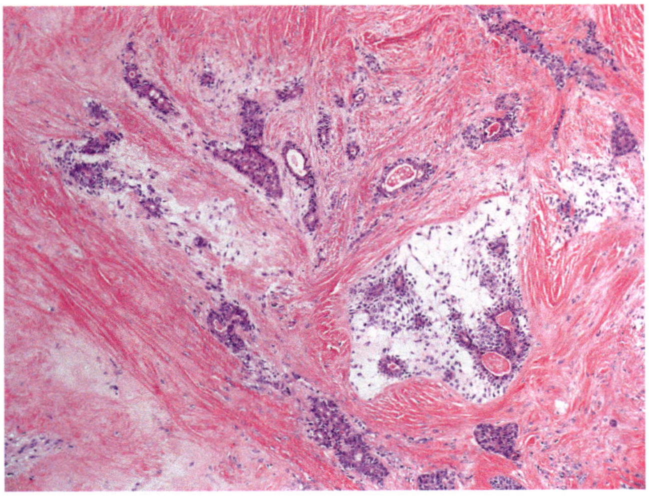

Fig. 22.24 (H&E, 100×) Pleomorphic adenoma, hyalinized

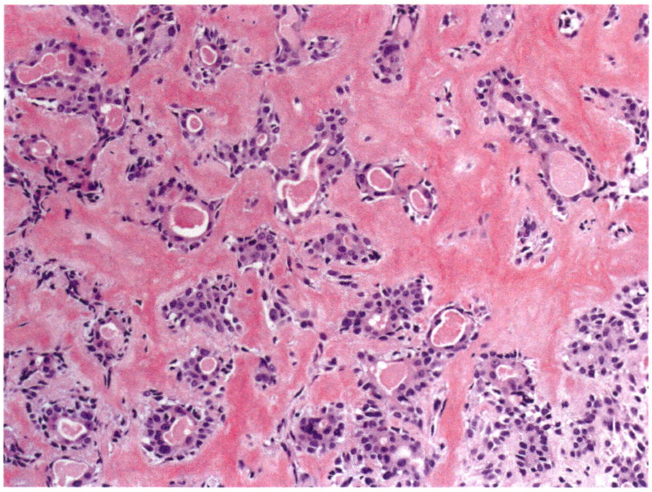

Fig. 22.25 (H&E, 200×) Pleomorphic adenoma, basement membrane-like material

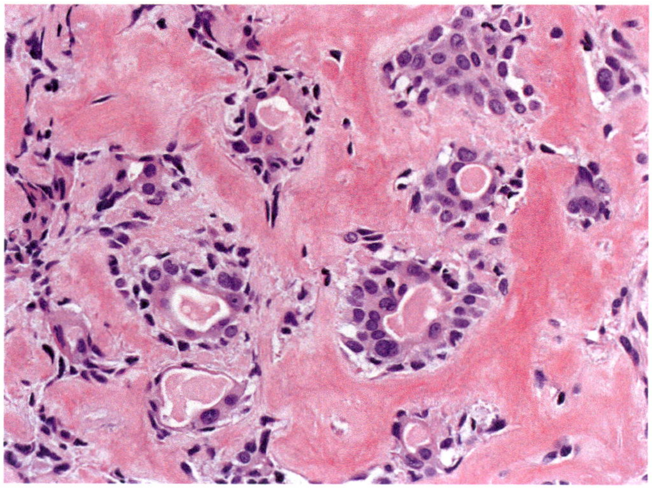

Fig. 22.26 (H&E, 400×) Pleomorphic adenoma, basement membrane-like material

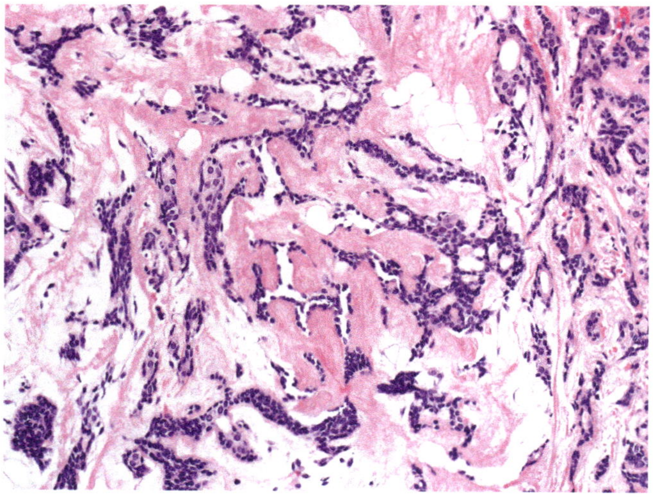

Fig. 22.27 (H&E, 200×) Pleomorphic adenoma, pseudo-vascular

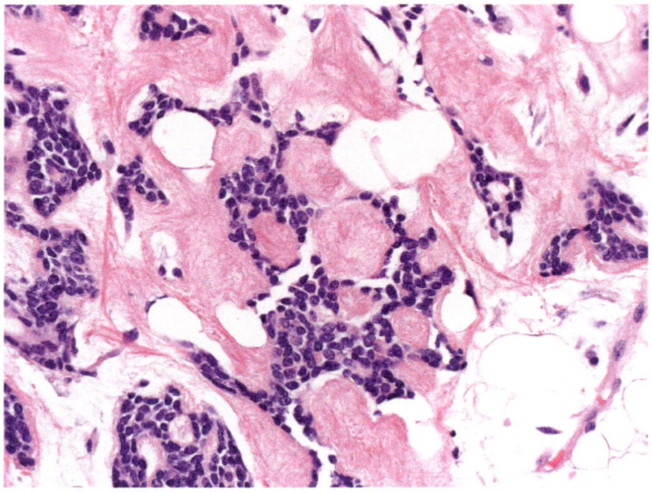

Fig. 22.28 (H&E, 400×) Pleomorphic adenoma, pseudo-vascular

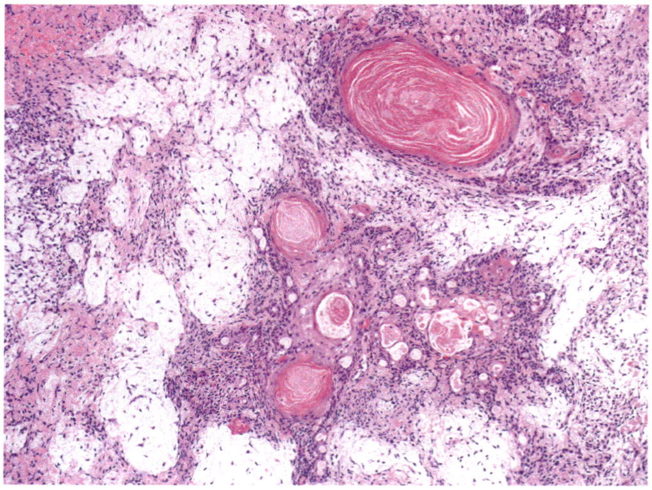

Fig. 22.29 (H&E, 100×) Pleomorphic adenoma, squamous metaplasia and keratinization

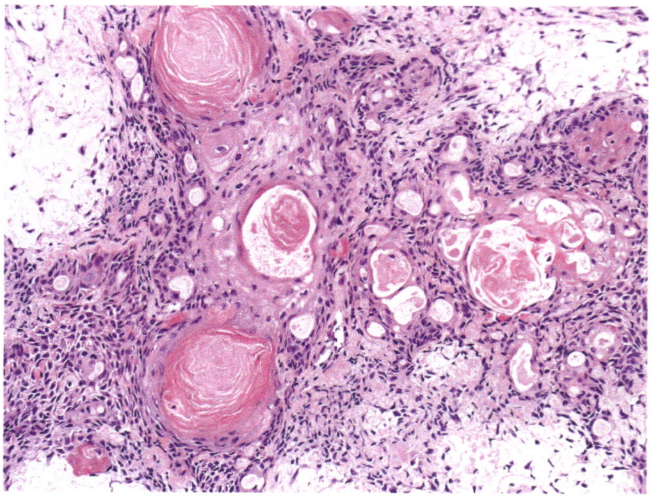

Fig. 22.30 (H&E, 200×) Pleomorphic adenoma, squamous metaplasia and keratinization

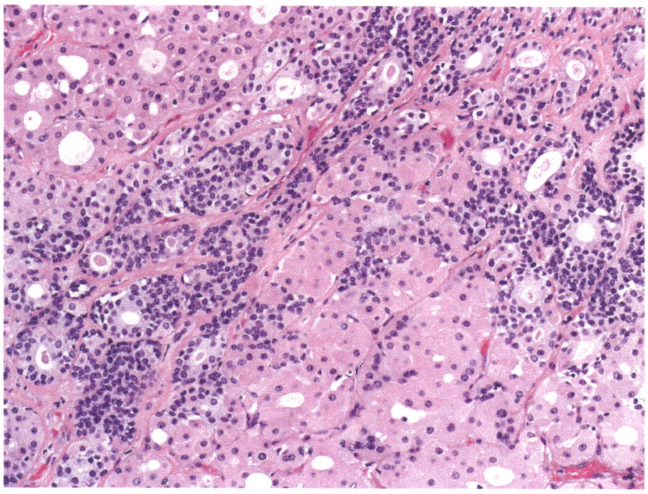

Fig. 22.31 (H&E, 200×) Pleomorphic adenoma, oncocytic metaplasia

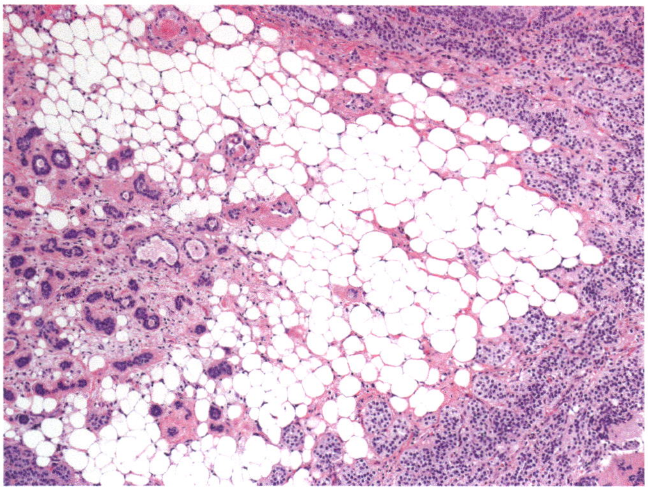

Fig. 22.32 (H&E, 100×) Pleomorphic adenoma, adipocytic metaplasia

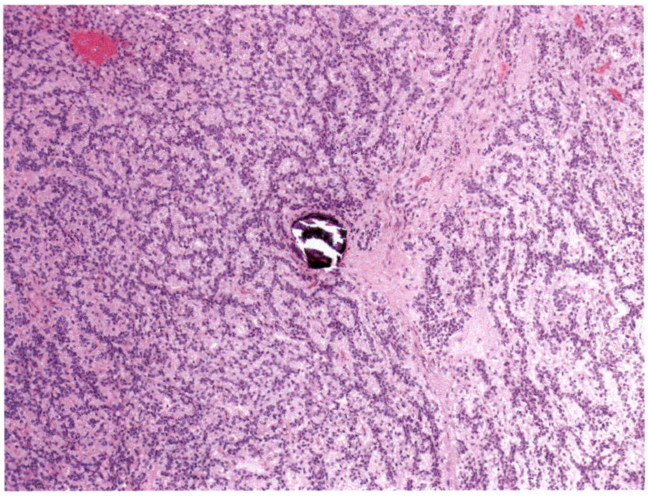

Fig. 22.33 (H&E, 100×) Pleomorphic adenoma, microcalcifications

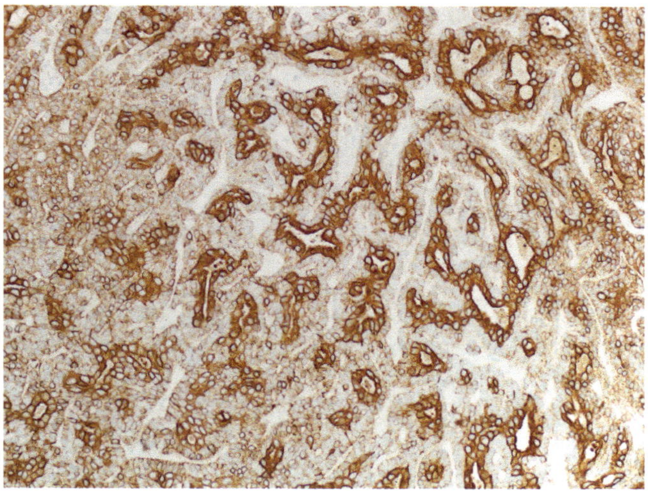

Fig. 22.34 (AE1/AE3, 200×) Pleomorphic adenoma, diffuse immunoreactivity

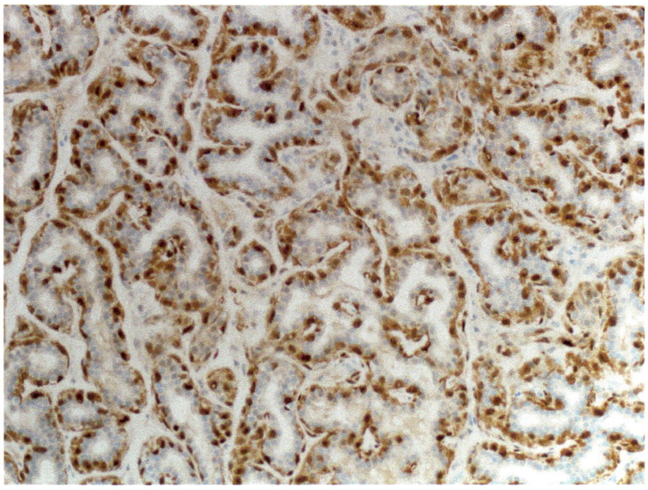

Fig. 22.35 (S-100, 200×) Pleomorphic adenoma, myoepithelial immunoreactivity

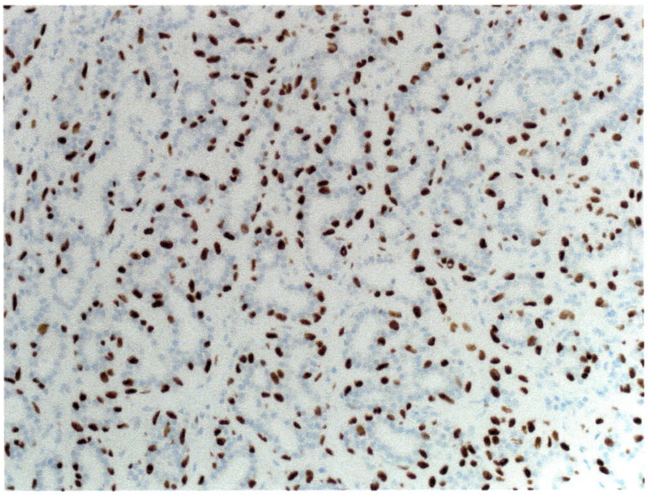

Fig. 22.36 (p63, 200×) Pleomorphic adenoma, myoepithelial immunoreactivity

Suggested Reading

Baldi A, Persichetti P, Di Marino MP, Nicoletti G, Baldi F. Pleomorphic adenoma of cervical heterotopic salivary glands. J Exp Clin Cancer Res. 2003;22(4):645–7.

Blevins NH, Jackler RK, Kaplan MJ, Boles R. Facial paralysis due to benign parotid tumors. Arch Otolaryngol Head Neck Surg. 1992;118:427–30.

Colella G, Cannavale R, Chiodini P. Meta-analysis of surgical approaches to the treatment of parotid pleomorphic adenomas and recurrence rates. J Craniomaxillofac Surg. 2015;43:738–45.

Coombes DM, Kaddour R, Shah N. Synchronous unilateral pleomorphic adenomas in the parotid gland: report of a case. Br J Oral Maxillofac Surg. 2009;47:155–6.

Eveson JW, Cawson RA. Salivary gland tumors. A review of 2410 cases with particular reference to histological types, site, age and sex distribution. J Pathol. 1985;146:51–8.

Gnepp DR. Malignant mixed tumors of the salivary glands: a review. Pathol Annu. 1993;28:279–328.

Gnepp DR, Schroeder W, Heffner D. Synchronous tumors arising in a single major salivary gland cancer. Cancer. 1989;63:1219–24.

Guntinas-Lichius O, Kick C, Klussmann JP, Jungehuelsing M, Stennert E. Pleomorphic adenoma of the parotid gland: a 13-year experience of consequent management by lateral or total parotidectomy. Eur Arch Otorhinolaryngol. 2004;261(3):143–6.

Huang JT, Li W, Chen XQ, Shi RH, Zhao YF. Synchronous bilateral pleomorphic adenomas of the parotid gland. J Investig Clin Dent. 2012;3:225–7.

Knight J, Ratnasingham K. Metastasizing pleomorphic adenoma: systematic review. Int J Surg. 2015;19:137–45.

Lam PW, Chan JK, Sin VC. Nasal pleomorphic adenoma with skeletal muscle differentiation: potential misdiagnosis as rhabdomyosarcoma. Hum Pathol. 1997;28(11):1299–302.

Manucha V, Ioffe OB. Metastasizing pleomorphic adenoma of the salivary gland. Arch Pathol Lab Med. 2008;132:1445–7.

Matsuyama A, Hisaoka M, Nagao Y, Hashimoto H. Aberrant PLAG1 expression in pleomorphic adenomas of the salivary gland: a molecular genetic and immunohistochemical study. Virchows Arch. 2011;458(5):583–92.

Miliauskas JR, Hunt JL. Primary unilateral multifocal pleomorphic adenoma of the parotid gland: molecular assessment and literature review. Head Neck Pathol. 2008;2:339–42.

Narozny W, Kuczkowski J, Mikaszewski B. Pleomorphic adenoma of the nasal cavity: clinical analysis of 8 cases. Am J Otolaryngol. 2005;26(3):218.

Perumal CJ, Meyer M, Mohamed A. A giant pleomorphic adenoma of the submandibular salivary gland: a case report. Craniomaxillofac Trauma Reconstr. 2012;5:185–8.

Phillips PP, Olsen KD. Recurrent pleomorphic adenoma of the parotid gland: report of 126 cases and a review of the literature. Ann Otol Rhinol Laryngol. 1995;104(2):100–4.

Pinkston JA, Cole P. Incidence rates of salivary gland tumors: results from a population-based study. Otolaryngol Head Neck Surg. 1999;20:834–40.

Riad MA, Abdel-Rahman H, Ezzat WF, Adly A, Dessouky O, Shehata M. Variables related to recurrence of pleomorphic adenomas: outcome of parotid surgery in 182 cases. Laryngoscope. 2011;121:1467–72.

Sataloff RT, Price DB, Roberts BR. Bilateral synchronous mixed tumors of the parotid glands. Arch Otolaryngol Head Neck Surg. 1987;113:880–1.

Skalova A, Altemani A, Di Palma S, Simpson RH, Hosticka L, Andrle P, et al. Pleomorphic adenoma of the salivary glands with intravascular tumor deposits: a diagnostic pitfall. Am J Surg Pathol. 2012;36:1674–82.

Spiro RH. Salivary neoplasms: overview of a 35-year experience with 2,807 patients. Head Neck Surg. 1986;8:177–84.

Triantafyllou A, Thompson LD, Devaney KO, Bell D, Hunt JL, Rinaldo A, et al. Functional histology of salivary gland Pleomophic adenoma: an appraisal. Head Neck Pathol. 2015;9:387–404.

Wittekindt C, Streubel K, Arnold G, Stennert E, Guntinas-Lichius O. Recurrent pleomorphic adenoma of the parotid gland: analysis of 108 consecutive patients. Head Neck. 2007;29:822–8.

23 Pleomorphic Adenoma, Carcinoma Ex

Carcinoma ex pleomorphic adenoma is the malignant counterpart of pleomorphic adenoma. Carcinoma ex pleomorphic adenoma affects primarily adults and presents at a mean age of approximately 60 years. Women are involved more than men. The majority of cases involve the parotid gland, presenting as single or multiple masses. Carcinoma ex pleomorphic adenoma may be circumscribed (*non-invasive*) or infiltrative (*invasive*), comprised of multiple cell types (ductal, myoepithelial, and mesenchymal), and exhibit a variety of architectural patterns (solid, trabecular, and cystic) (Figs. 23.1–23.40).

J. J. García, *Atlas of Salivary Gland Pathology*, https://doi.org/10.1007/978-3-319-09021-4_23

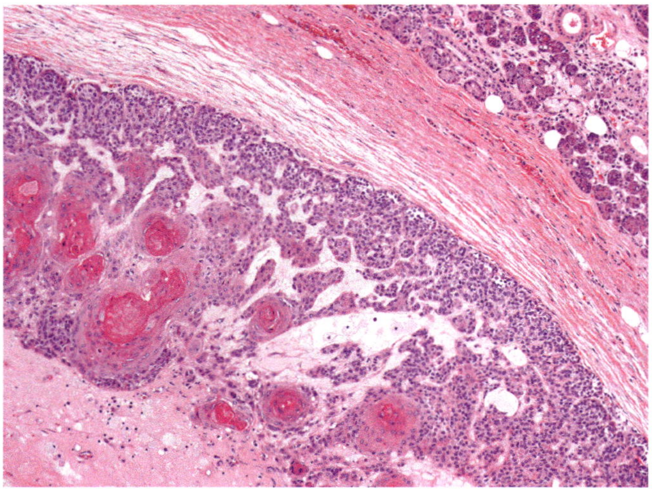

Fig. 23.1 (H&E, 100×) Carcinoma ex pleomorphic adenoma, encapsulated

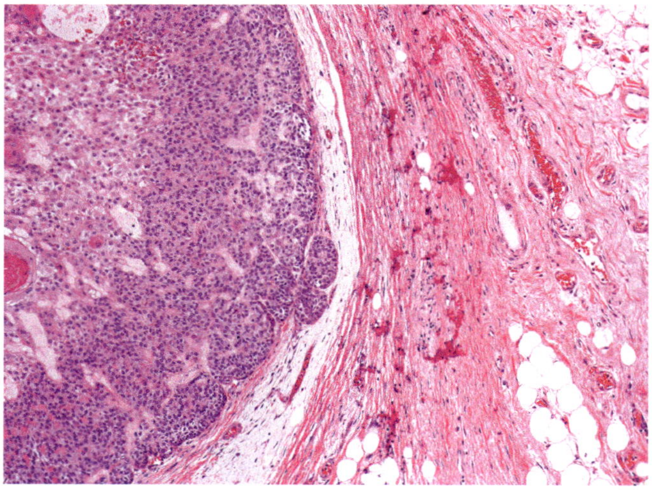

Fig. 23.2 (H&E, 100×) Carcinoma ex pleomorphic adenoma, circumscribed

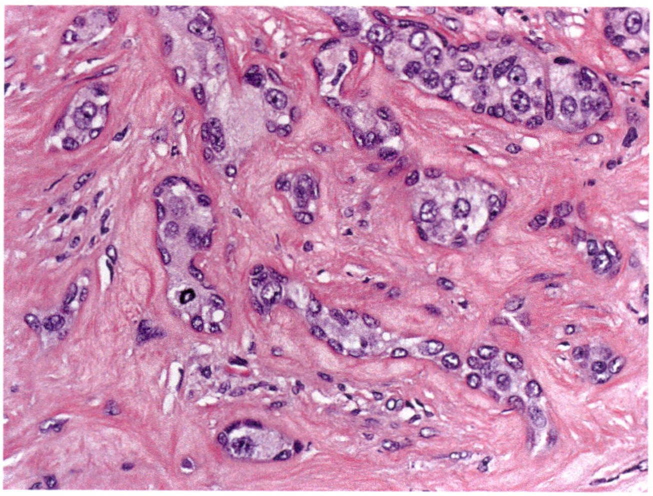

Fig. 23.3 (H&E, 400×) Carcinoma ex pleomorphic adenoma, infiltrative

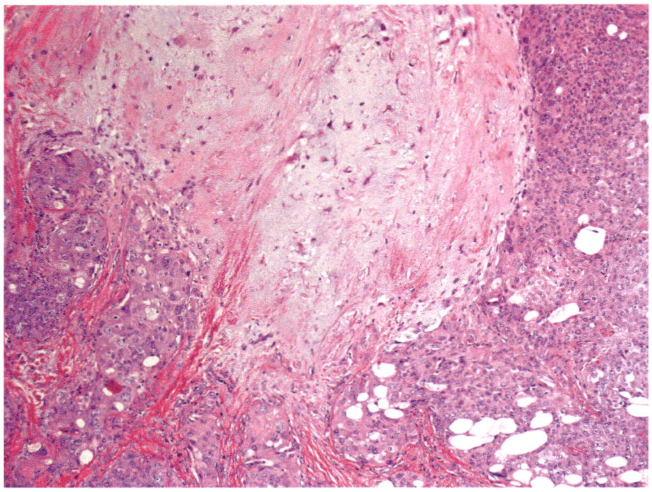

Fig. 23.4 (H&E, 100×) Carcinoma ex pleomorphic adenoma, triphasic or more

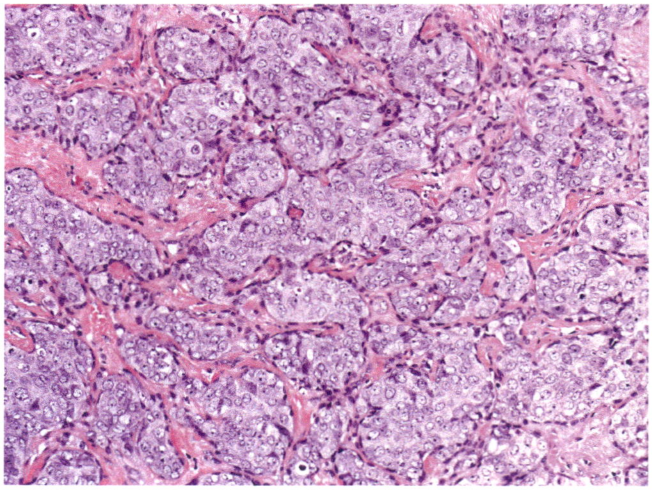

Fig. 23.5 (H&E, 200×) Carcinoma ex pleomorphic adenoma, ducts

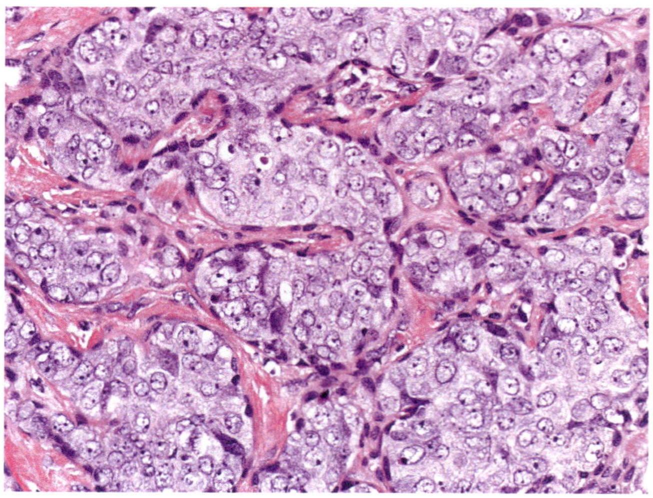

Fig. 23.6 (H&E, 400×) Carcinoma ex pleomorphic adenoma, ducts

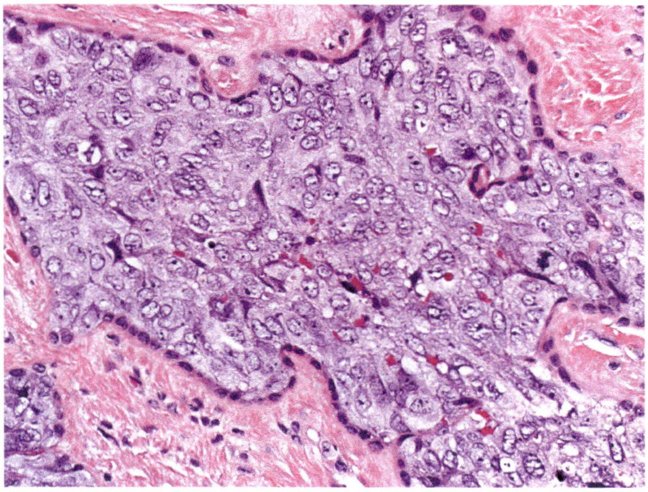

Fig. 23.7 (H&E, 400×) Carcinoma ex pleomorphic adenoma, ducts

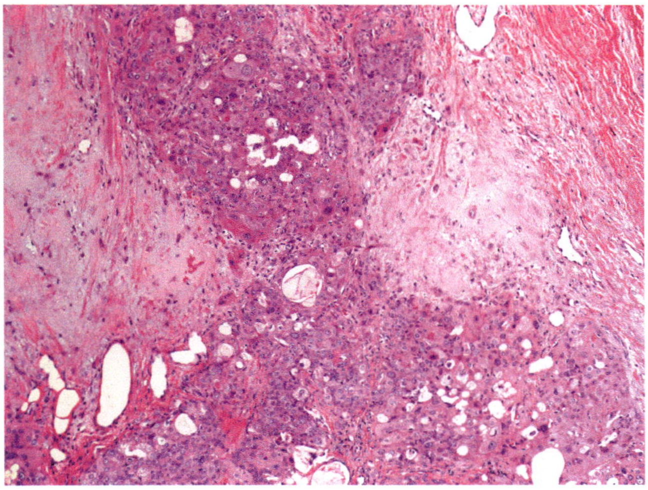

Fig. 23.8 (H&E, 100×) Carcinoma ex pleomorphic adenoma, chondroid differentiation

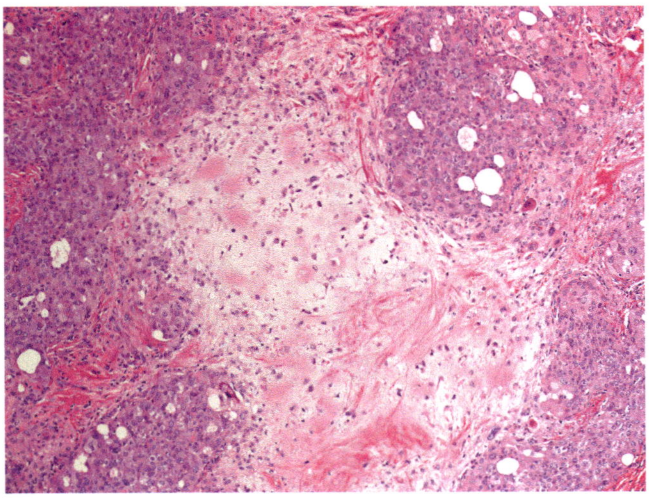

Fig. 23.9 (H&E, 100×) Carcinoma ex pleomorphic adenoma, chondroid differentiation

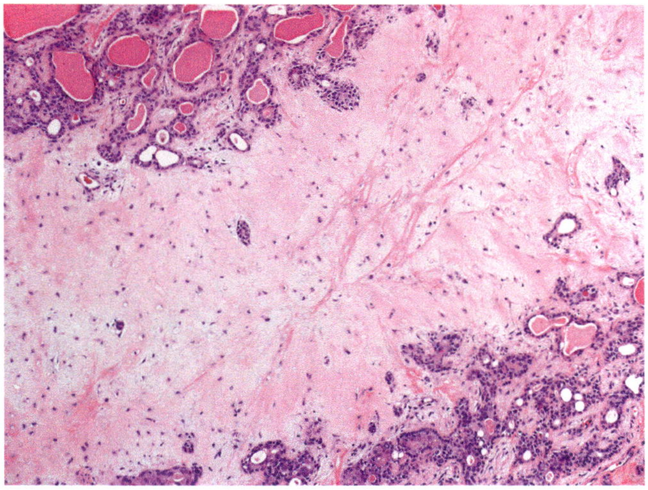

Fig. 23.10 (H&E, 100×) Carcinoma ex pleomorphic adenoma, chondroid differentiation

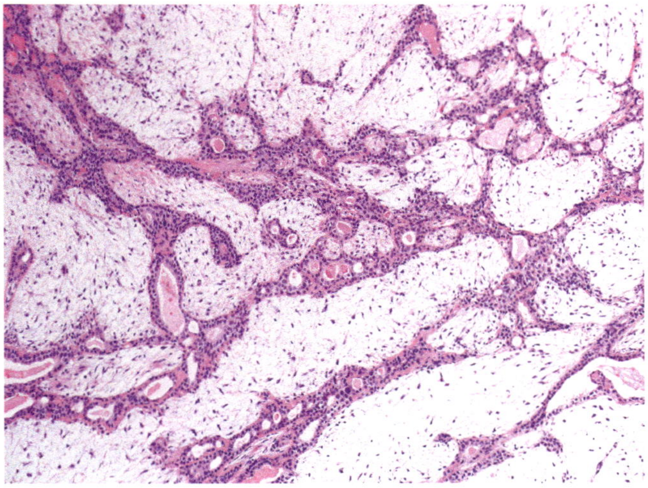

Fig. 23.11 (H&E, 100×) Carcinoma ex pleomorphic adenoma, myxoid

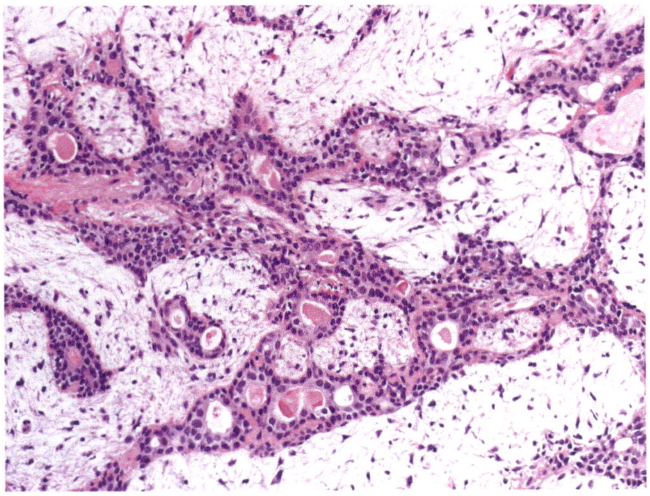

Fig. 23.12 (H&E, 200×) Carcinoma ex pleomorphic adenoma, myxoid

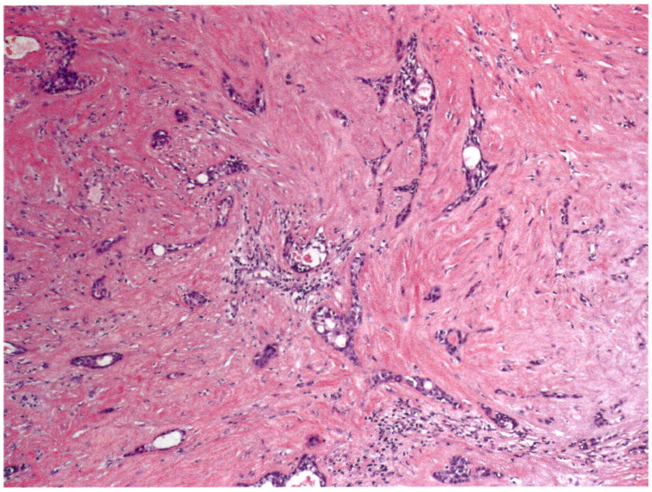

Fig. 23.13 (H&E, 100×) Carcinoma ex pleomorphic adenoma, hyalinized

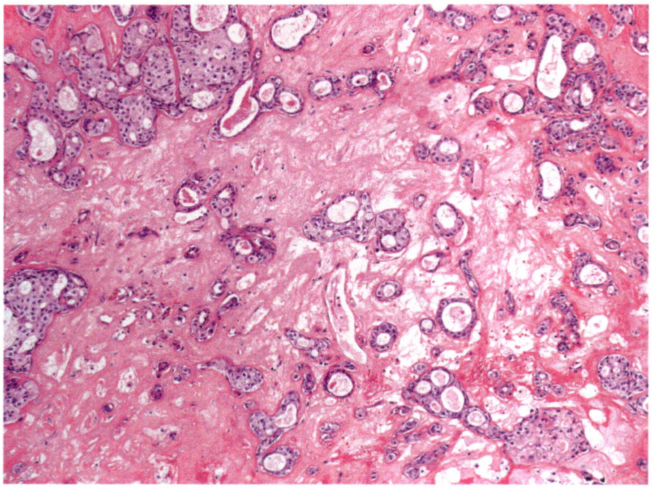

Fig. 23.14 (H&E, 100×) Carcinoma ex pleomorphic adenoma, salivary duct carcinoma

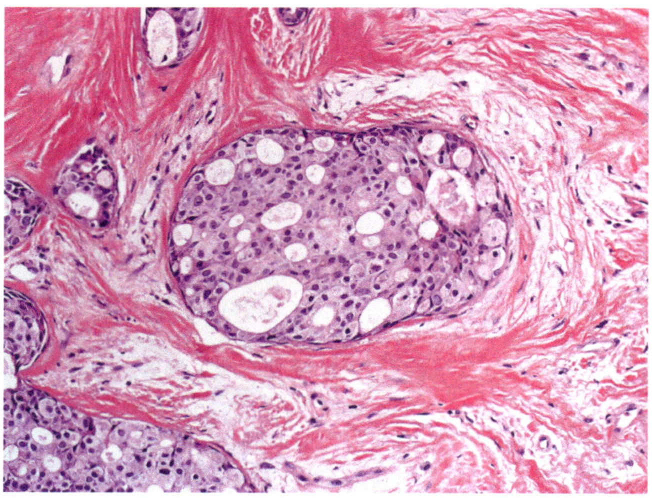

Fig. 23.15 (H&E, 200×) Carcinoma ex pleomorphic adenoma, salivary duct carcinoma

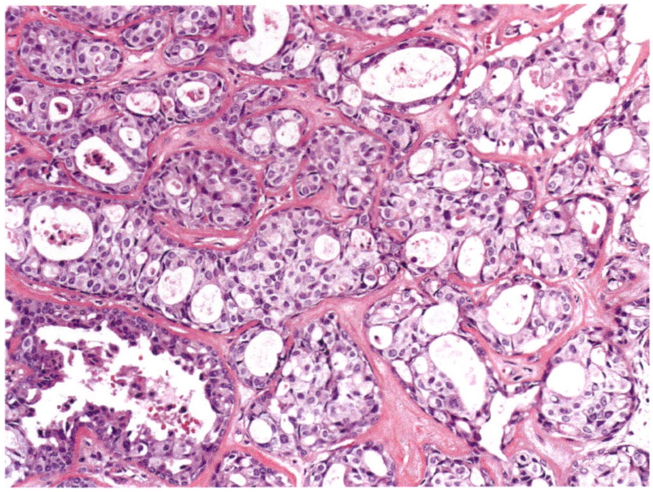

Fig. 23.16 (H&E, 200×) Carcinoma ex pleomorphic adenoma, salivary duct carcinoma

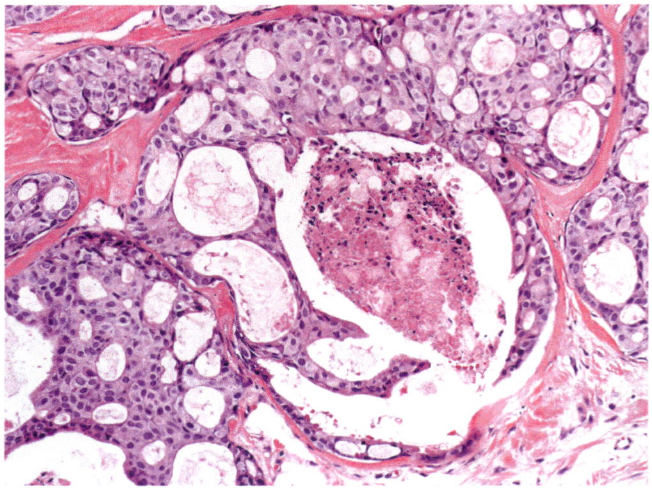

Fig. 23.17 (H&E, 200×) Carcinoma ex pleomorphic adenoma, salivary duct carcinoma

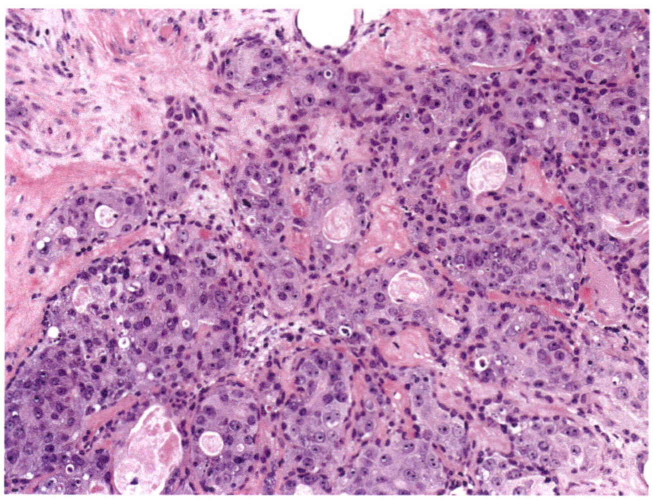

Fig. 23.18 (H&E, 200×) Carcinoma ex pleomorphic adenoma, cytomorphologic atypia

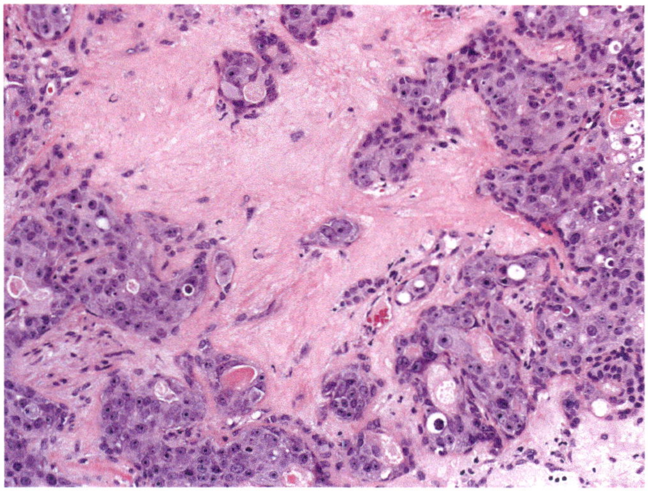

Fig. 23.19 (H&E, 200×) Carcinoma ex pleomorphic adenoma, cytomorphologic atypia

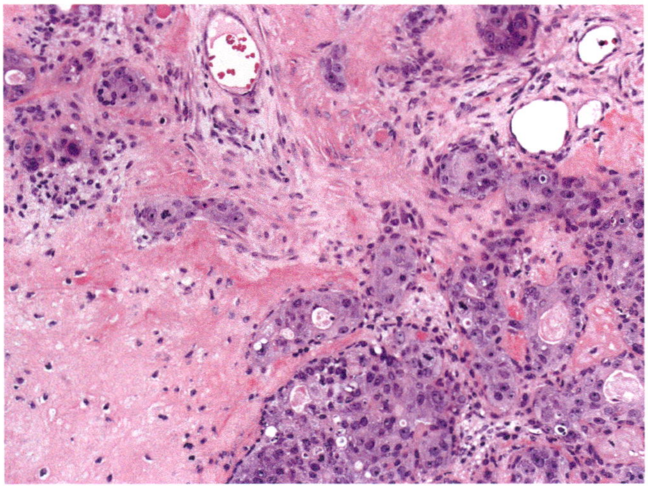

Fig. 23.20 (H&E, 200×) Carcinoma ex pleomorphic adenoma, cytomorphologic atypia

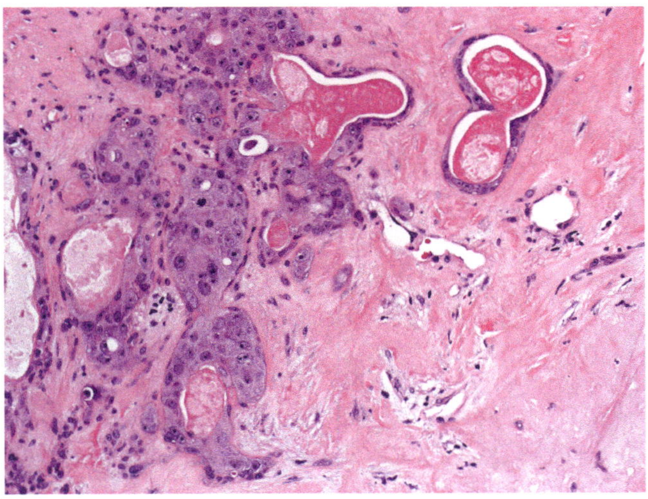

Fig. 23.21 (H&E, 200×) Carcinoma ex pleomorphic adenoma, cytomorphologic atypia

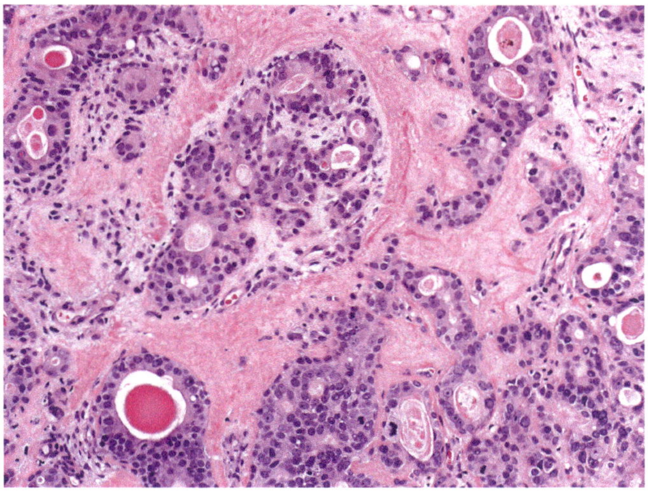

Fig. 23.22 (H&E, 200×) Carcinoma ex pleomorphic adenoma, cytomorphologic atypia

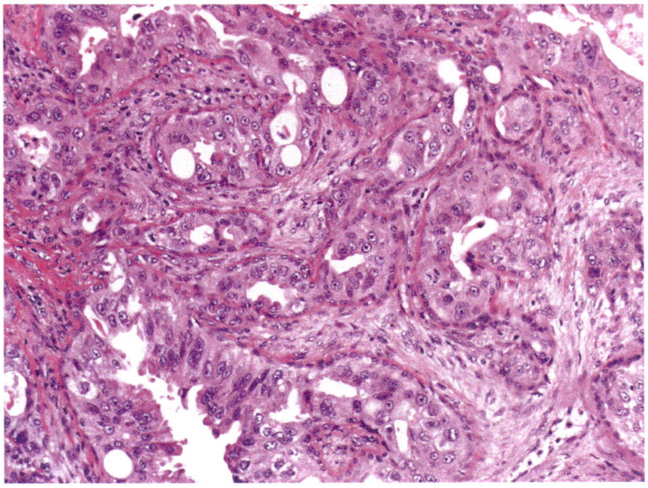

Fig. 23.23 (H&E, 200×) Carcinoma ex pleomorphic adenoma, cytomorphologic atypia

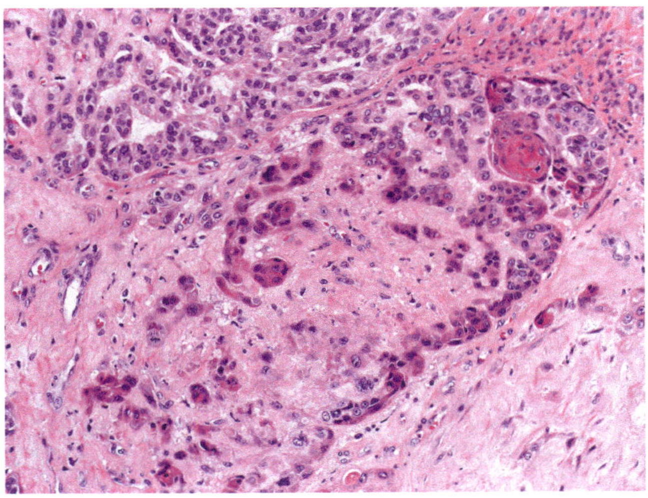

Fig. 23.24 (H&E, 200×) Carcinoma ex pleomorphic adenoma, cytomorphologic atypia

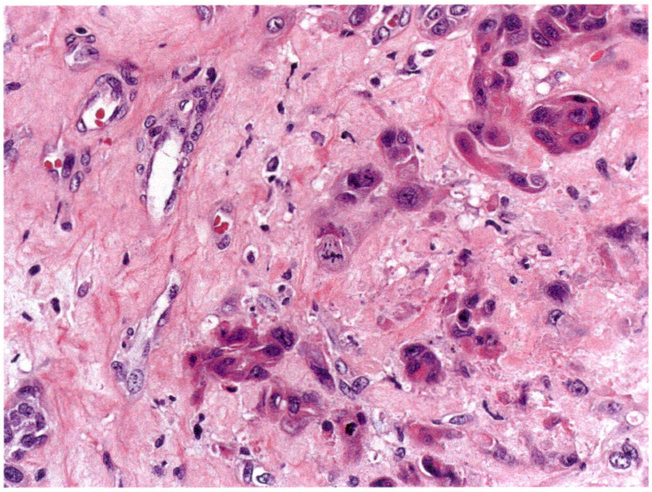

Fig. 23.25 (H&E, 400×) Carcinoma ex pleomorphic adenoma, cytomorphologic atypia

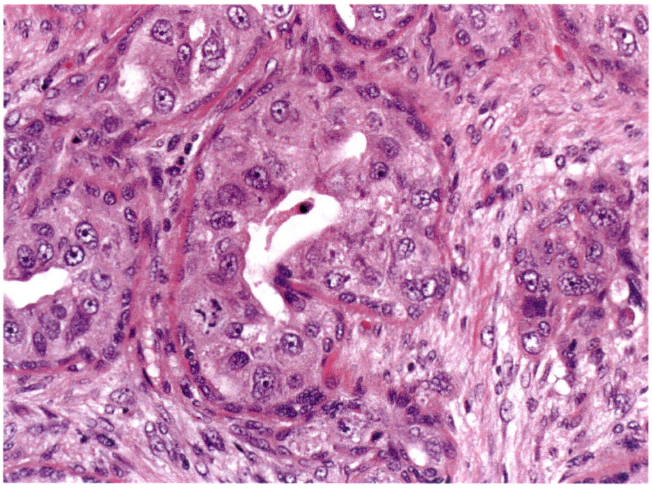

Fig. 23.26 (H&E, 400×) Carcinoma ex pleomorphic adenoma, cytomorphologic atypia

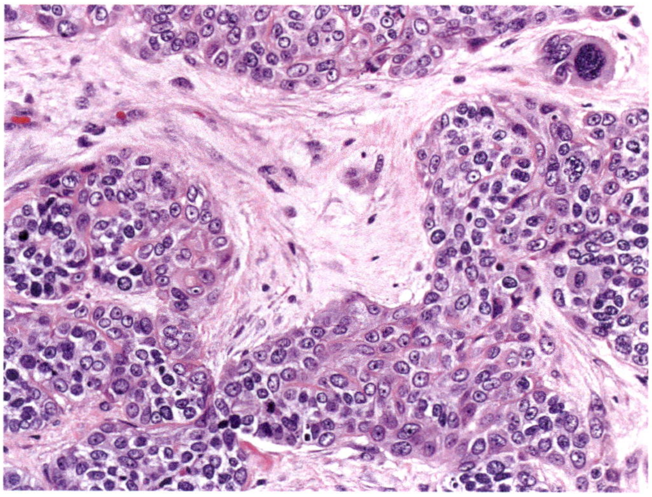

Fig. 23.27 (H&E, 400×) Carcinoma ex pleomorphic adenoma, cytomorphologic atypia

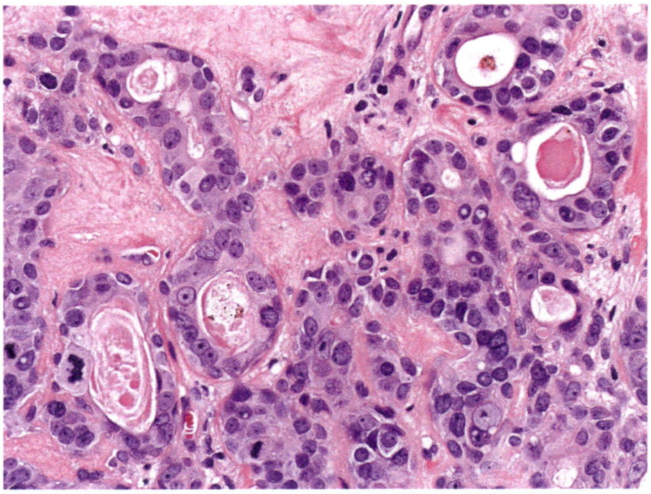

Fig. 23.28 (H&E, 400×) Carcinoma ex pleomorphic adenoma, mitotic activity

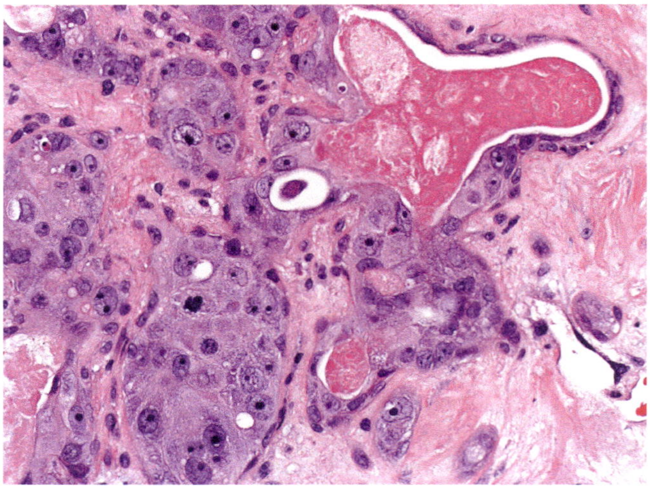

Fig. 23.29 (H&E, 400×) Carcinoma ex pleomorphic adenoma, mitotic activity

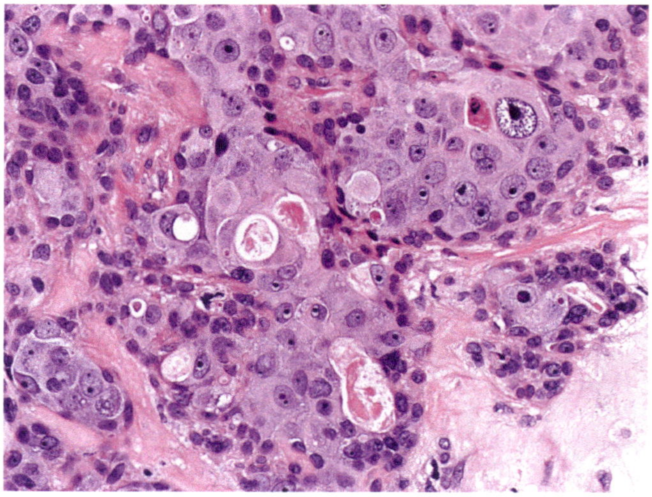

Fig. 23.30 (H&E, 400×) Carcinoma ex pleomorphic adenoma, mitotic activity

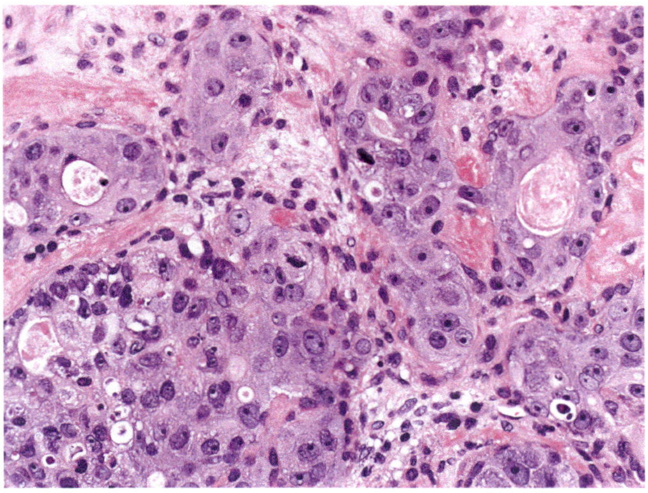

Fig. 23.31 (H&E, 400×) Carcinoma ex pleomorphic adenoma, mitotic activity

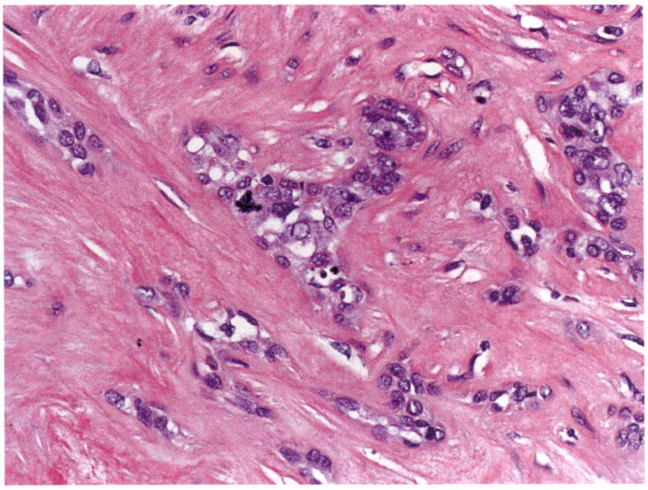

Fig. 23.32 (H&E, 400×) Carcinoma ex pleomorphic adenoma, mitotic activity

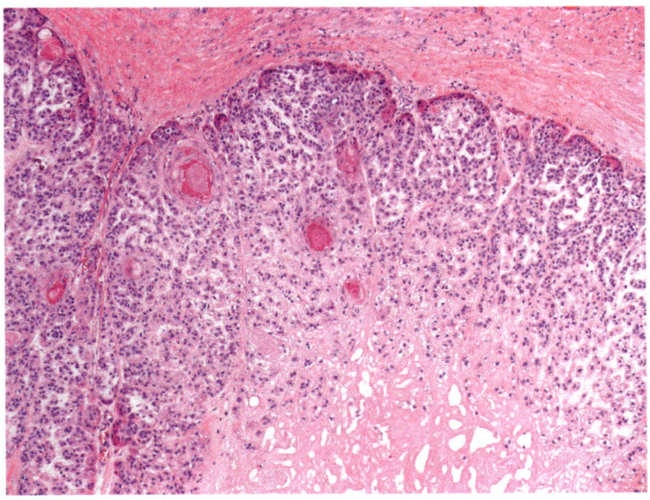

Fig. 23.33 (H&E, 100×) Carcinoma ex pleomorphic adenoma, squamous metaplasia and keratinization

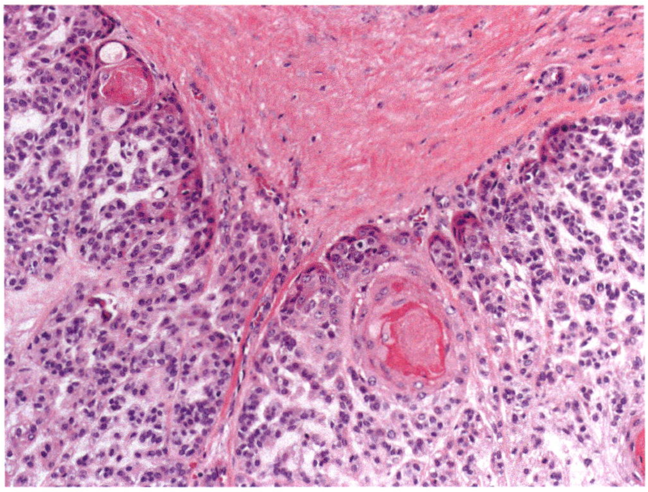

Fig. 23.34 (H&E, 200×) Carcinoma ex pleomorphic adenoma, squamous metaplasia and keratinization

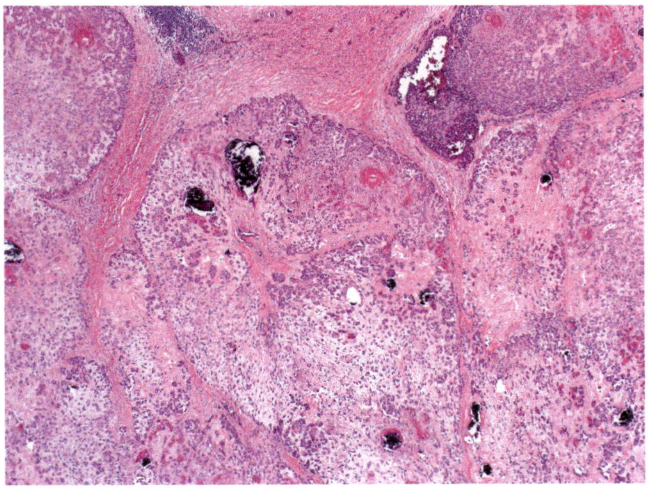

Fig. 23.35 (H&E 40×) Carcinoma ex pleomorphic adenoma, microcalcifications

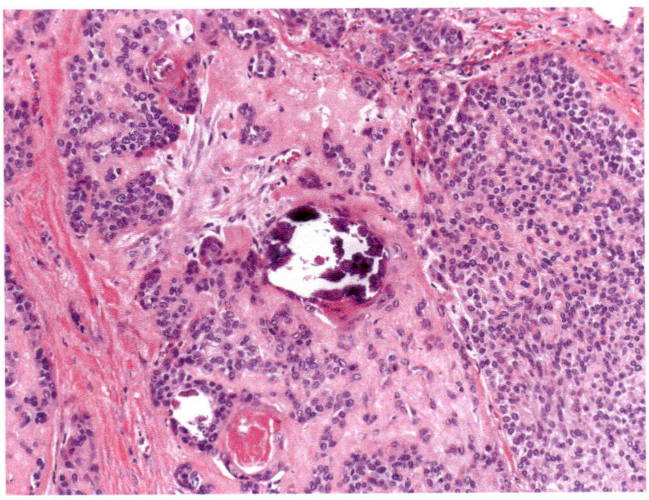

Fig. 23.36 (H&E, 200×) Carcinoma ex pleomorphic adenoma, microcalcifications

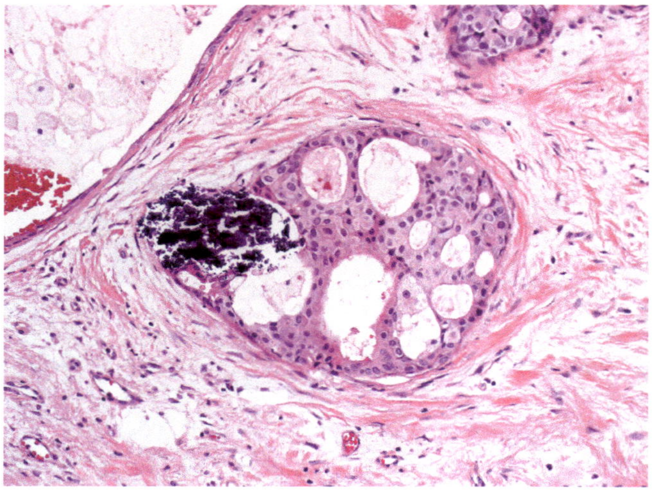

Fig. 23.37 (H&E, 200×) Carcinoma ex pleomorphic adenoma, microcalcifications

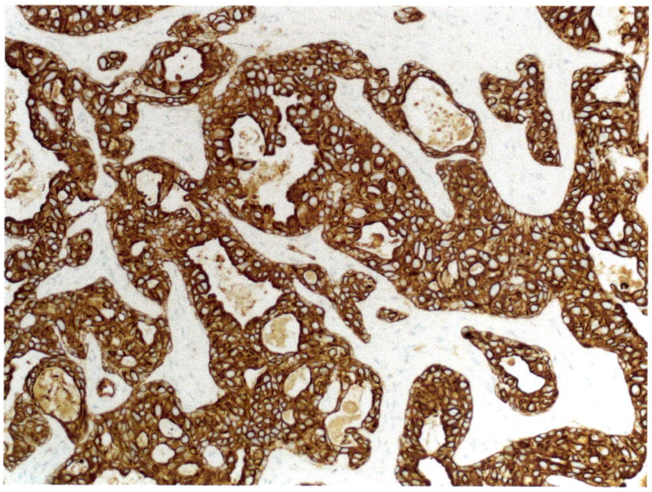

Fig. 23.38 (AE1/AE3, 200×) Carcinoma ex pleomorphic adenoma, diffuse immunoreactivity

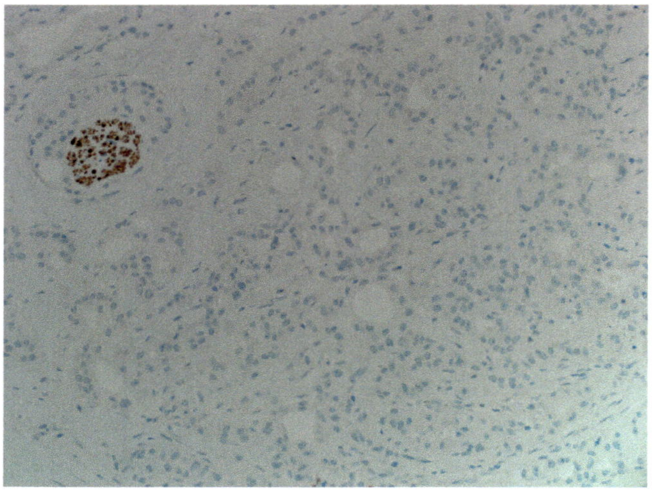

Fig. 23.39 (S-100, 200×) Carcinoma ex pleomorphic adenoma, negative immunoreactivity

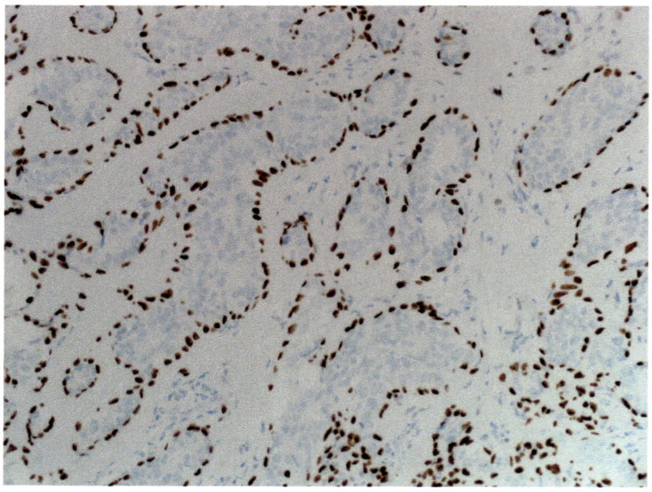

Fig. 23.40 (p63, 200×) Carcinoma ex pleomorphic adenoma, myoepithelial immunoreactivity

Suggested Reading

Altemani A, Martins MT, Freitas L, Soares F, Araujo NS, Araujo VC. Carcinoma ex pleomorphic adenoma (CXPA): immunoprofile of the cells involved in carcinomatous progression. Histopathology. 2005;46:635–41.

Antony J, Gopalan V, Smith RA, Lam AK. Carcinoma ex pleomorphic adenoma: a comprehensive review of clinical, pathological and molecular data. Head Neck Pathol. 2012;6(1):1–9.

Auclair PL, Ellis GL. Atypical features in salivary gland mixed tumors: their relationship to malignant transformation. Mod Pathol. 1996;9:652–7.

Cohn ML, Callender DL, El-Naggar AK. Sebaceous carcinoma ex-pleomorphic adenoma: a rare phenotypic occurrence. Ann Diagn Pathol. 2004;8(4):224–6.

Di Palma S. Carcinoma ex pleomorphic adenoma, with particular emphasis on early lesions. Head Neck Pathol. 2013;7(Suppl 1):S68–76.

Di Palma S, Skalova A, Vanieek T, Simpson RH, Starek I, Leivo I. Non-invasive (intracapsular) carcinoma ex pleomorphic adenoma: recognition of focal carcinoma by HER-2/neu and MIB1 immunohistochemistry. Histopathology. 2005;46(2):144–52.

Griffith CC, Thompson LD, Assaad A, Purgina BM, Lai C, Bauman JE, et al. Salivary duct carcinoma and the concept of early carcinoma ex pleomorphic adenoma. Histopathology. 2014;65:854–60.

Katabi N, Ghossein R, Ho A, Dogan S, Zhang L, Sung YS, et al. Consistent PLAG1 and HMGA2 abnormalities distinguish carcinoma ex-pleomoprhic adenoma from its de novo counterparts. Hum Pathol. 2015;46:26–33.

Katabi N, Gomez D, Klimstra DS, Carlson DL, Lee N, Ghossein R. Prognostic factors of recurrence in salivary carcinoma ex pleomorphic adenoma, with emphasis on the carcinoma histologic subtype: a clinicopathologic study of 43 cases. Hum Pathol. 2010;41:927–34.

Kim JW, Kwon GY, Roh JL, Choi SH, Nam SY, Kim SY, et al. Carcinoma ex pleomorphic adenoma of the salivary glands: distinct clinicopathologic features and immunoprofiles between subgroups according to cellular differentiation. J Korean Med Sci. 2011;26:1277–85.

Klijanienko J, El-Naggar AK, Servois V, Rodriguez J, Validire P, Vielh P. Mucoepidermoid carcinoma ex pleomorphic adenoma: nonspecific preoperative cytologic findings in six cases. Cancer. 1998;84:231–4.

Klijanienko J, El-Naggar AK, Vielh P. Fine-needle sampling findings in 26 carcinoma ex pleomorphic adenomas. Diagn Cytopathol. 1999;21:163–6.

Lewis JE, Olsen KD, Sebo TJ. Carcinoma ex pleomorphic adenoma: pathologic analysis of 73 cases. Hum Pathol. 2001;32:596–604.

Li Volsi VA, Perzin KH, LiVolsi VA. Malignant mixed tumors arising in salivary glands I. Carcinomas arising in benign mixed tumors: a clinicopathologic study. Cancer. 1977;39:2209–30.

Nakamori K, Ohuchi T, Hasegawa T, Hiratsuka H. Carcinoma ex pleomorphic adenoma of the buccal region is composed of salivary duct carcinoma and squamous cell carcinoma components. Int J Oral Maxillofac Surg. 2009;38(10):1116–8.

Nigam S, Kumar N, Jain S. Cytomorphologic spectrum of carcinoma ex pleomorphic adenoma. Acta Cytol. 2004;48(3):309–14.

Tortoledo ME, Luna MA, Batsakis JG. Carcinomas ex pleomorphic adenoma and malignant mixed tumors. Histomorphologic indexes. Arch Otolaryngol. 1984;110:172–6.

Weiler C, Zengel P, van der Wal JE, Guntinas-Lichius O, Schwarz S, Harrison JD, et al. Carcinoma ex pleomorphic adenoma with special reference to the prognostic significance of histological progression: a clinicopathological investigation of 41 cases. Histopathology. 2011;59(4):741–50.

24 Polymorphous Adenocarcinoma

Polymorphous adenocarcinoma affects children and adults and presents at a mean age of approximately 60 years. Women are involved more than men. The majority of cases involve minor salivary glands, presenting as single or multiple masses. Most cases of polymorphous adenocarcinoma behave as low to intermediate-grade malignancies. Polymorphous adenocarcinoma may be circumscribed or infiltrative, comprised almost exclusively of one cell type (ductal), and exhibit a variety of architectural patterns (solid, trabecular, cribriform, and cystic) (Figs. 24.1–24.28).

J. J. García, *Atlas of Salivary Gland Pathology*, https://doi.org/10.1007/978-3-319-09021-4_24

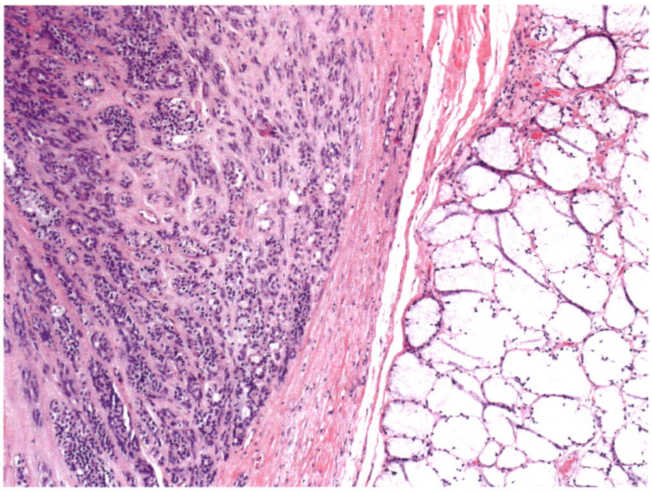

Fig. 24.1 (H&E, 100×) Polymorphous adenocarcinoma, circumscribed

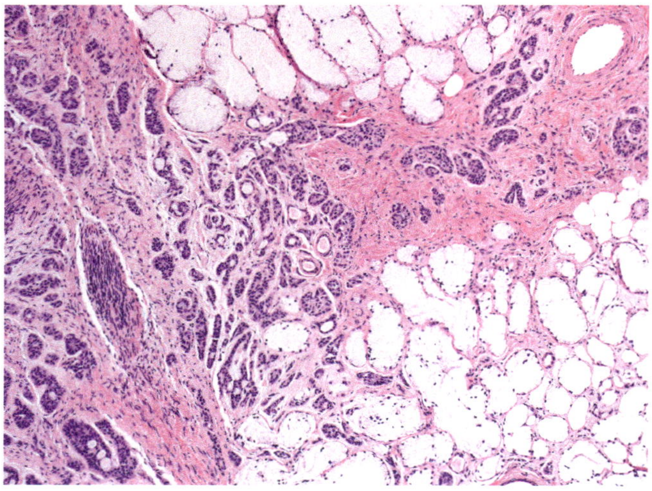

Fig. 24.2 (H&E, 100×) Polymorphous adenocarcinoma, infiltrative

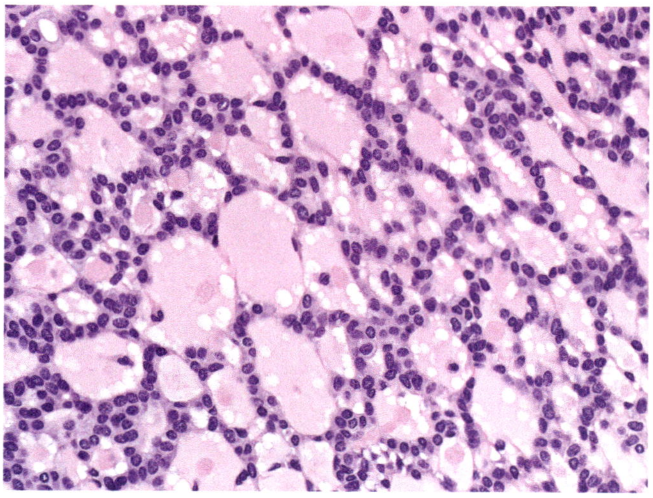

Fig. 24.3 (H&E, 400×) Polymorphous adenocarcinoma, monophasic

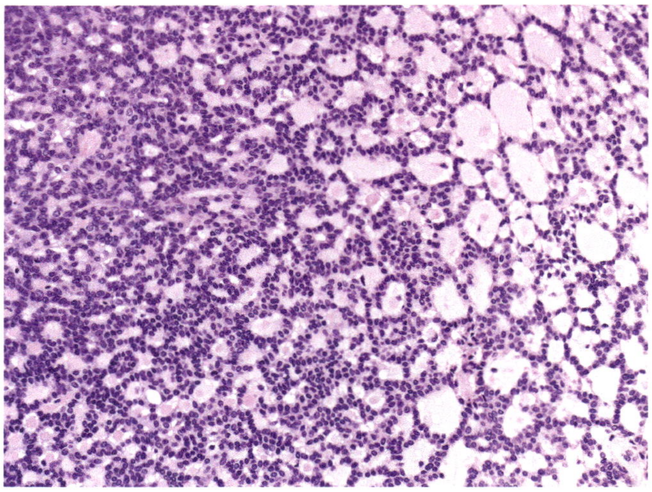

Fig. 24.4 (H&E, 200×) Polymorphous adenocarcinoma, ducts

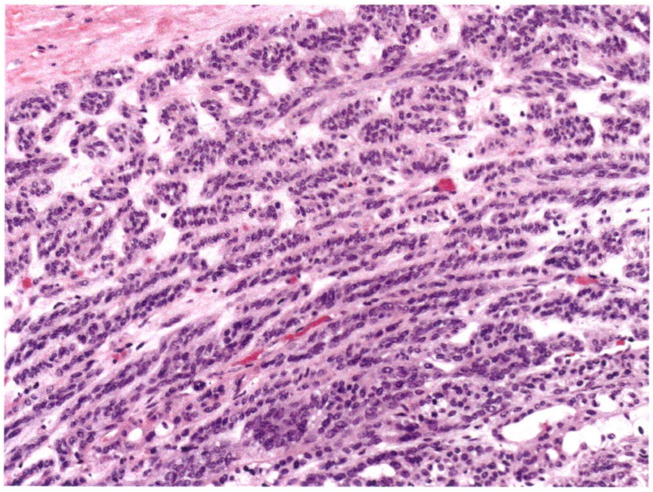

Fig. 24.5 (H&E, 200×) Polymorphous adenocarcinoma, ducts

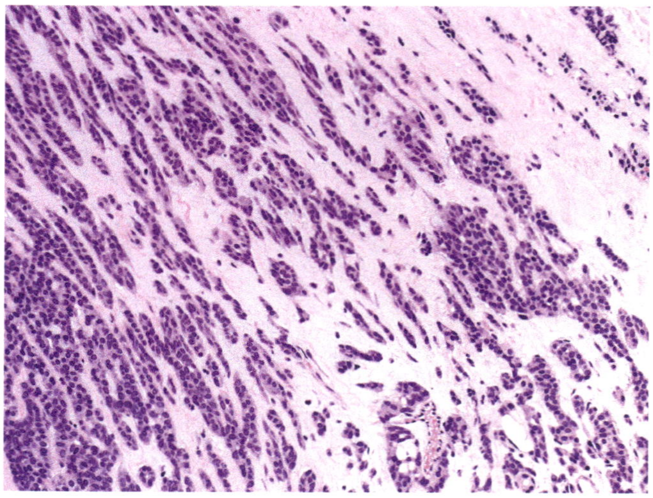

Fig. 24.6 (H&E, 200×) Polymorphous adenocarcinoma, ducts

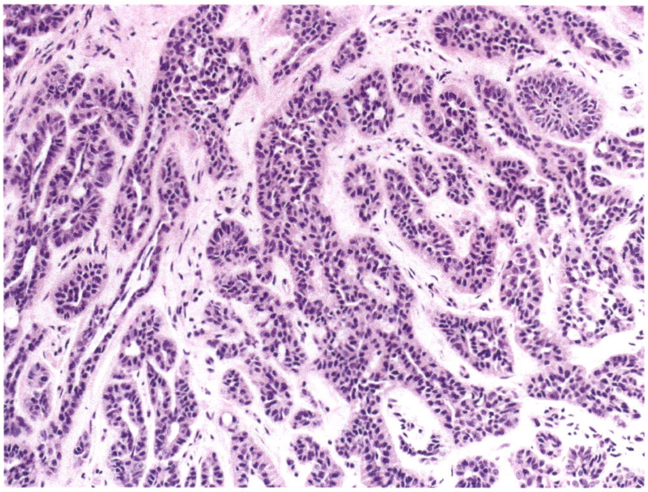

Fig. 24.7 (H&E, 200×) Polymorphous adenocarcinoma, ducts

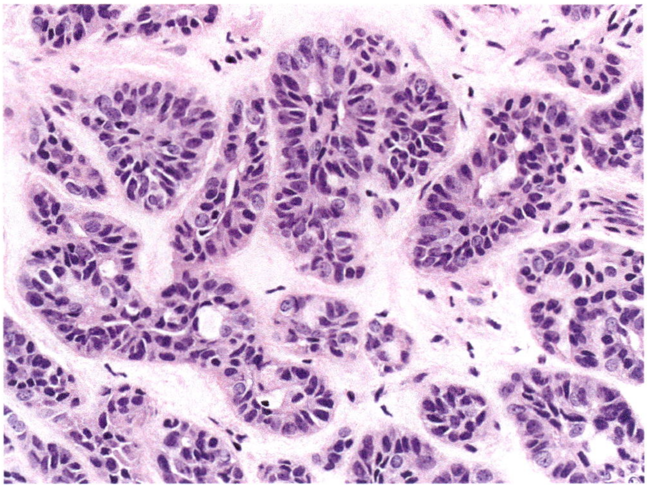

Fig. 24.8 (H&E, 400×) Polymorphous adenocarcinoma, ducts

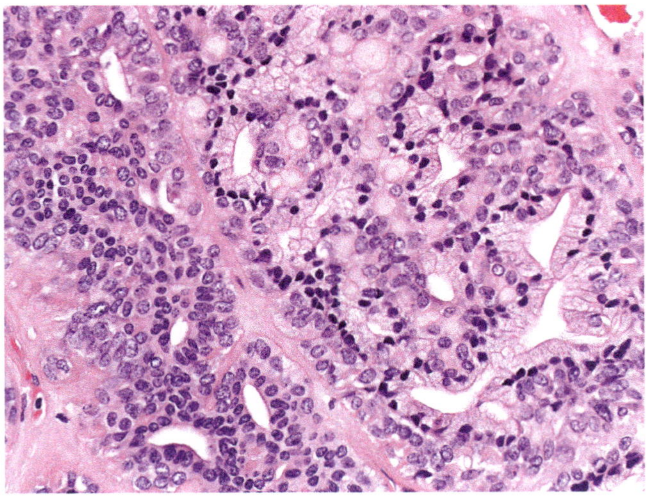

Fig. 24.9 (H&E, 400×) Polymorphous adenocarcinoma, ducts

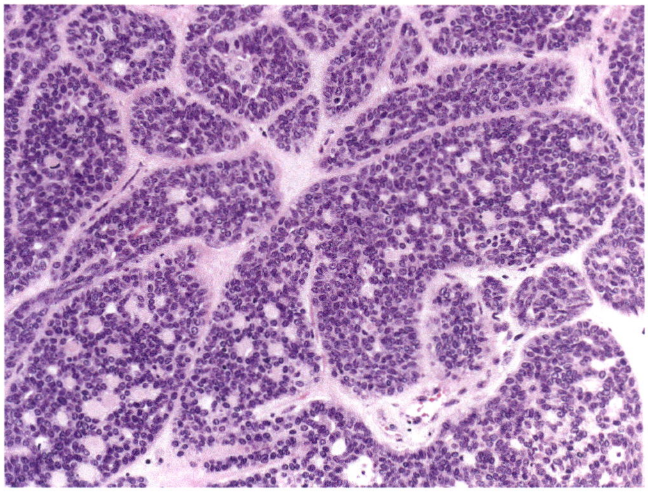

Fig. 24.10 (H&E, 100×) Polymorphous adenocarcinoma, cribriform

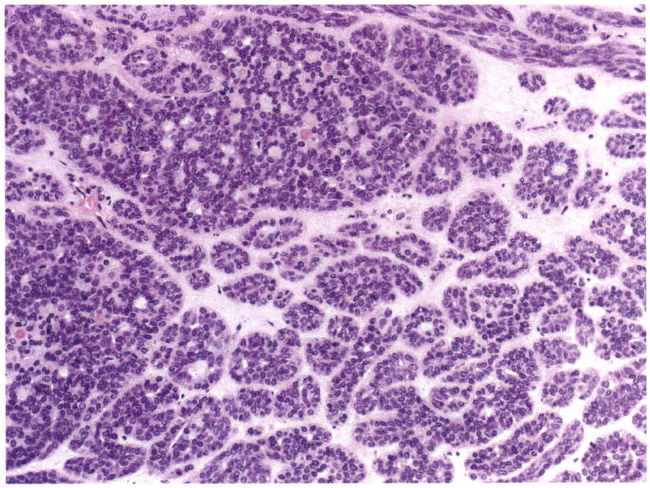

Fig. 24.11 (H&E, 200×) Polymorphous adenocarcinoma, cribriform

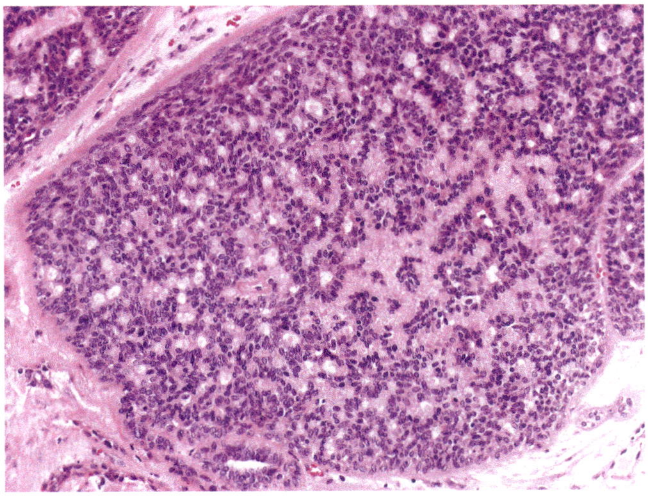

Fig. 24.12 (H&E, 200×) Polymorphous adenocarcinoma, cribriform

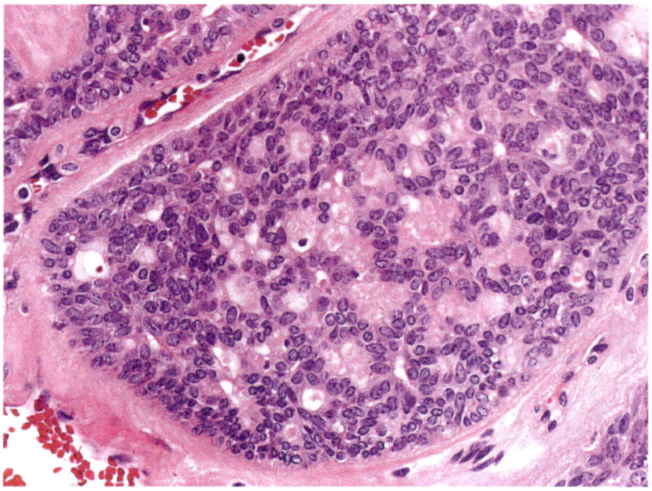

Fig. 24.13 (H&E, 400×) Polymorphous adenocarcinoma, cribriform

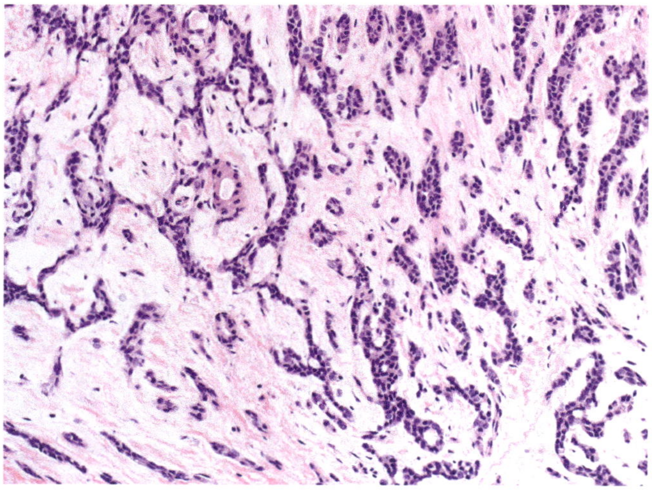

Fig. 24.14 (H&E, 200×) Polymorphous adenocarcinoma, myxoid

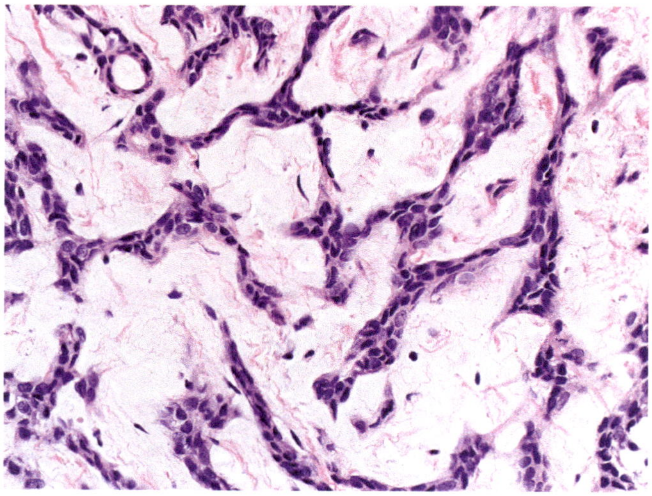

Fig. 24.15 (H&E, 400×) Polymorphous adenocarcinoma, myxoid

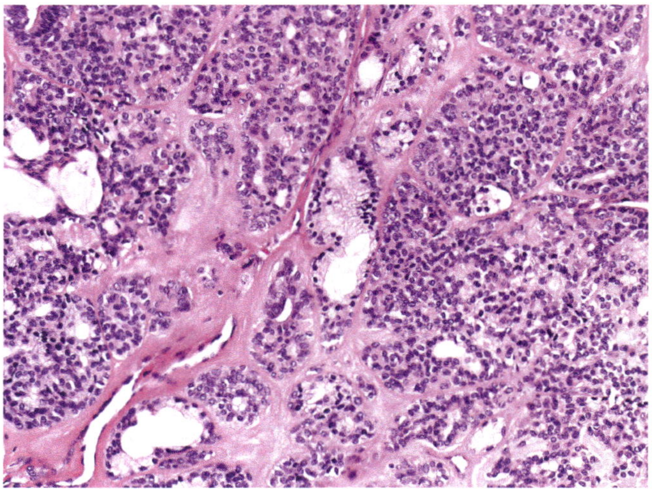

Fig. 24.16 (H&E, 200×) Polymorphous adenocarcinoma, mucinous metaplasia

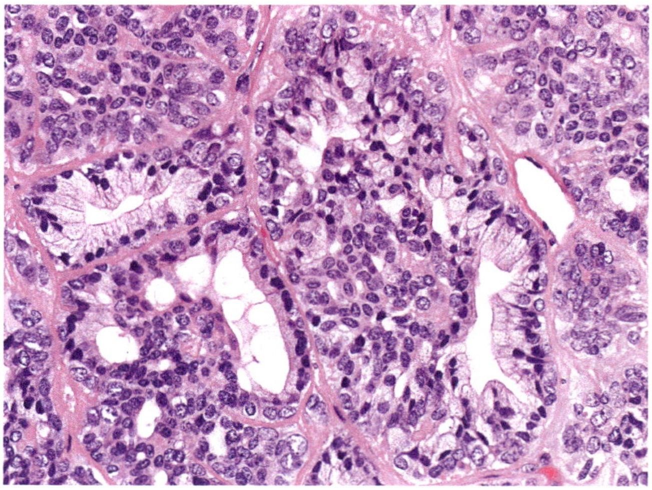

Fig. 24.17 (H&E, 400×) Polymorphous adenocarcinoma, mucinous metaplasia

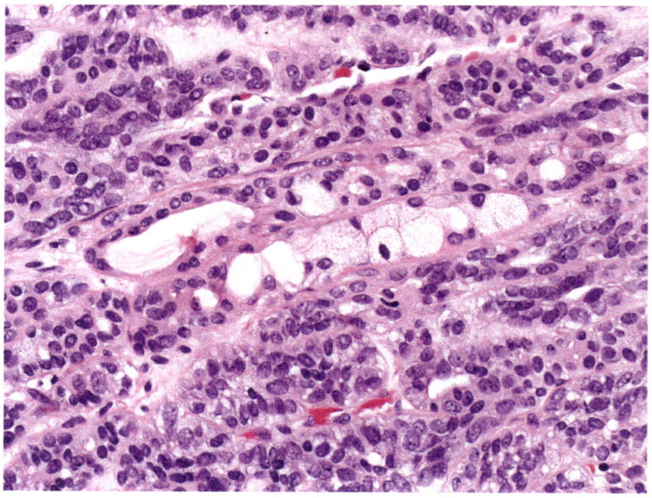

Fig. 24.18 (H&E, 400×) Polymorphous adenocarcinoma, mucinous metaplasia

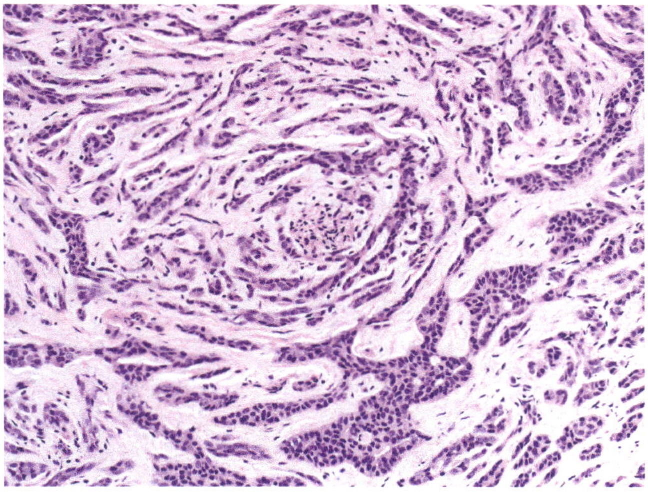

Fig. 24.19 (H&E, 200×) Polymorphous adenocarcinoma, neurotropism

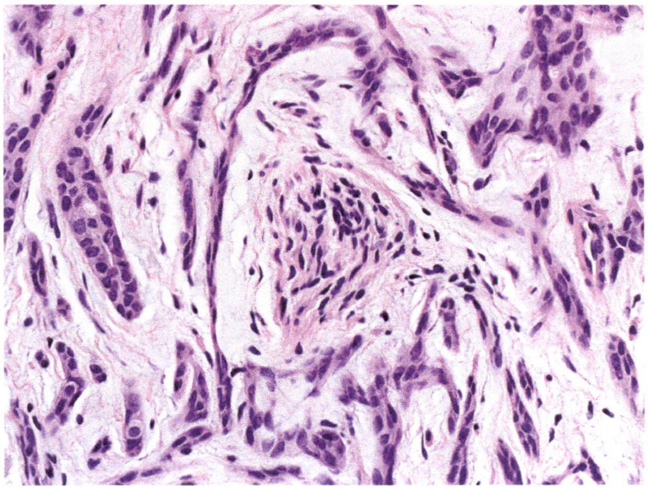

Fig. 24.20 (H&E, 400×) Polymorphous adenocarcinoma, neurotropism

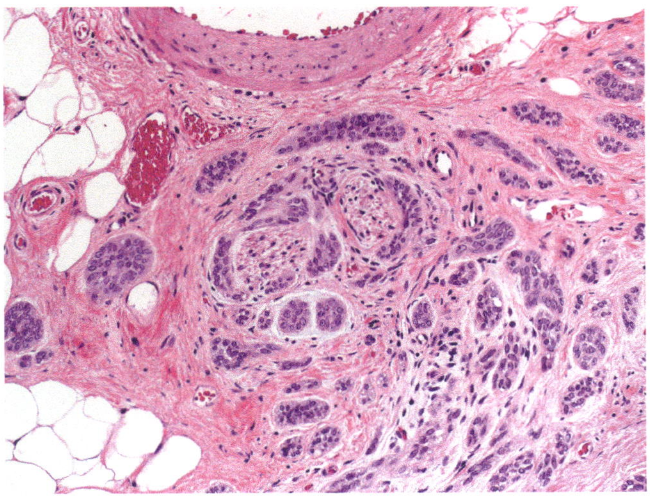

Fig. 24.21 (H&E, 200×) Polymorphous adenocarcinoma, perineural invasion

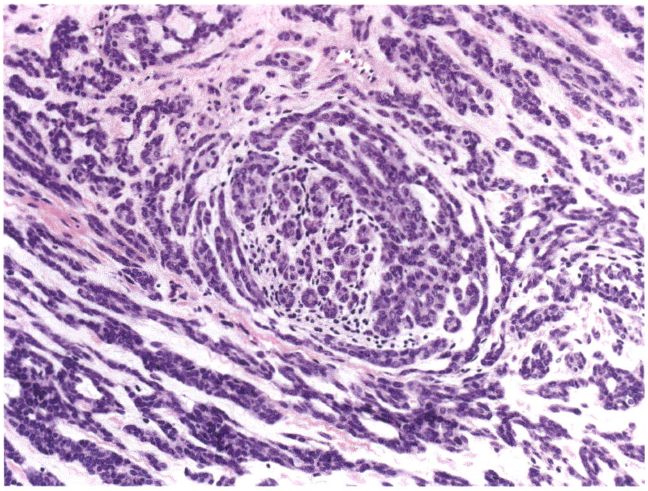

Fig. 24.22 (H&E, 200×) Polymorphous adenocarcinoma, perineural invasion

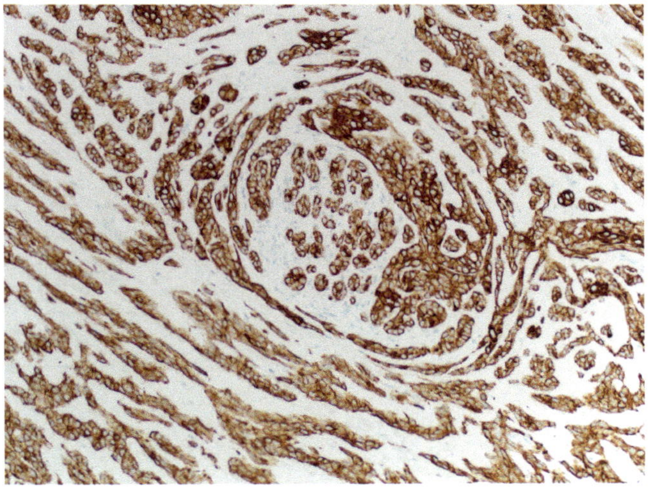

Fig. 24.23 (AE1/AE3, 200×) Polymorphous adenocarcinoma, diffuse immunoreactivity

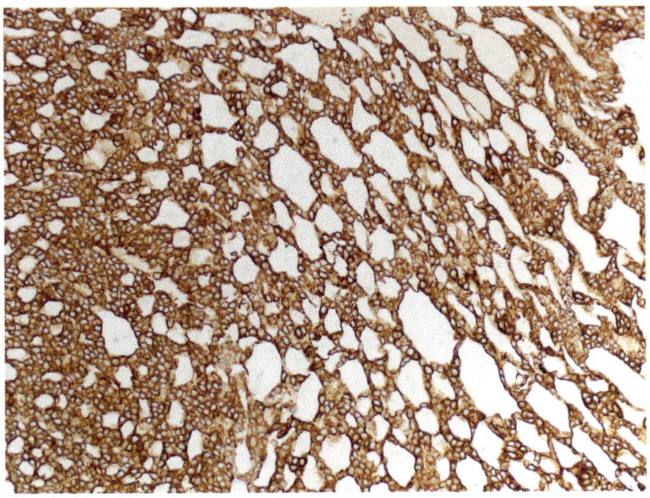

Fig. 24.24 (AE1/AE3, 200×) Polymorphous adenocarcinoma, diffuse immunoreactivity

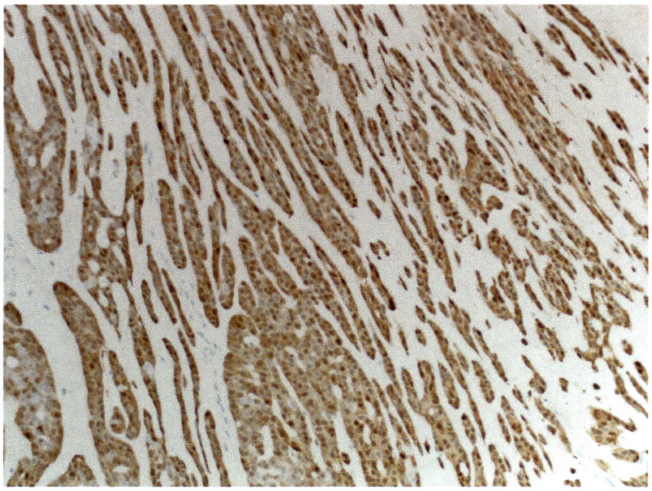

Fig. 24.25 (S-100, 200×) Polymorphous adenocarcinoma, diffuse immunoreactivity

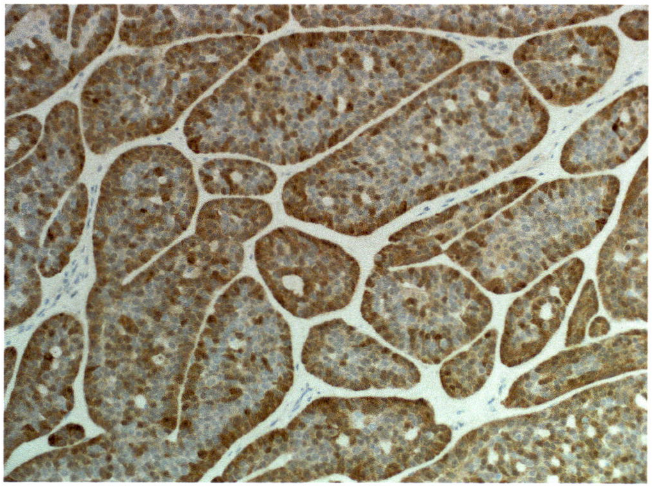

Fig. 24.26 (S-100, 200×) Polymorphous adenocarcinoma, diffuse immunoreactivity

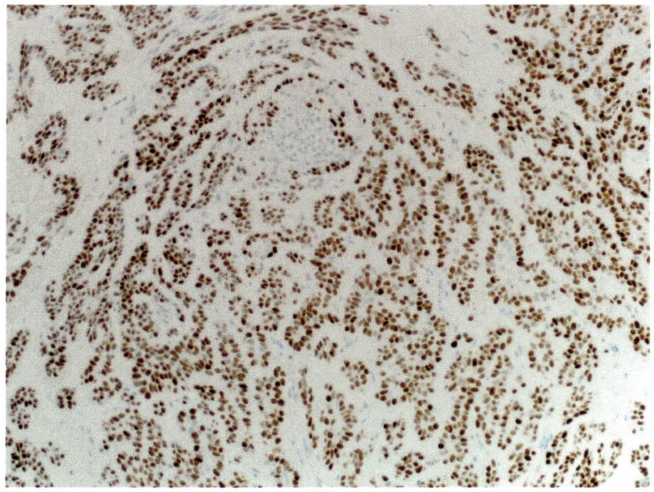

Fig. 24.27 (p63, 200×) Polymorphous adenocarcinoma, diffuse immunoreactivity

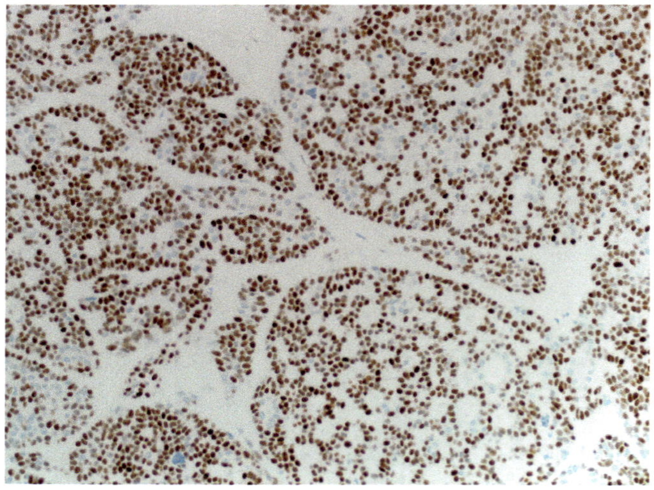

Fig. 24.28 (p63, 200×) Polymorphous adenocarcinoma, focal immunoreactivity

Suggested Reading

Darling MR, Schneider JW, Phillips VM. Polymorphous low-grade adenocarcinoma and adenoid cystic carcinoma: a review and comparison of immunohistochemical markers. Oral Oncol. 2002;38(7):641–5.

Edwards PC, Bhuiya T, Kelsch RD. C-kit expression in the salivary gland neoplasms adenoid cystic carcinoma, polymorphous low-grade adenocarcinoma, and monomorphic adenoma. Oral Surg Oral Med Oral Pathol Oral Radiol Endod. 2003;95(5):586–93.

Edwards PC, Bhuiya T, Kelsch RD. Assessment of p63 expression in the salivary gland neoplasms adenoid cystic carcinoma, polymorphous low-grade adenocarcinoma, and basal cell and canalicular adenomas. Oral Surg Oral Med Oral Pathol Oral Radiol Endod. 2004;97(5):613–9.

Evans HL, Luna MA. Polymorphous low-grade adenocarcinoma: a study of 40 cases with long-term follow up and an evaluation of the importance of papillary areas. Am J Surg Pathol. 2000;24(10):1319–28.

Martins C, Fonseca I, Roque L, Ribeiro C, Soares J. Cytogenetic similarities between two types of salivary gland carcinomas: adenoid cystic carcinoma and polymorphous low-grade adenocarcinoma. Cancer Genet Cytogenet. 2001;128(2):130–6.

Penner CR, Folpe AL, Budnick SD. C-kit expression distinguishes salivary gland adenoid cystic carcinoma from polymorphous low-grade adenocarcinoma. Mod Pathol. 2002;15(7):687–91.

Saenz-Santamaria J, Catalina-Fernandez I. Polymorphous low-grade adenocarcinoma of the salivary gland. Diagnosis by fine needle aspiration cytology. Acta Cytol. 2004;48(1):52–6.

Simpson RH, Pereira EM, Ribeiro AC, Abdulkadir A, Reis-Filho JS. Polymorphous low-grade adenocarcinoma of the salivary glands with transformation to high-grade carcinoma. Histopathology. 2002;41(3):250–9.

Salivary Duct Carcinoma

25

Salivary duct carcinoma affects primarily adults and presents at a mean age of approximately 60 years. Women are involved less than men. The majority of cases involve the parotid gland, presenting as single or multiple masses. Most cases of salivary duct carcinoma behave as high-grade malignancies. Salivary duct carcinoma is infiltrative, comprised almost exclusively of one cell type (ductal), and may exhibit a variety of architectural patterns (solid, trabecular, cribriform, papillary, and cystic) (Figs. 25.1–25.27).

J. J. García, *Atlas of Salivary Gland Pathology*, https://doi.org/10.1007/978-3-319-09021-4_25

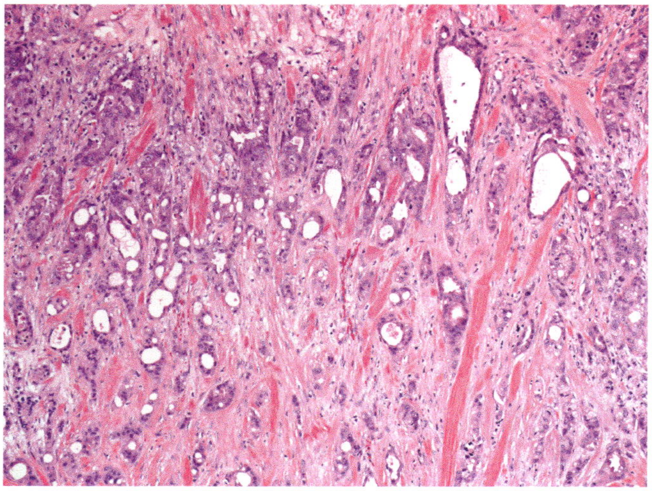

Fig. 25.1 (H&E, 100×) Salivary duct carcinoma, infiltrative

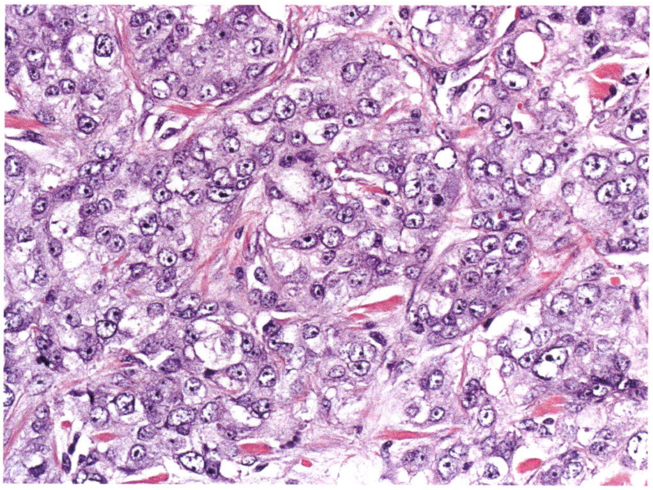

Fig. 25.2 (H&E, 400×) Salivary duct carcinoma, monophasic

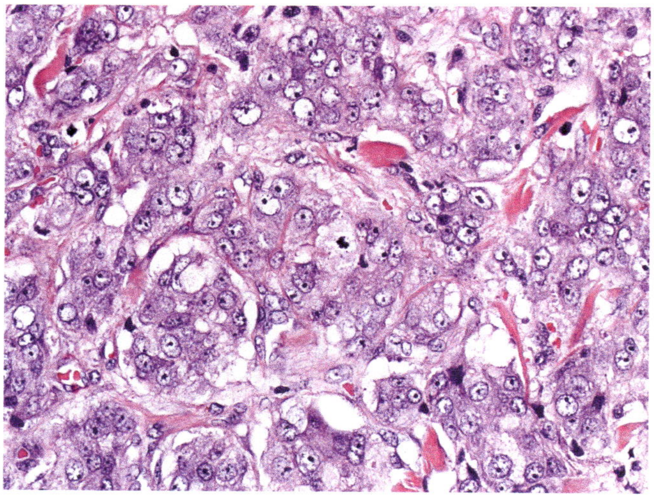

Fig. 25.3 (H&E, 400×) Salivary duct carcinoma, solid

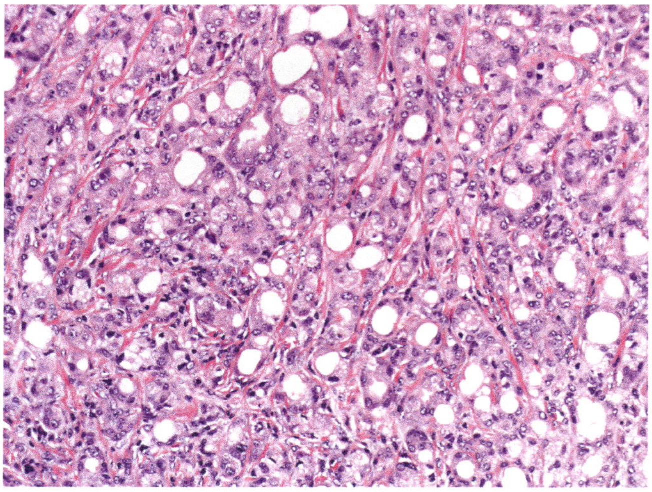

Fig. 25.4 (H&E, 200×) Salivary duct carcinoma, microcystic

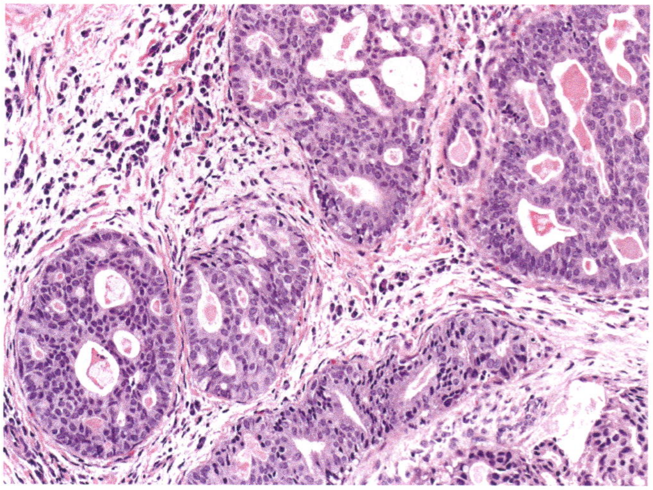

Fig. 25.5 (H&E, 200×) Salivary duct carcinoma, cribriform

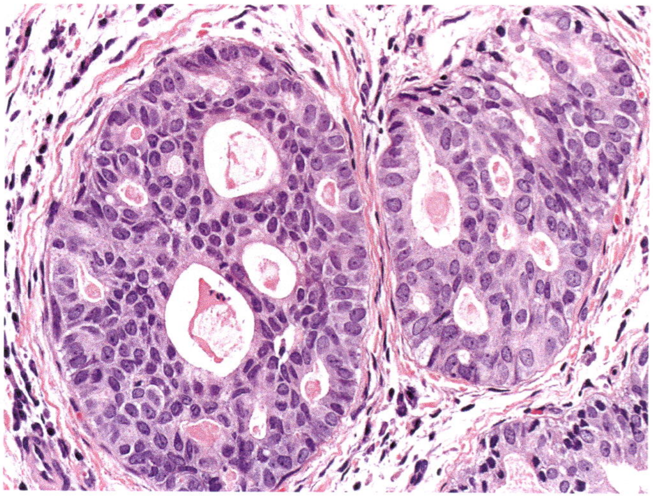

Fig. 25.6 (H&E, 400×) Salivary duct carcinoma, cribriform

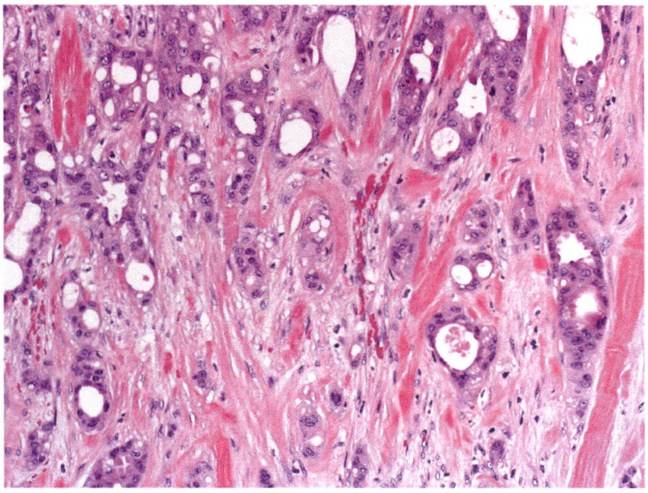

Fig. 25.7 (H&E, 200×) Salivary duct carcinoma, trabecular

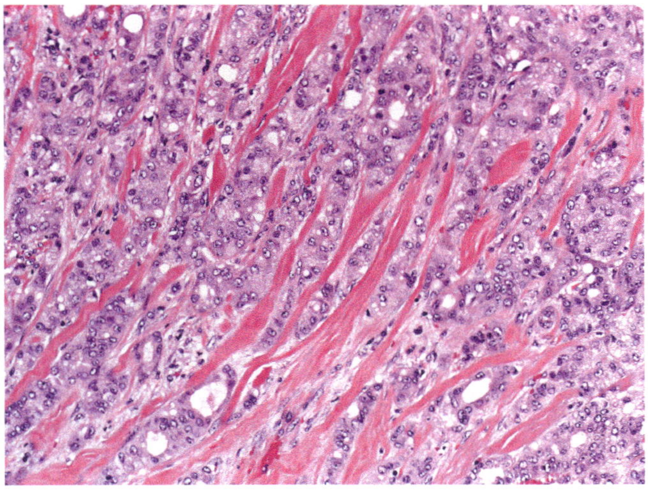

Fig. 25.8 (H&E, 200×) Salivary duct carcinoma, trabecular

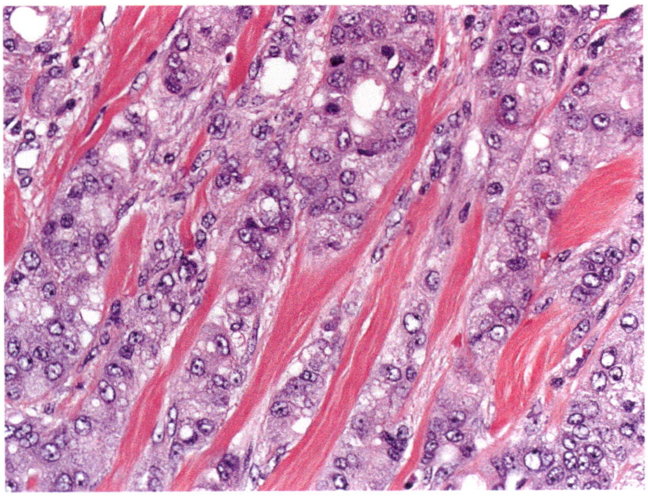

Fig. 25.9 (H&E, 400×) Salivary duct carcinoma, trabecular

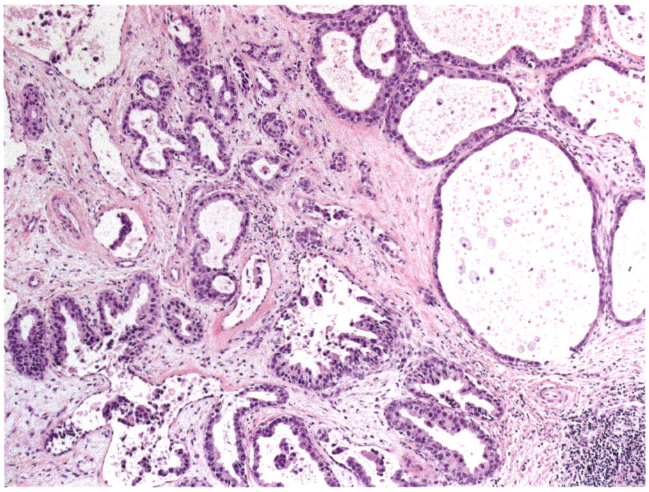

Fig. 25.10 (H&E, 100×) Salivary duct carcinoma, micropapillary

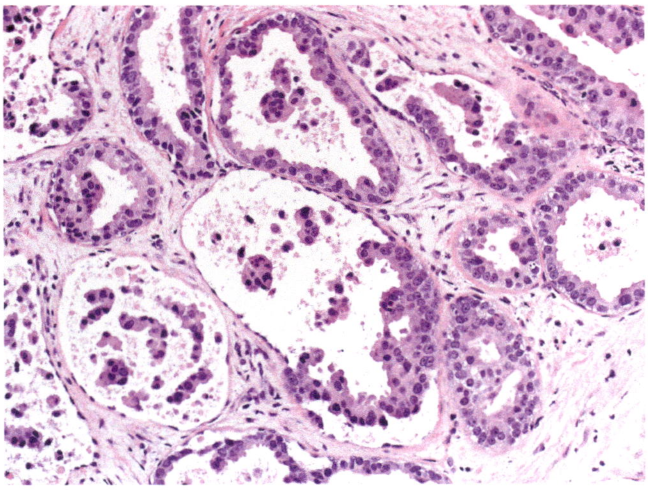

Fig. 25.11 (H&E, 200×) Salivary duct carcinoma, micropapillary

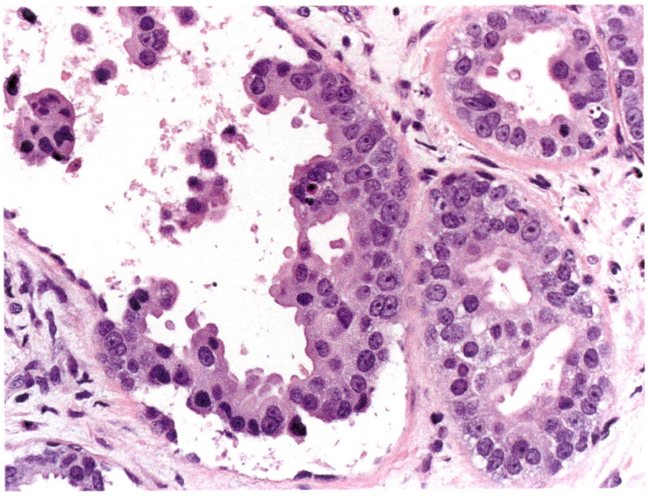

Fig. 25.12 (H&E, 400×) Salivary duct carcinoma, micropapillary

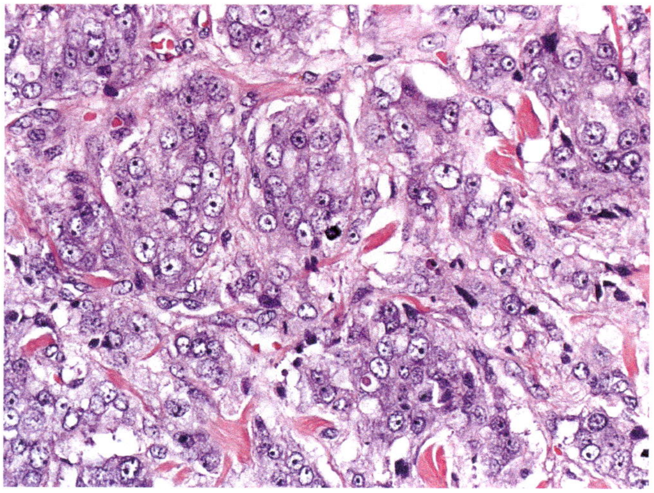

Fig. 25.13 (H&E, 400×) Salivary duct carcinoma, mitotic activity

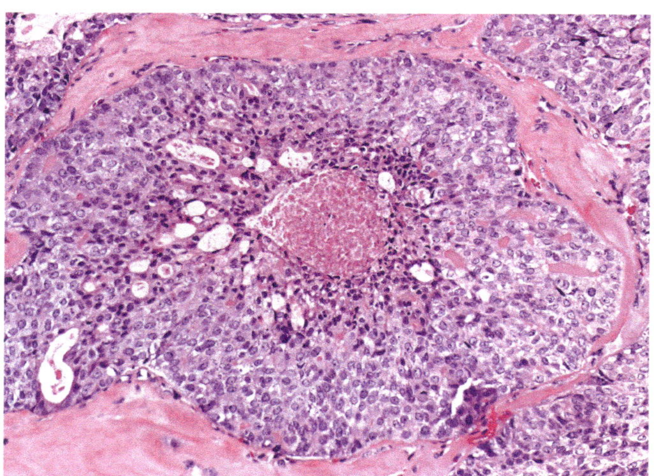

Fig. 25.14 (H&E, 200×) Salivary duct carcinoma, necrosis

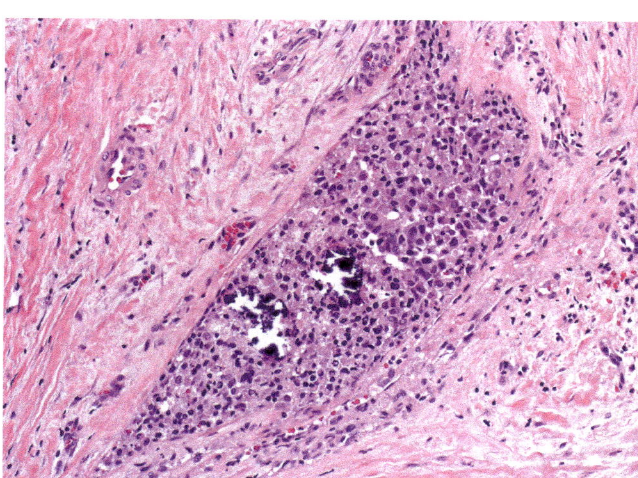

Fig. 25.15 (H&E, 200×) Salivary duct carcinoma, microcalcifications

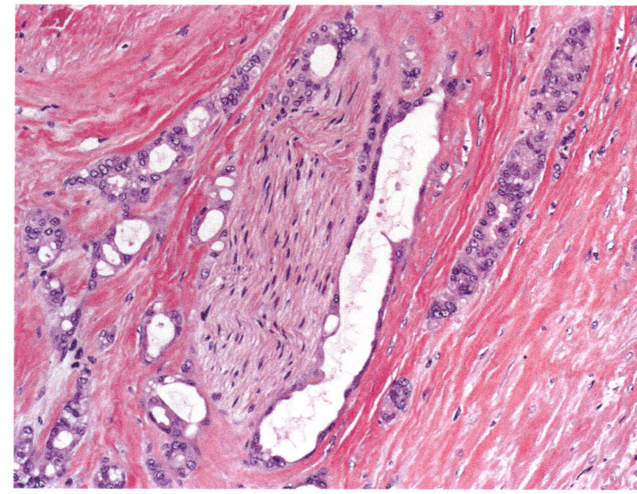

Fig. 25.16 (H&E, 200×) Salivary duct carcinoma, perineural invasion

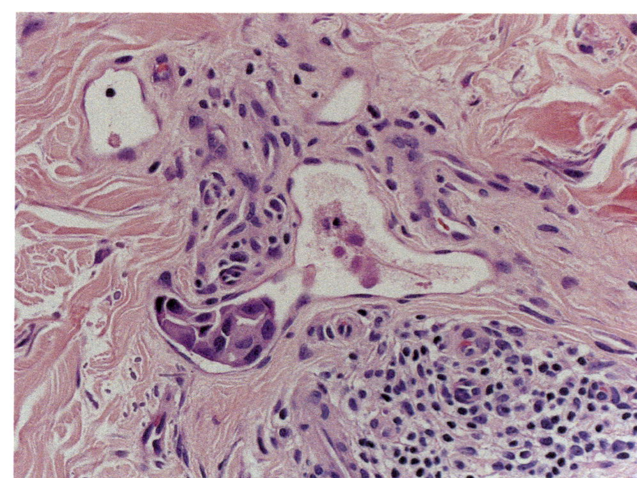

Fig. 25.17 (H&E, 400×) Salivary duct carcinoma, angiolymphatic invasion

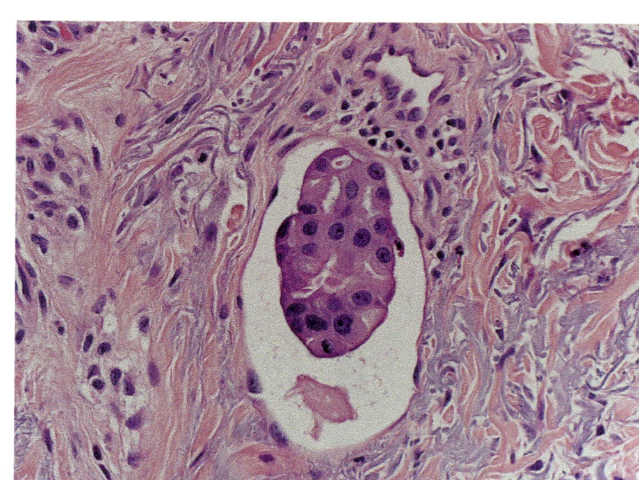

Fig. 25.18 (H&E, 400×) Salivary duct carcinoma, angiolymphatic invasion

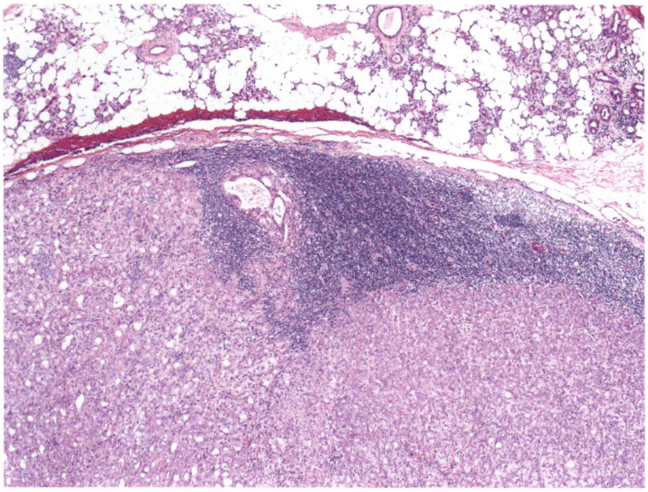

Fig. 25.19 (H&E, 40×) Salivary duct carcinoma, intraparotid lymph node metastasis

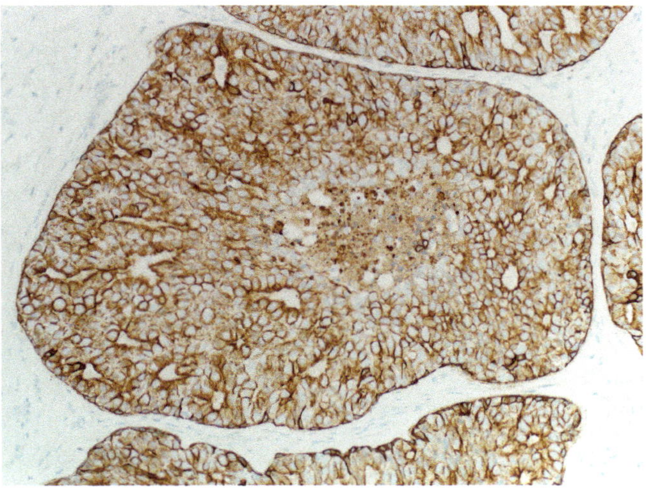

Fig. 25.20 (AE1/AE3, 200×) Salivary duct carcinoma, diffuse immunoreactivity

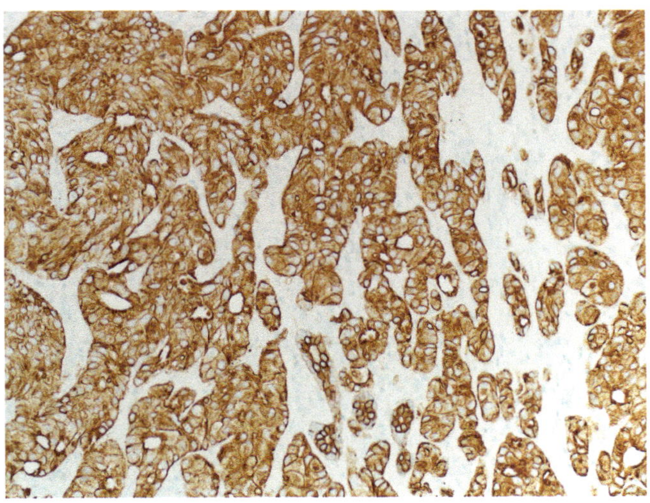

Fig. 25.21 (AE1/AE3, 200×) Salivary duct carcinoma, diffuse immunoreactivity

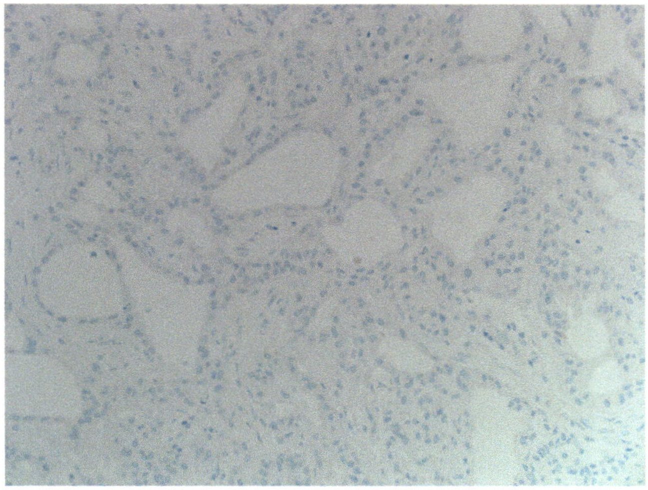

Fig. 25.22 (S-100, 200×) Salivary duct carcinoma, negative immunoreactivity

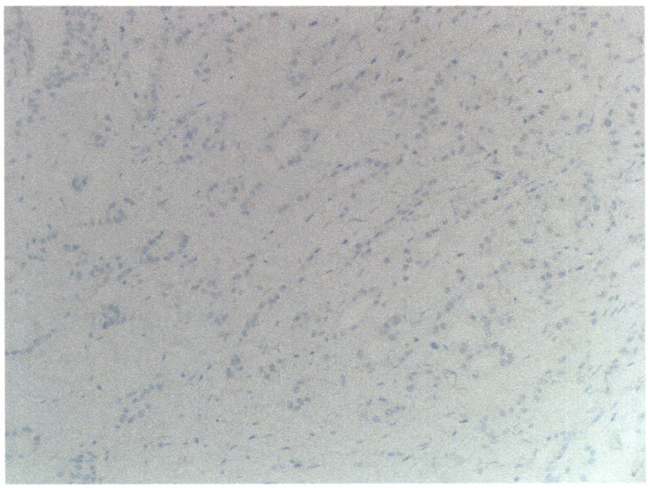

Fig. 25.23 (p63, 200×) Salivary duct carcinoma, negative immunoreactivity

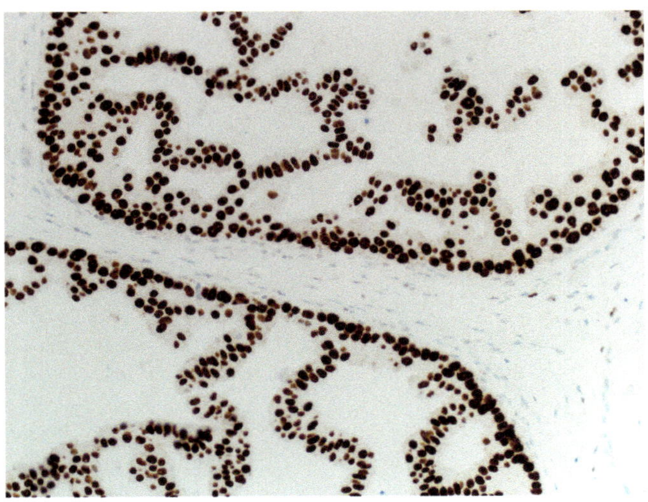

Fig. 25.24 (Androgen receptor, 200×) Salivary duct carcinoma, diffuse immunoreactivity

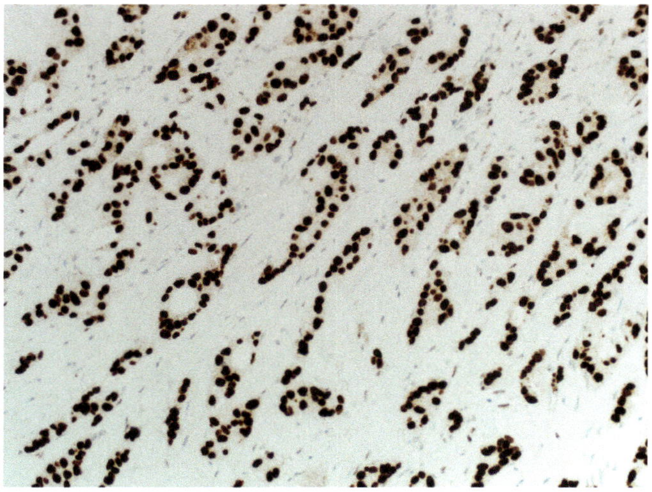

Fig. 25.25 (Androgen receptor, 200×) Salivary duct carcinoma, diffuse immunoreactivity

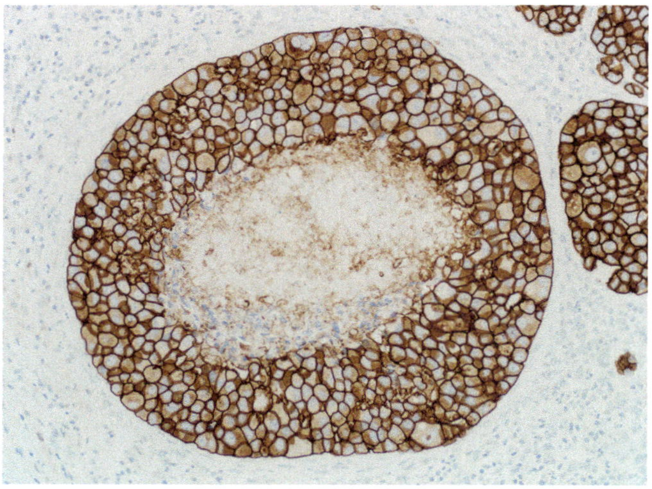

Fig. 25.26 (HER2, 200×) Salivary duct carcinoma, membranous immunoreactivity

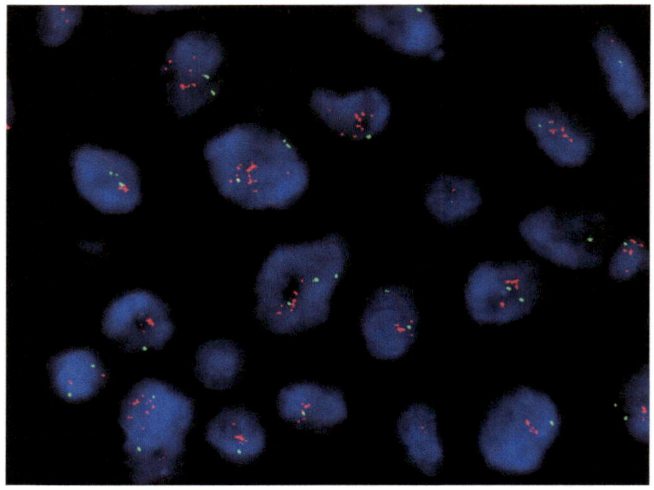

Fig. 25.27 (Fluorescent in situ hybridization, 600X) Salivary duct carcinoma, *HER2* amplification

Suggested Reading

Salivary duct carcinoma in major and minor salivary glands. J Craniomaxillofac Surg. 1989;17(8):373.

Barnes L, Rao U, Contis L, Krause J, Schwartz A, Scalamogna P. Salivary duct carcinoma. Part II. Immunohistochemical evaluation of 13 cases for estrogen and progesterone receptors, cathepsin D, and c-erbB-2 protein. Oral Surg Oral Med Oral Pathol. 1994a;78(1):74–80.

Barnes L, Rao U, Krause J, Contis L, Schwartz A, Scalamogna P. Salivary duct carcinoma. Part I. A clinicopathologic evaluation and DNA image analysis of 13 cases with review of the literature. Oral Surg Oral Med Oral Pathol. 1994b;78(1):64–73.

Brandwein MS, Jagirdar J, Patil J, Biller H, Kaneko M. Salivary duct carcinoma (cribriform salivary carcinoma of excretory ducts). A clinicopathologic and immunohistochemical study of 12 cases. Cancer. 1990;65(10):2307–14.

Delgado R, Vuitch F, Albores-Saavedra J. Salivary duct carcinoma. Cancer. 1993;72(5):1503–12.

Etges A, Pinto DS Jr, Kowalski LP, Soares FA, Araujo VC. Salivary duct carcinoma: immunohistochemical profile of an aggressive salivary gland tumour. J Clin Pathol. 2003;56(12):914–8.

Fan CY, Wang J, Barnes EL. Expression of androgen receptor and prostatic specific markers in salivary duct carcinoma: an immunohistochemical analysis of 13 cases and review of the literature. Am J Surg Pathol. 2000;24(4):579–86.

Fan CY, Melhem MF, Hosal AS, Grandis JR, Barnes EL. Expression of androgen receptor, epidermal growth factor receptor, and transforming growth factor alpha in salivary duct carcinoma. Arch Otolaryngol Head Neck Surg. 2001;127(9):1075–9.

Fayemi AO, Toker C. Salivary duct carcinoma. Arch Otolaryngol. 1974;99(5):366–8.

Garland TA, Innes DJ Jr, Fechner RE. Salivary duct carcinoma: an analysis of four cases with review of literature. Am J Clin Pathol. 1984;81(4):436–41.

Henley JD, Seo IS, Dayan D, Gnepp DR. Sarcomatoid salivary duct carcinoma of the parotid gland. Hum Pathol. 2000;31:208–13.

Jaehne M, Dippel A, Sagowski C. Salivary duct carcinoma of the submandibular gland. HNO. 2005a;53(11):940–4.

Jaehne M, Roeser K, Jaekel T, Schepers JD, Albert N, Loning T. Clinical and immunohistologic typing of salivary duct carcinoma: a report of 50 cases. Cancer. 2005b;103(12):2526–33.

Jayaprakash V, Merizanu M, Warren GW, Arshad H, Hicks WL Jr, Rigual NR, et al. Survival rates and prognostic factors for infiltrating salivary duct carcinoma: analysis of 228 cases from the surveillance, epidemiology, and end results database. Head Neck. 2014;36:694–701.

Kusafuka K, Onitsuka T, Muramatsu K, Miki T, Murai C, Suda T, et al. Salivary duct carcinoma with rhabdoid features: report of 2 cases with immunohistochemical and ultrastructural analyses. Head Neck. 2014;36:E28–35.

Lewis JE, McKinney BC, Weiland LH, Ferreiro JA, Olsen KD. Salivary duct carcinoma. Clinicopathologic and immunohistochemical review of 26 cases. Cancer. 1996;77(2):223–30.

Martinez-Barba E, Cortes-Guardiola JA, Minguela-Puras A, Torroba-Caron A, Mendez-Trujillo S, Bermejo-Lopez J. Salivary duct carcinoma: clinicopathological and immunohistochemical studies. J Craniomaxillofac Surg. 1997;25(6):328–34.

Masubuchi T, Tada Y, Maruya SI, Osamura Y, Kamata SE, Miura K, et al. Clinicopathological significance of androgen receptor, HER2, Ki-67 and EGFR expressions in salivary duct carcinoma. Int J Clin Oncol. 2015;20(1):35–44.

Moriki T, Ueta S, Takahashi T, Mitani M, Ichien M. Salivary duct carcinoma: cytologic characteristics and application of androgen receptor immunostaining for diagnosis. Cancer. 2001;93(5):344–50.

Nabili V, Tan JW, Bhuta S, Sercarz JA, Head CS. Salivary duct carcinoma: a clinical and histologic review with implications for trastuzumab therapy. Head Neck. 2007;29(10):907–12.

Nagao T, Gaffey TA, Visscher DW, Kay PA, Minato H, Serizawa H, et al. Invasive micropapillary salivary duct carcinoma: a distinct histologic variant with biologic significance. Am J Surg Pathol. 2004;28(3):319–26.

Ponniah I, Murali GM, SureshKumar P, Kumaran MG, Shaheen A. Salivary duct carcinoma of the palate. Indian J Dent Res. 2005;16(4):167–70.

Roh JL, Cho KJ, Kwon GY, Choi SH, Nam SY, Kim SY. Prognostic values of pathologic findings and hypoxia markers in 21 patients with salivary duct carcinoma. J Surg Oncol. 2008;97(7):596–600.

Shimizu A, Yamane M, Ito H, Araki S, Yoshida T, Suzuki M. Clinicopathological study of salivary duct carcinoma. Nihon Jibiinkoka Gakkai Kaiho. 2002;105(6):727–31.

Simpson RH. Salivary duct carcinoma: new developments-morphological variants including pure in situ high-grade lesions: proposed molecular classification. Head Neck Pathol. 2013;7(Suppl 1):S48–58.

Simpson RHW, Desai S, Di Palma S. Salivary duct carcinoma in situ of the parotid gland. Histopathology. 2008;53(4):416–25.

Skalova A. Starek, Kucerova V, Szepe P, plank L. salivary duct carcinoma—a highly aggressive salivary gland tumor with HER-2/neu oncoprotein overexpression. Pathol Res Pract. 2001;197(9):621–6.

Skalova A, Starek I, Vanecek T, Kucerova V, Plank L, Szepe P. Amplification and overexpression of HER-2/neu in parotid gland salivary duct carcinoma. Immunohistochemical study and fluorescence in situ hybridization. Cesk Patol. 2002;38(Suppl 1):27–34.

Williams L, Thompson LD, Seethala RR, Weinreb I, Assaad AM, Tuluc M, et al. Salivary duct carcinoma: the predominance of apocrine morphology, prevalence of histologic variants, and androgen receptor expression. Am J Surg Pathol. 2015;39:705–13.

26 Secretory Carcinoma

Secretory carcinoma affects children and adults and presents at a mean age of approximately 45 years. Women and men are involved with similar frequency. The majority of cases involve the parotid gland, presenting as single or multiple masses. Most cases of secretory carcinoma behave as low to intermediate-grade malignancies; however, a subset of cases with high-grade transformation (necrosis, elevated mitotic activity, and cytomorphologic atypia) are predisposed to recurrence, lymph node involvement, and distant metastasis. Secretory carcinoma may be circumscribed or infiltrative, comprised of multiple cell types, and exhibit a variety of architectural patterns (solid, follicular, papillary, and cystic) (Figs. 26.1–26.30).

J. J. García, *Atlas of Salivary Gland Pathology*, https://doi.org/10.1007/978-3-319-09021-4_26

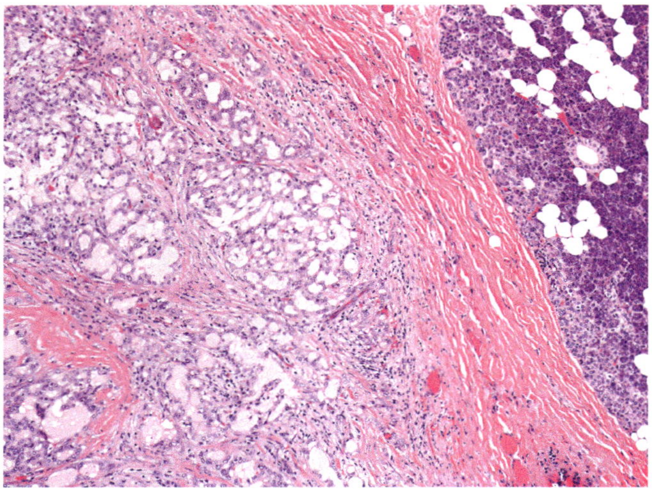

Fig. 26.1 (H&E, 100×) Secretory carcinoma, circumscribed

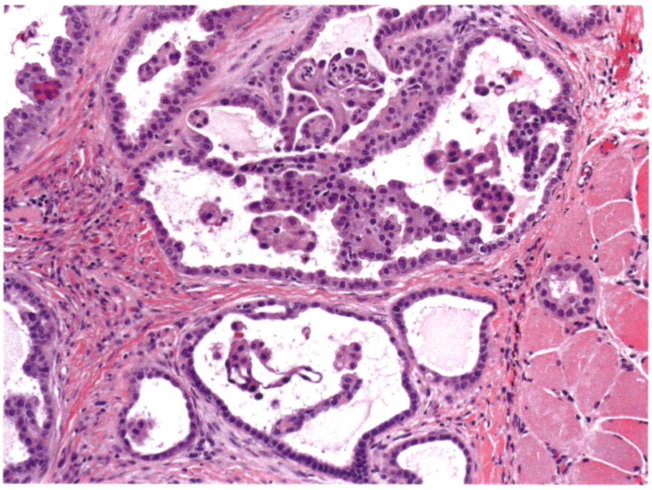

Fig. 26.2 (H&E, 200×) Secretory carcinoma, infiltrative

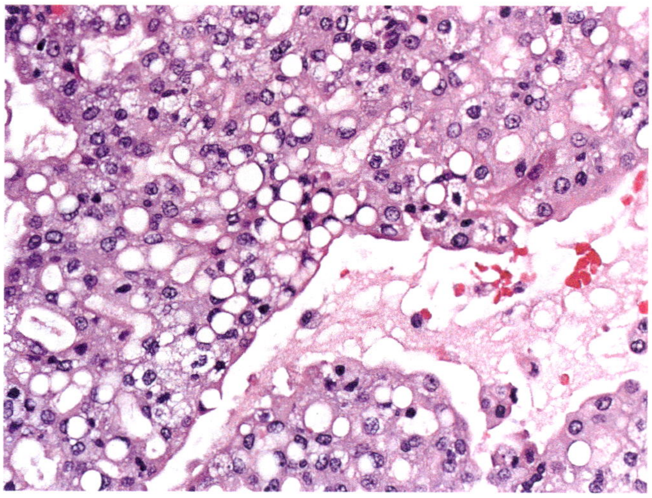

Fig. 26.3 (H&E, 400×) Secretory carcinoma, triphasic or more

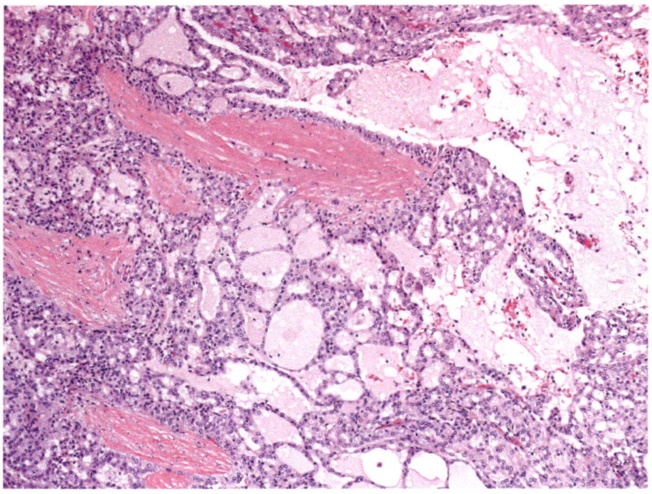

Fig. 26.4 (H&E, 100×) Secretory carcinoma, follicular

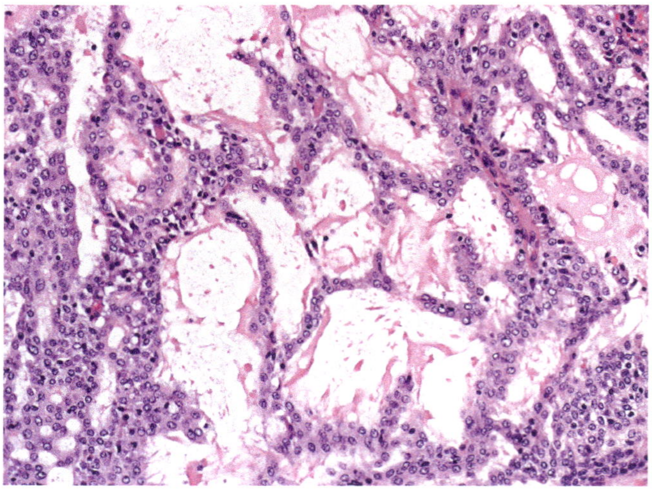

Fig. 26.5 (H&E, 200×) Secretory carcinoma, follicular

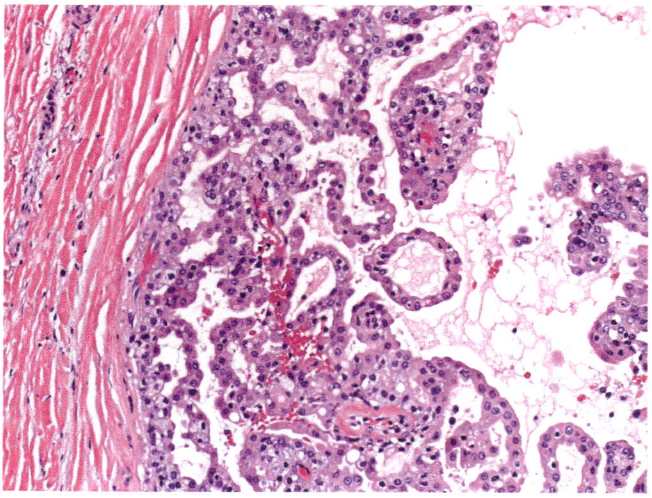

Fig. 26.6 (H&E, 200×) Secretory carcinoma, micropapillary

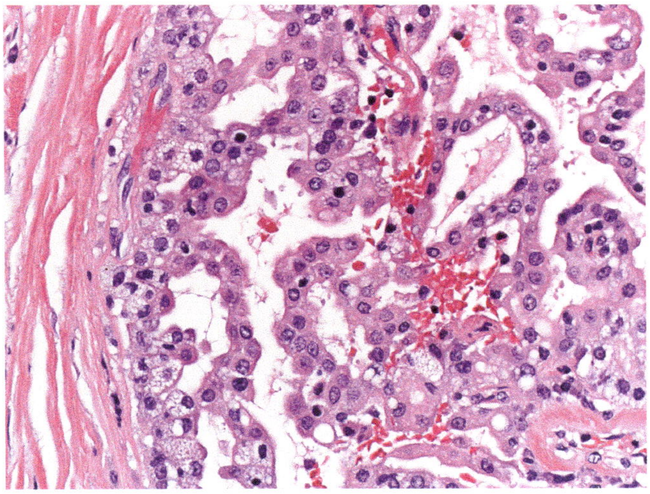

Fig. 26.7 (H&E, 400×) Secretory carcinoma, micropapillary

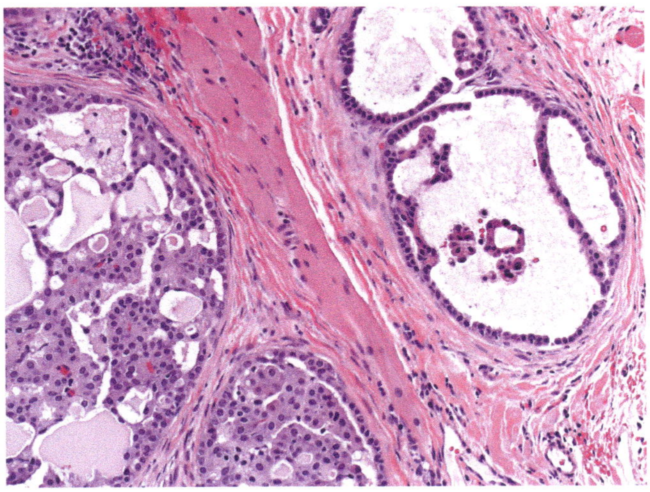

Fig. 26.8 (H&E, 200×) Secretory carcinoma, micropapillary

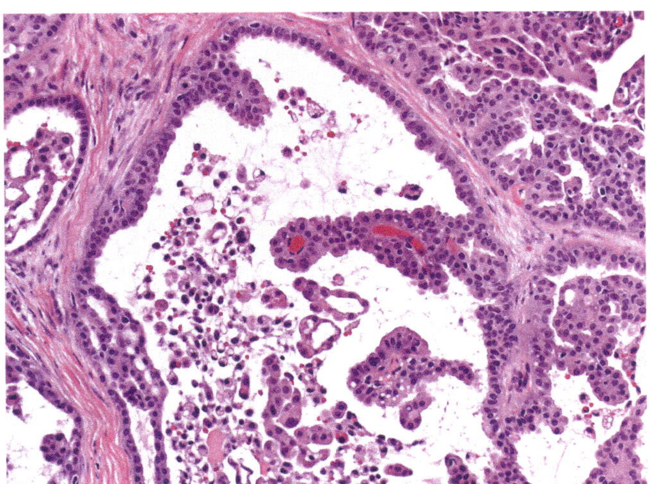

Fig. 26.9 (H&E, 200×) Secretory carcinoma, micropapillary

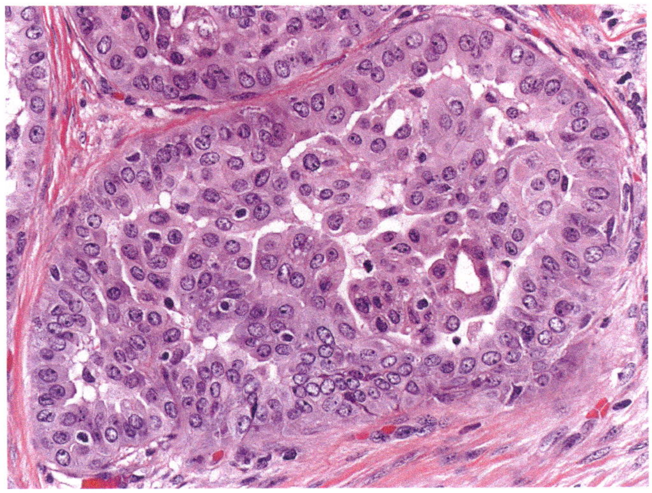

Fig. 26.10 (H&E, 400×) Secretory carcinoma, micropapillary

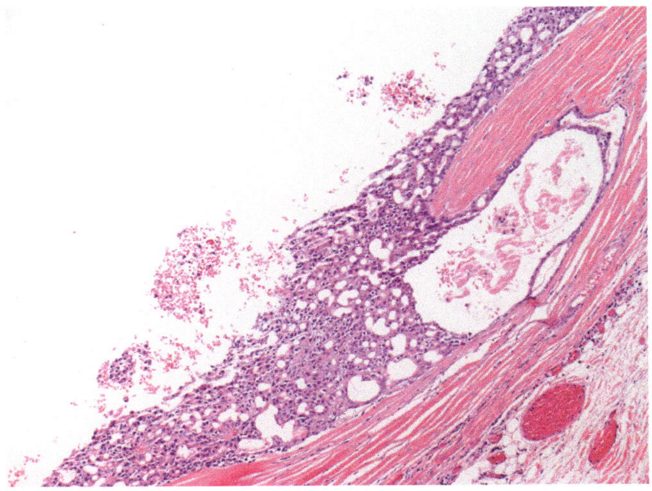

Fig. 26.11 (H&E, 100×) Secretory carcinoma, cystic

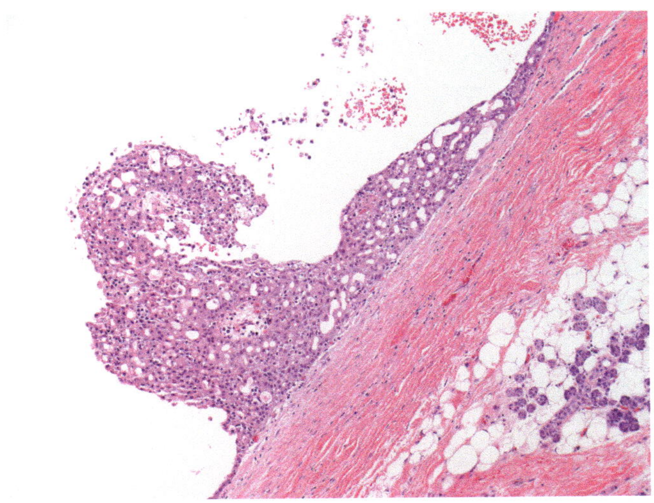

Fig. 26.12 (H&E, 100×) Secretory carcinoma, cystic

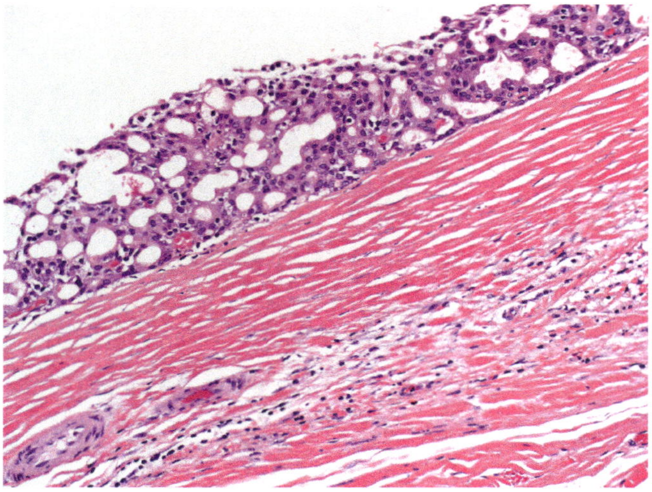

Fig. 26.13 (H&E, 200×) Secretory carcinoma, cystic

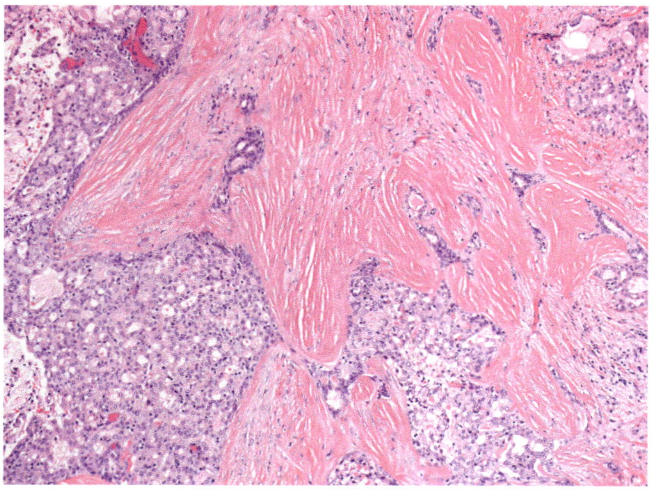

Fig. 26.14 (H&E, 100×) Secretory carcinoma, microcystic

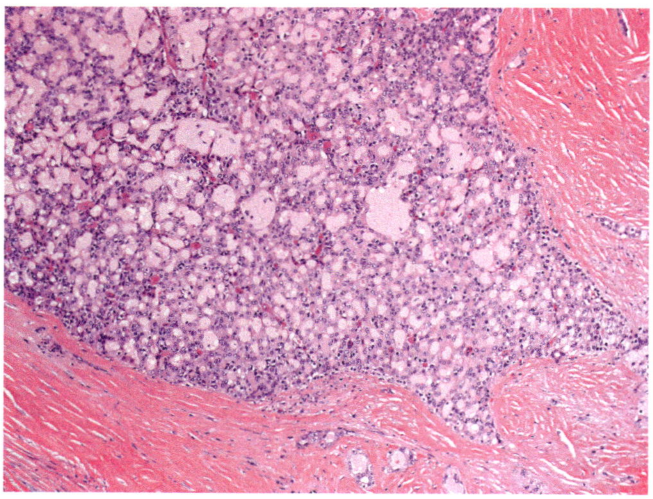

Fig. 26.15 (H&E, 100×) Secretory carcinoma, microcystic

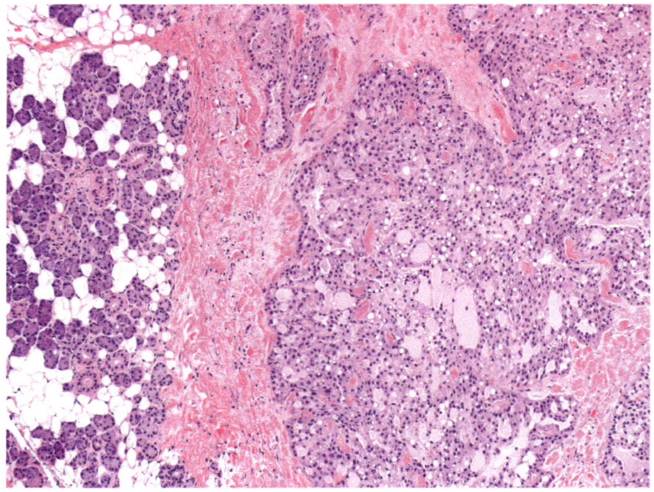

Fig. 26.16 (H&E, 100×) Secretory carcinoma, microcystic

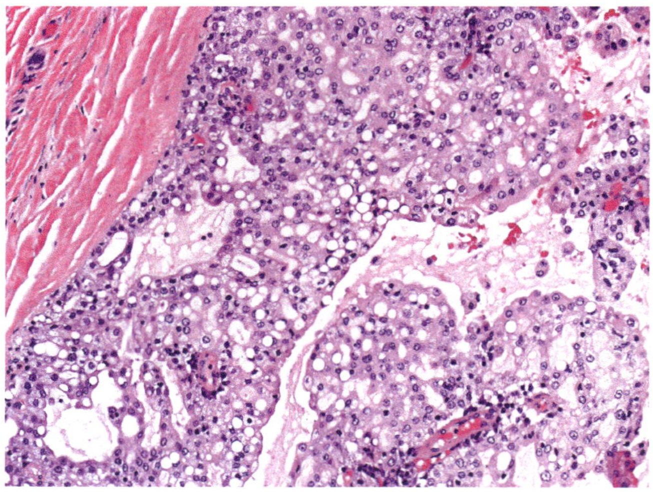

Fig. 26.17 (H&E, 200×) Secretory carcinoma, microcystic

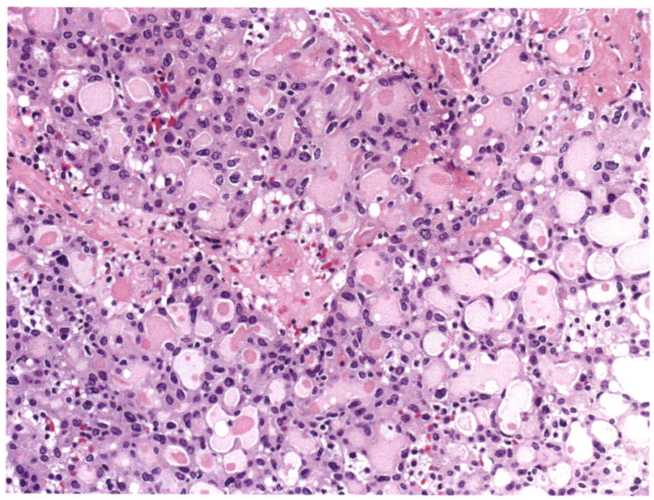

Fig. 26.18 (H&E, 200×) Secretory carcinoma, microcystic

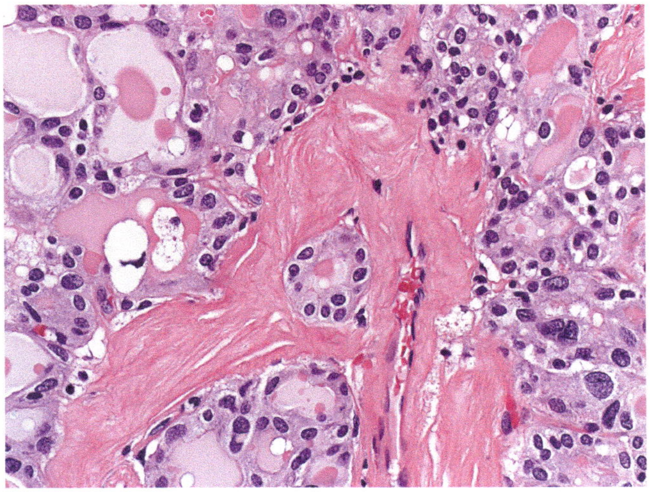

Fig. 26.19 (H&E, 400×) Secretory carcinoma, microcystic

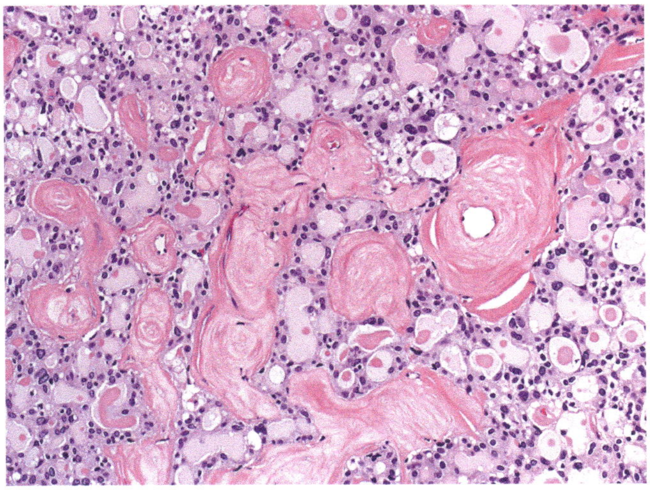

Fig. 26.20 (H&E, 200×) Secretory carcinoma, hyalinized

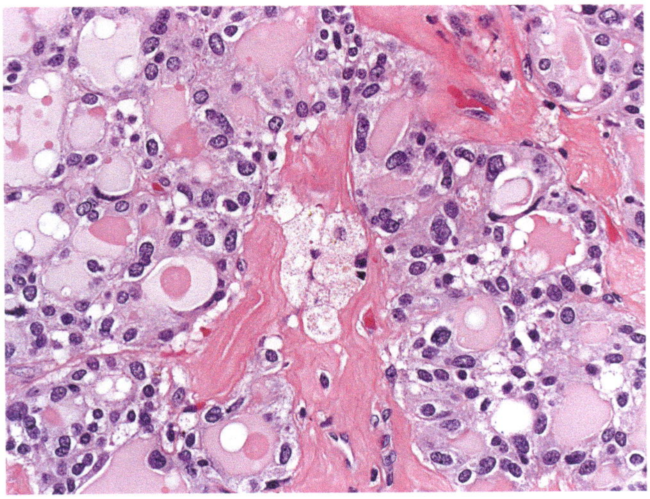

Fig. 26.21 (H&E, 400×) Secretory carcinoma, hyalinized

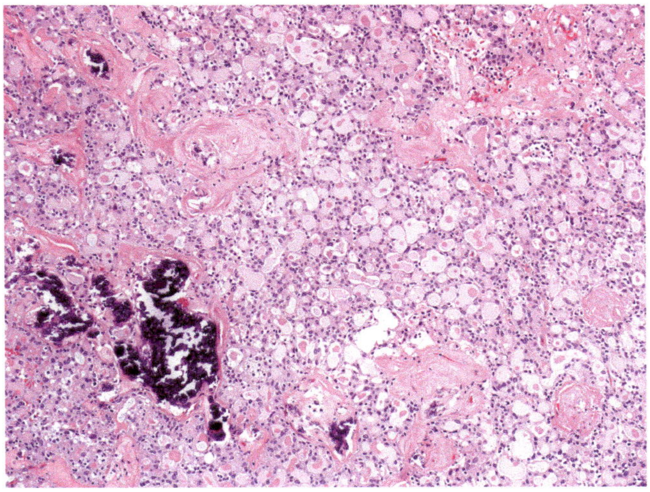

Fig. 26.22 (H&E, 100×) Secretory carcinoma, microcalcifications

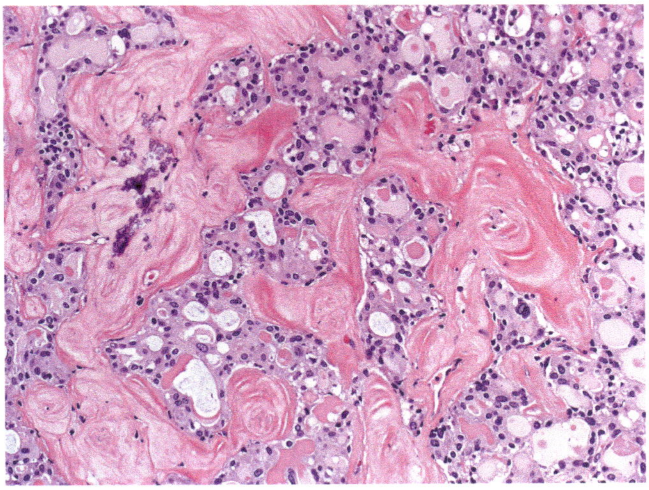

Fig. 26.23 (H&E, 200×) Secretory carcinoma, microcalcifications

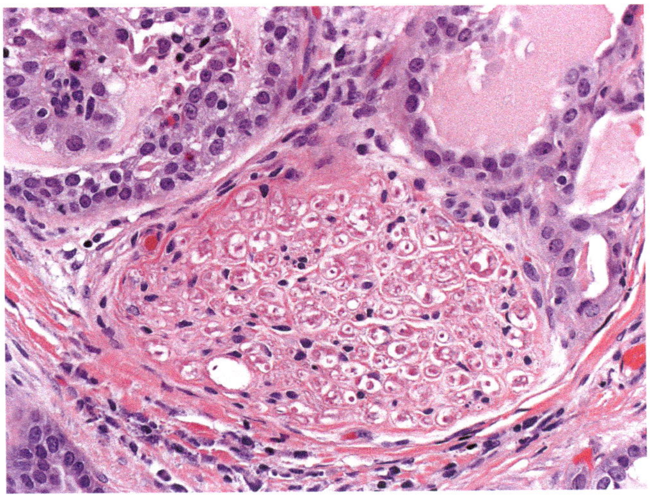

Fig. 26.24 (H&E, 400×) Secretory carcinoma, perineural invasion

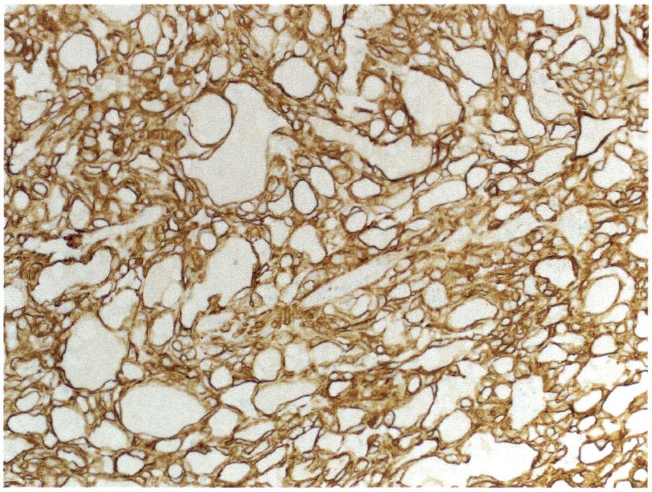

Fig. 26.25 (AE1/AE3, 200×) Secretory carcinoma, diffuse immunoreactivity

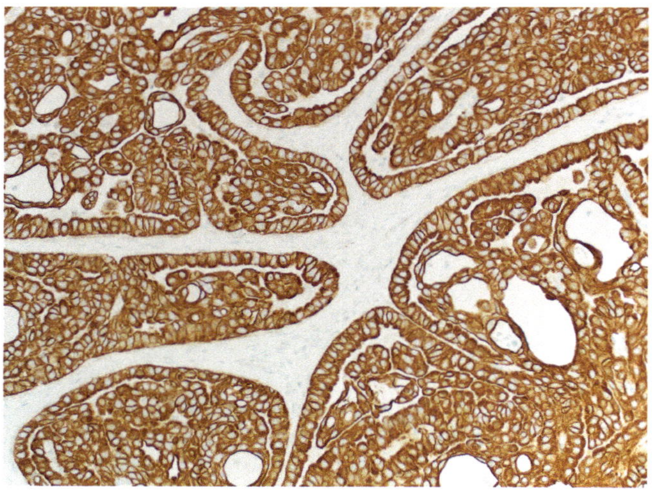

Fig. 26.26 (AE1/AE3, 200×) Secretory carcinoma, diffuse immunoreactivity

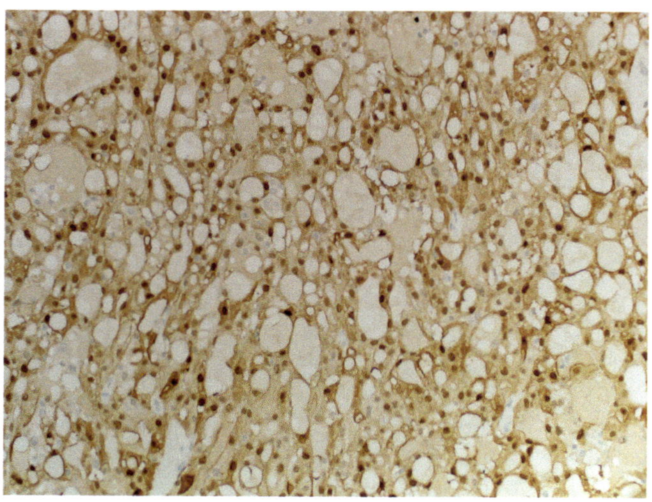

Fig. 26.27 (S-100, 200×) Secretory carcinoma, diffuse immunoreactivity

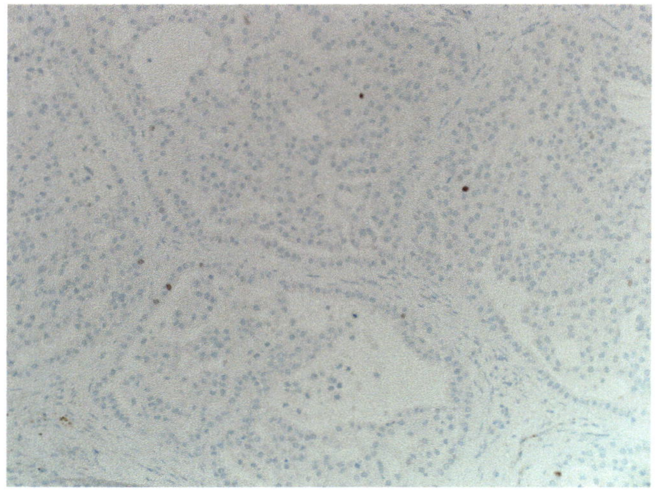

Fig. 26.28 (p63, 200×) Secretory carcinoma, rare immunoreactivity

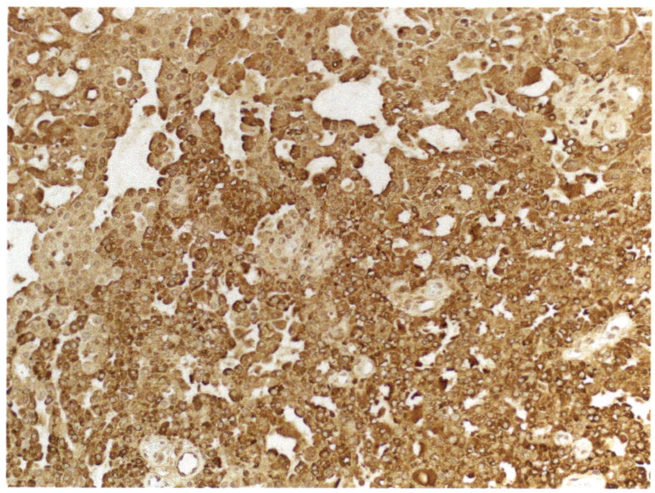

Fig. 26.29 (Mammaglobin, 200×) Secretory carcinoma, diffuse immunoreactivity

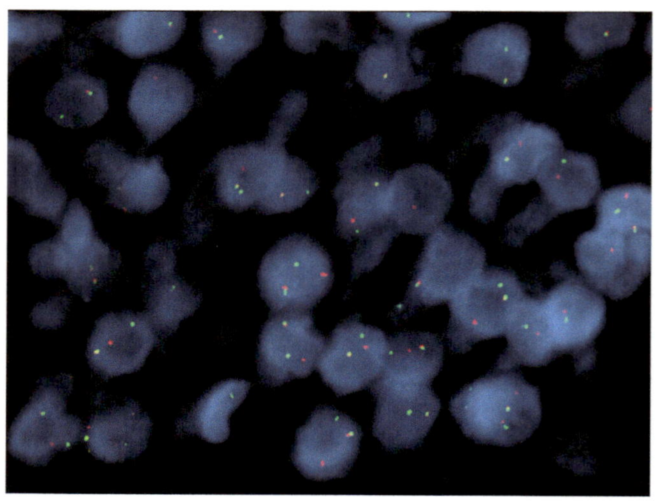

Fig. 26.30 (Fluorescent in situ hybridization, 600×) Secretory carcinoma, *ETV6* rearrangement

Suggested Reading

Bishop JA. Unmasking MASC; bringing to light the unique morphologic, immunohistochemical and genetic features of the newly recognized mammary analogue secretory carcinoma of salivary glands. Head Neck Pathol. 2013;7:35–9.

Bishop JA, Yonescu R, Batista DA, Westra WH, Ali SZ. Cytopathologic features of mammary analogue secretory carcinoma. Cancer Cytopathol. 2013a;121:228–33.

Bishop JA, Yonescu R, Batista D, Eisele DW, Westra WH. Most nonparotid "acinic cell carcinomas" represent mammary analog secretory carcinomas. Am J Surg Pathol. 2013b;37:1053–7.

Chenevert J, Duvvuri U, Chiosea S, Dacic S, Cieply K, Kim J, et al. DOG1: a novel marker of salivary acinar and intercalated duct differentiation. Mod Pathol. 2012;25:919–29.

Chiosea SI, Griffith C, Assaad A, Seethala RR. The profile of acinic cell carcinoma after recognition of mammary analog secretory carciona. Am J Surg Pathol. 2012a;36:343–50.

Chiosea SI, Griffith C, Assaad A, Seethala RR. Clinicopathological characterization of mammary analogue secretory carcinoma of salivary glands. Histopathology. 2012b;61:387–94.

Griffith CC, Stelow EB, Saqi A, Khalbuss WE, Schneider F, Chiosea SI, et al. The cytological features of mammary analogue secretory carcinoma: a series of 6 molecularly confirmed cases. Cancer Cytopathol. 2013;121:234–41.

Majewska H, Skalova A, Stodulski D, Klimkova A, Steiner P, Stankiewicz C, et al. Mammary analogue secretory carcinoma of salivary glands: a new entity associated with ETV6 gene rearrangement. Virchows Arch. 2015;466:245–54.

Pusztaszeri MP, Faquin WC. Update in salivary gland cytopathology: recent molecular advances and diagnostic applications. Semin Diagn Pathol. 2015;32:264–74.

Samulski TD, LiVolsi VA, Baloch Z. The cytopathologic features of mammary analog secretory carcinoma and its mimics. Cytojournal. 2014;11:24.

Sethi R, Kozin E, Remenschneider A, Meier J, VanderLaan P, Faquin W, et al. Mammary analogue secretory carcinoma: update on a new diagnosis of salivary gland malignancy. Laryngoscope. 2014;124:188–95.

Shah AA, Wenig BM, LeGallo RD, Mills SE, Stelow EB. Morphology in conjunction with immunohistochemistry is sufficient for the diagnosis of mammary analogue secretory carcinoma. Head Neck Pathol. 2015;9:85–95.

Skalova A. Mammary analogue secretory carcinoma of salivary gland origin: an update and expanded morphologic and immunohistochemical spectrum of a recently described entity. Head Neck Pathol. 2013;7(Suppl 1):S30–6.

Skalova A, Vanecek T, Sima R, Laco J, Weinreb I, Perez-Ordonez B, et al. Mammary analogue secretory carcinoma of salivary glands, containing the ETV6-NTRK3 fusion gene: a hitherto undescribed salivary gland tumor entity. Am J Surg Pathol. 2010;34:599–608.

Skalova A, Vanecek T, Majewska H, Laco J, Grossmann P, Simpson RH, et al. Mammary analogue secretory carcinoma of salivary glands with high-grade transformation: report of 3 cases with the ETV6-NTRK3 gene fusion and analysis of TP53, B-catenin, EGFR, and CCND1 genes. Am J Surg Pathol. 2014;38:23–33.

Urano M, Nagao T, Miyabe S, Ishibashi K, Higuchi K, Kuroda M. Characterization of mammary analogue secretory carcinoma of the salivary gland: discrimination from its mimics by the presence of the ETV6-NTRK3 translocation and novel surrogate markers. Hum Pathol. 2015;46:94–103.

27 Small Cell Neuroendocrine Carcinoma

Small cell neuroendocrine carcinoma affects children and adults and presents at a mean age of approximately 65 years. Women are involved more than men. The majority of cases involve the parotid gland, presenting as single or multiple masses. Most cases of small cell neuroendocrine carcinoma behave as high-grade malignancies. Small cell neuroendocrine carcinoma may be circumscribed or infiltrative, comprised almost exclusively of one cell type (neuroendocrine), and may exhibit a variety of architectural patterns (solid, organoid, and cords) (Figs. 27.1–27.25).

J. J. García, *Atlas of Salivary Gland Pathology*, https://doi.org/10.1007/978-3-319-09021-4_27

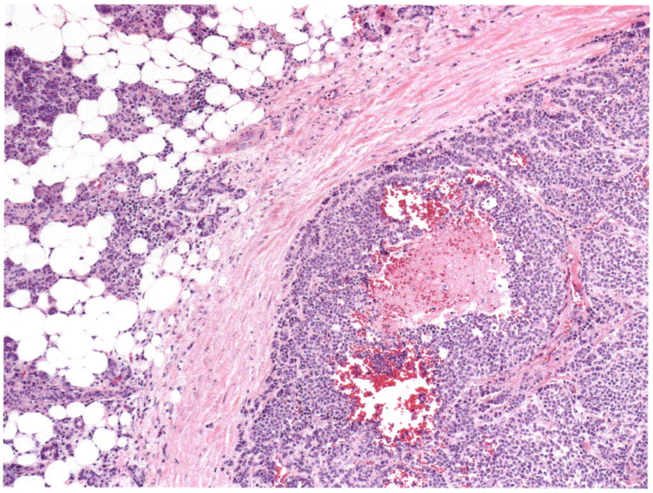

Fig. 27.1 (H&E, 100×) Small cell neuroendocrine carcinoma, circumscribed

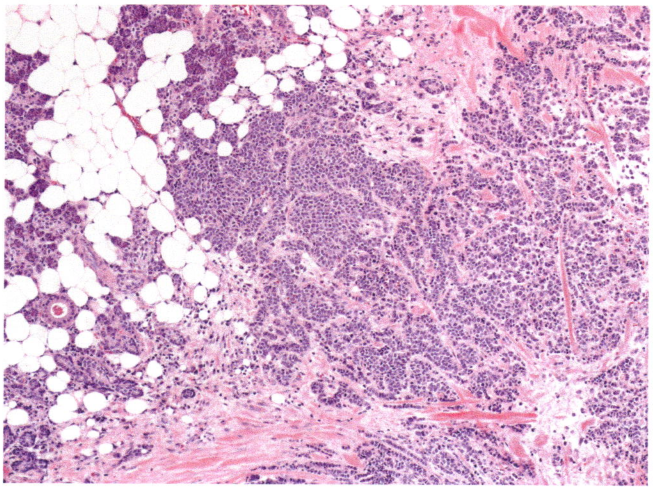

Fig. 27.2 (H&E, 100×) Small cell neuroendocrine carcinoma, infiltrative

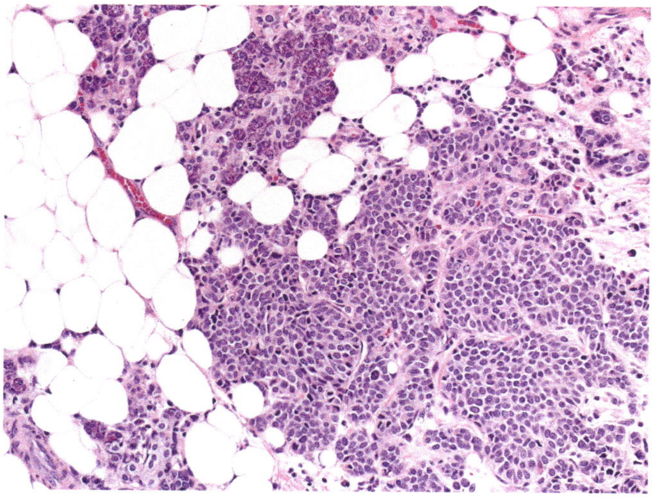

Fig. 27.3 (H&E, 200×) Small cell neuroendocrine carcinoma, monophasic

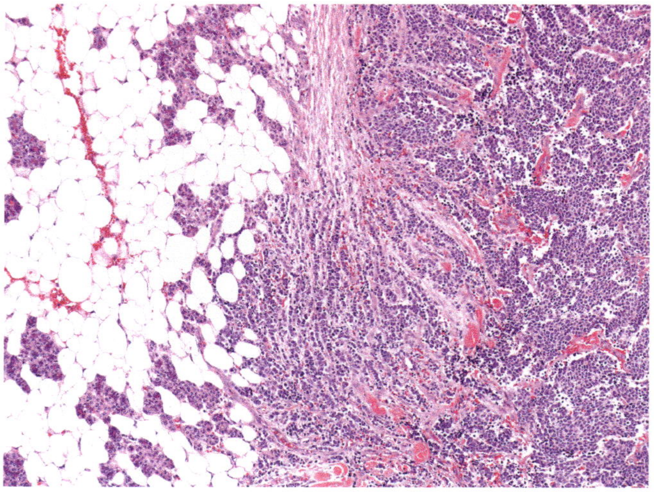

Fig. 27.4 (H&E, 100×) Small cell neuroendocrine carcinoma, cords

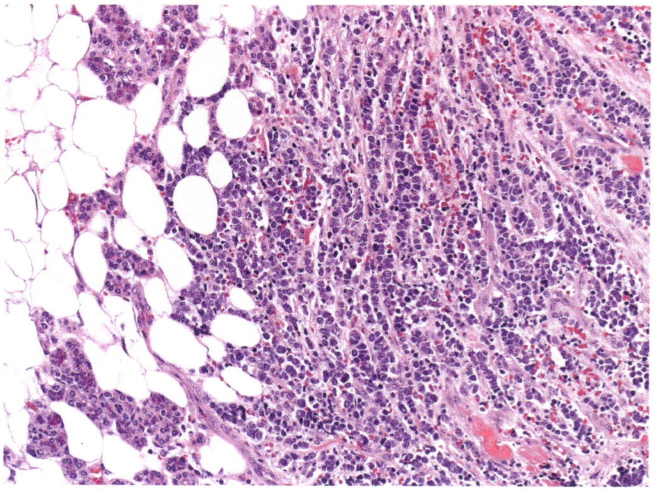

Fig. 27.5 (H&E, 200×) Small cell neuroendocrine carcinoma, cords

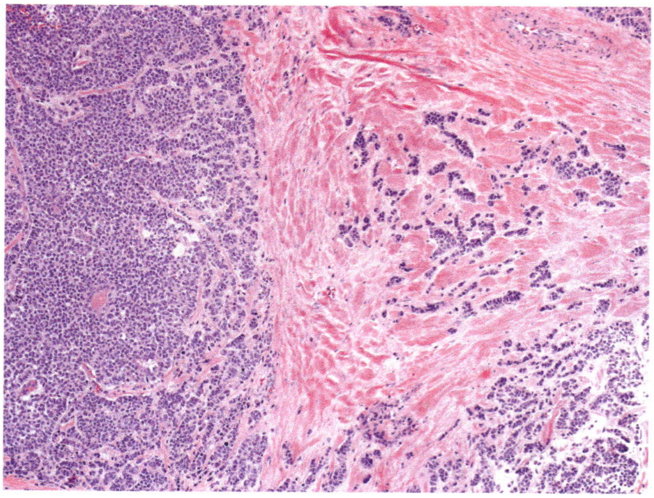

Fig. 27.6 (H&E, 100×) Small cell neuroendocrine carcinoma, cords

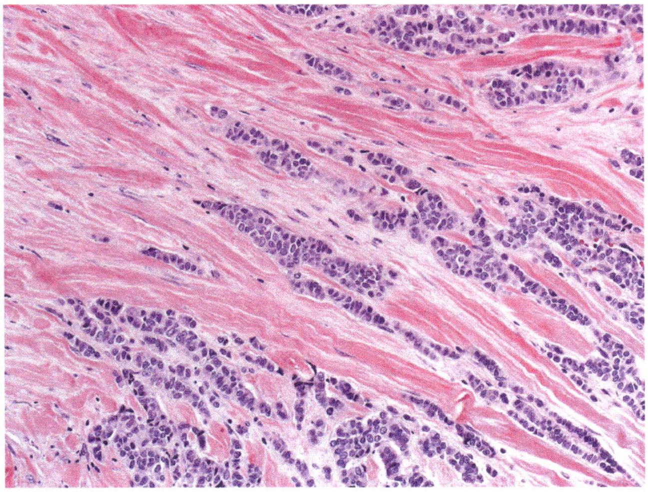

Fig. 27.7 (H&E, 200×) Small cell neuroendocrine carcinoma, cords

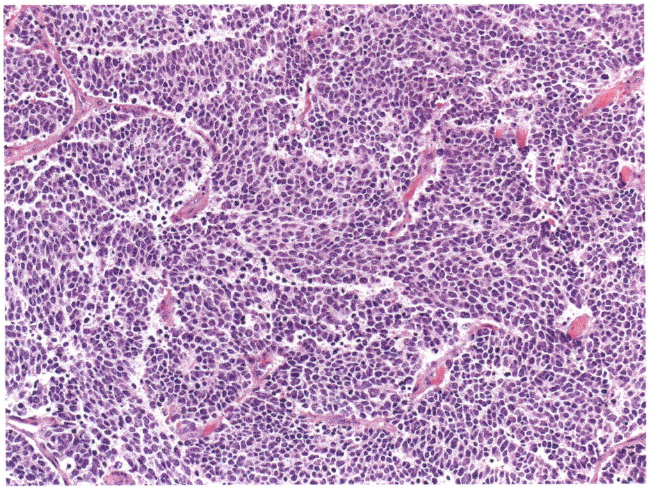

Fig. 27.8 (H&E, 200×) Small cell neuroendocrine carcinoma, solid

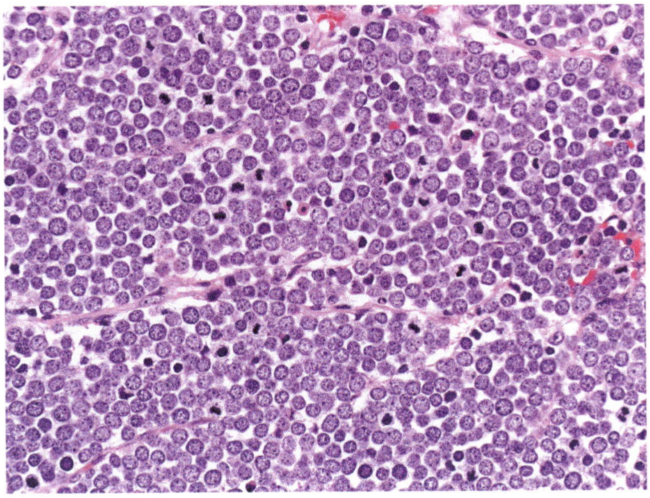

Fig. 27.9 (H&E, 400×) Small cell neuroendocrine carcinoma, solid

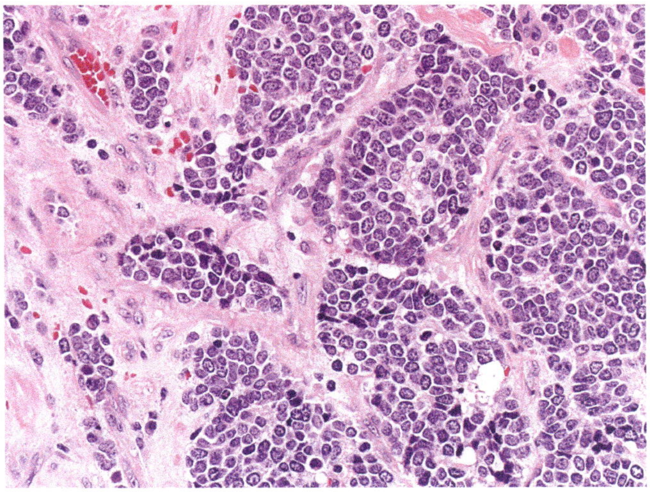

Fig. 27.10 (H&E, 400×) Small cell neuroendocrine carcinoma, cytomorphologic atypia

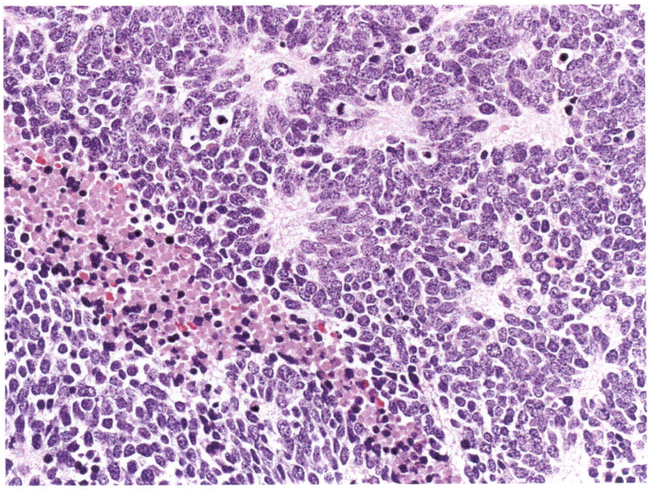

Fig. 27.11 (H&E, 400×) Small cell neuroendocrine carcinoma, mitotic activity

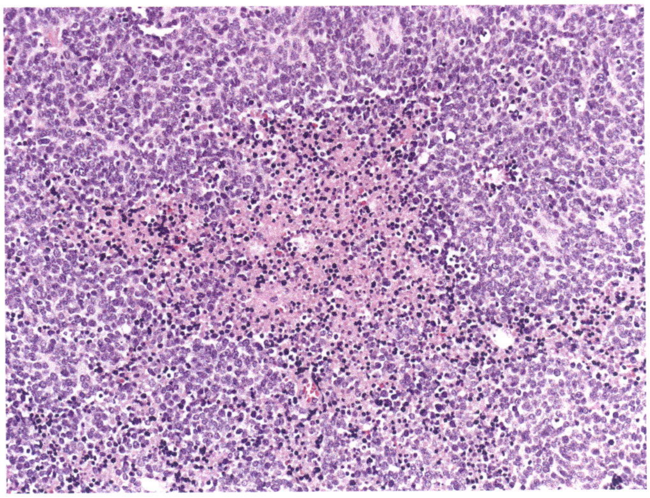

Fig. 27.12 (H&E, 200×) Small cell neuroendocrine carcinoma, necrosis

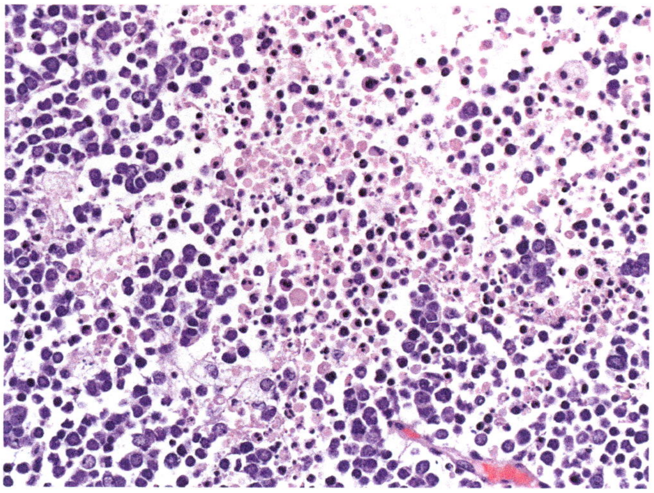

Fig. 27.13 (H&E, 400×) Small cell neuroendocrine carcinoma, necrosis

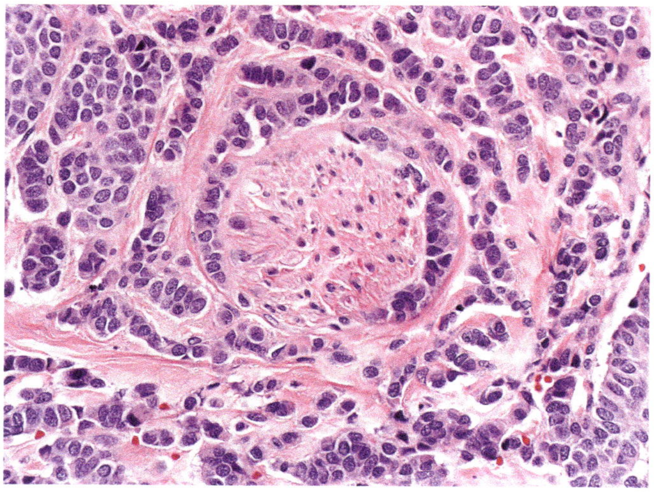

Fig. 27.14 (H&E, 400×) Small cell neuroendocrine carcinoma, perineural invasion

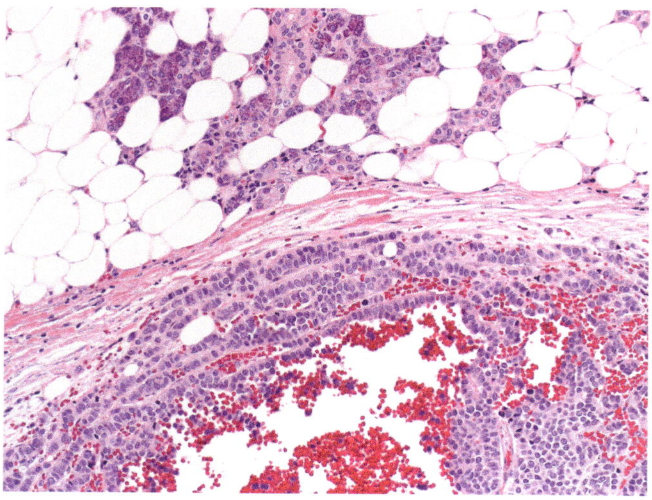

Fig. 27.15 (H&E, 200×) Small cell neuroendocrine carcinoma, hemorrhagic

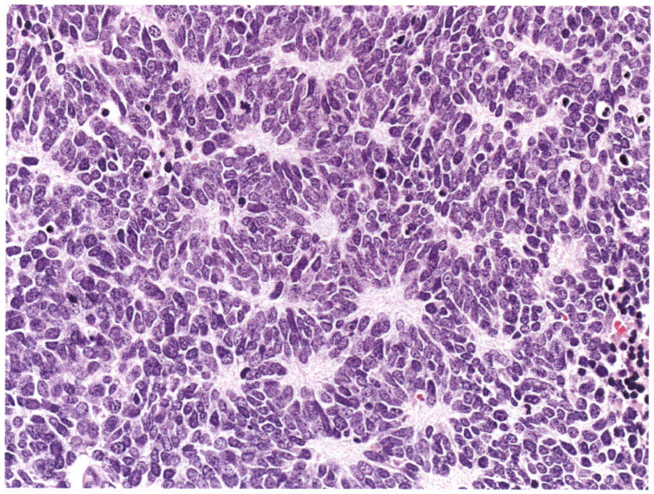

Fig. 27.16 (H&E, 400×) Small cell neuroendocrine carcinoma, Homer Wright pseudorosettes

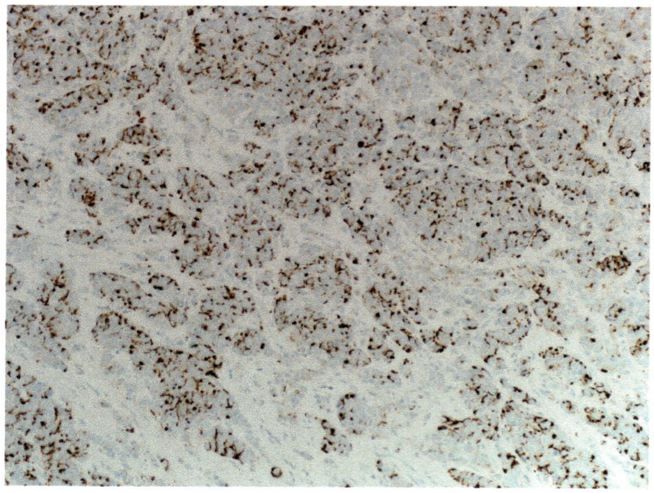

Fig. 27.17 (AE1/AE3, 400×) Small cell neuroendocrine carcinoma, diffuse immunoreactivity

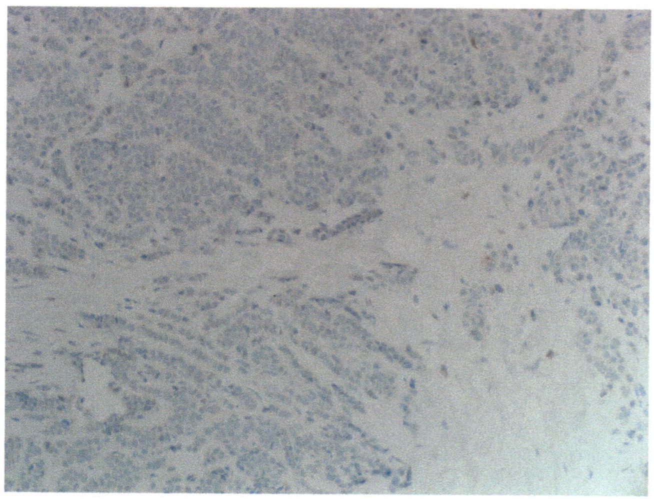

Fig. 27.18 (S-100, 200×) Small cell neuroendocrine carcinoma, negative immunoreactivity

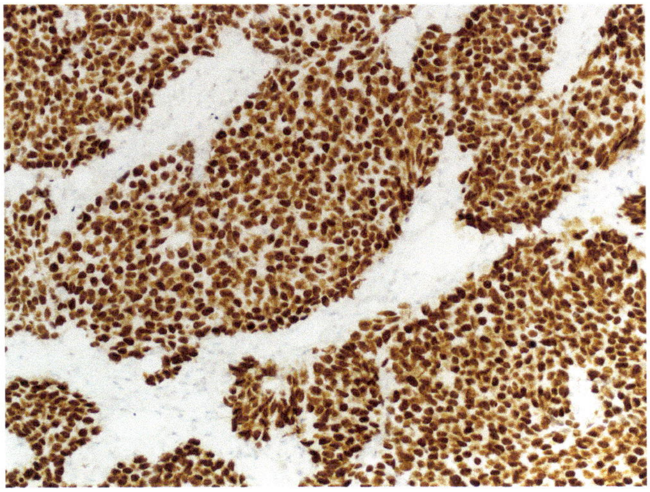

Fig. 27.19 (p63, 200×) Small cell neuroendocrine carcinoma, diffuse immunoreactivity

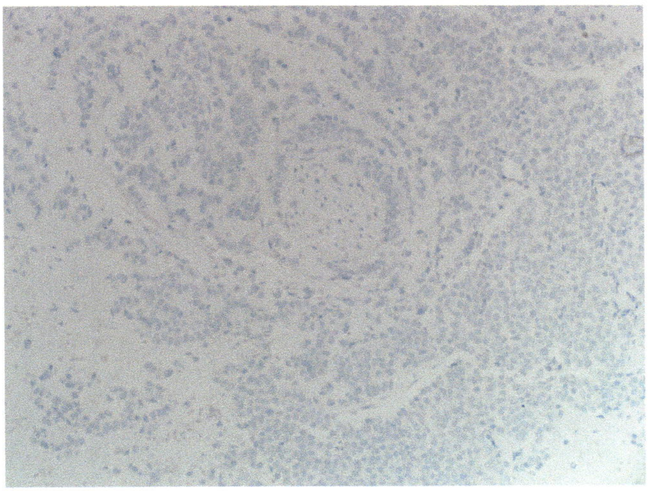

Fig. 27.20 (p63, 200×) Small cell neuroendocrine carcinoma, negative immunoreactivity

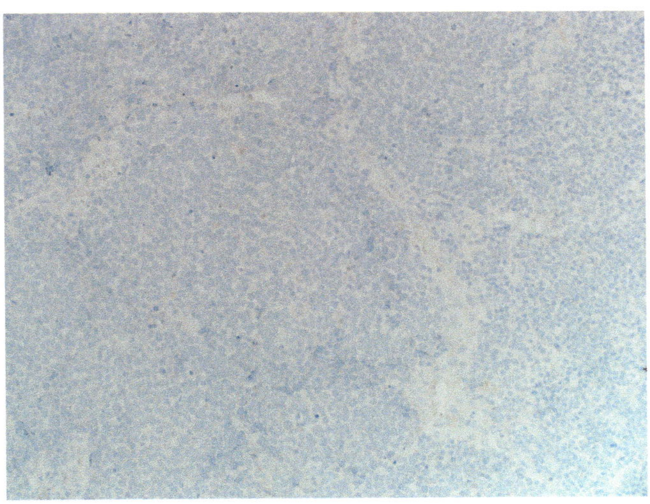

Fig. 27.21 (CK7, 200×) Small cell neuroendocrine carcinoma, negative immunoreactivity

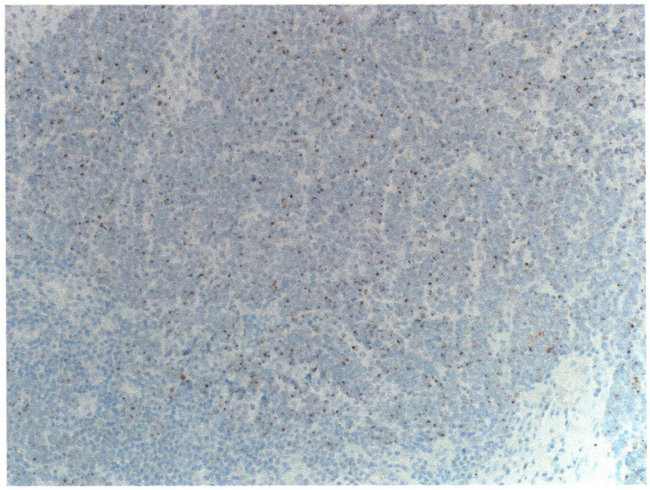

Fig. 27.22 (CK20, 200×) Small cell neuroendocrine carcinoma, diffuse immunoreactivity

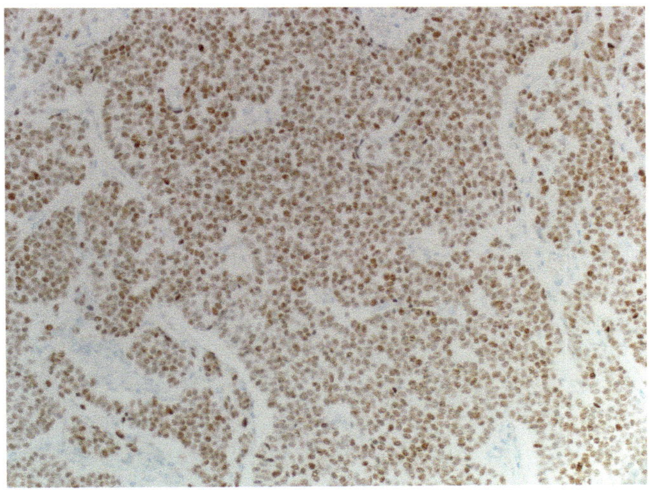

Fig. 27.23 (TTF-1, 200×) Small cell neuroendocrine carcinoma, diffuse immunoreactivity

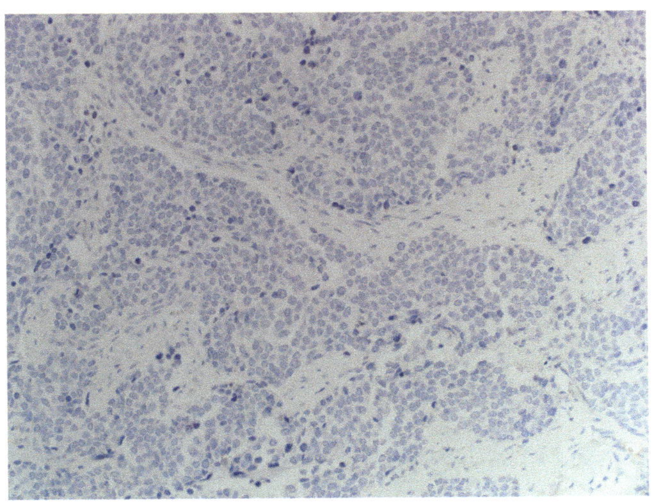

Fig. 27.24 (TTF-1, 200×) Small cell neuroendocrine carcinoma, negative immunoreactivity

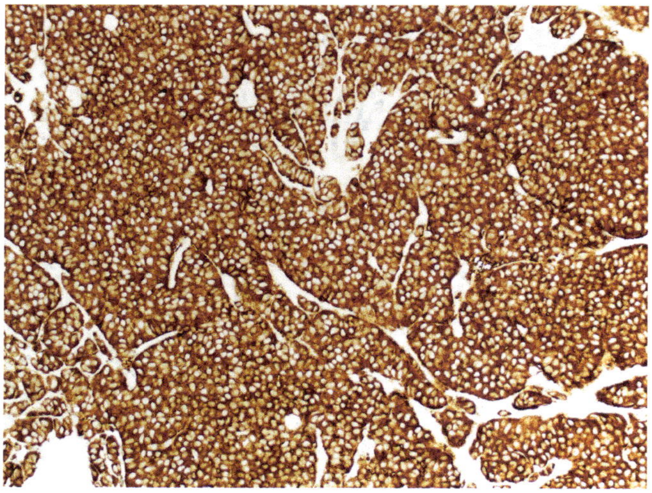

Fig. 27.25 (Synaptophysin, 200×) Small cell neuroendocrine carcinoma, diffuse immunoreactivity

Suggested Reading

Casas P, Bernaldez R, Patron M, Lopez-Ferrer P, Garcia-Cabezas MA. Large cell neuroendocrine carcinoma of the parotid gland: case report and literature review. Auris Nasus Larynx. 2005;32: 89–93.

Chernock RD, Duncavage EJ, Gnepp DR, El-Mofty SK, Lewis JS Jr. Absence of Merkel cell polyomavirus in primary parotid high-grade neuroendocrine carcinomas regardless of cytokeratin 20 immunophenotype. Am J Surg Pathol. 2011;35:1806–11.

Cheuk W, Kwan MY, Suster S, Chan JK. Immunostaining for thyroid transcription factor 1 and cytokeratin 20 aids the distinction of small cell carcinoma from Merkel cell carcinoma, but not pulmonary from extrapulmonary small cell carcinomas. Arch Pathol Lab Med. 2001;125(2):228–31.

Cimino-Matthews A, Lin BM, Chang SS, Boahene KD, Bishop JA. Small cell carcinoma ex-pleomorphic adenoma of the parotid gland. Head Neck Pathol. 2012;6:502–6.

Galanis E, Frytak S, Lloyd RV. Extrapulmonary small cell carcinoma. Cancer. 1997;79(9):1729–36.

Gnepp DR, Wick MR. Small cell carcinoma of the major salivary glands. An immunohistochemical study. Cancer. 1990;66(1):185–92.

Kao HL, Chang WC, Li WY, Chia-Heng Li A, Fen-Yau LA. Head and neck large cell neuroendocrine carcinoma should be separated from atypical carcinoid on the basis of different clinical features, overall survival, and pathogenesis. Am J Surg Pathol. 2012;36:185–92.

Kawaratani H, Tsujimoto T, Yoshikawa M, Kawanami F, Shirai Y, Yoshiji H, et al. Large cell neuroendocrine carcinoma presenting with neck swelling in the submandibular gland: a case report. J Med Case Rep. 2013;7:81.

Nagao T, Gaffey TA, Olsen KD, Serizawa H, Lewis JE. Small cell carcinoma of the major salivary glands: clinicopathologic study with emphasis on cytokeratin 20 immunoreactivity and clinical outcome. Am J Surg Pathol. 2004;28(6):762–70.

Nagao T, Sugano I, Ishida Y, Tajima Y, Munakata S, Asoh A, et al. Primary large-cell neuroendocrine carcinoma of the parotid gland: immunohistochemical and molecular analysis of two cases. Mod Pathol. 2000;13:554–61.

Pang B, Leong CC, Salto-Tellez M, Petersson F. Desmoplastic small round cell tumor of major salivary glands: report of 1 case and a review of the literature. Appl Immunhistochem Mol Morphol. 2011;19:70–5.

Said-Al-Naief N, Sciandra K, Gnepp DR. Moderately differentiated neuroendocrine carcinoma (atypical carcinoid) of the parotid gland: report of three cases with contemporary review of salivary neuroendocrine carcinomas. Head Neck Pathol. 2013;7:295–303.

Servato JP, da Silva SJ, de Faria PR, Cardoso SV, Loyola AM. Small cell carcinoma of the salivary gland: a systematic literature review and two case reports. Int J Oral Maxillofac Surg. 2013;42:89–98.

Walters DM, Little SC, Hessler RB, Gourin CG. Small cell carcinoma of the submandibular gland: a rare small round blue cell tumor. Am J Otolaryngol. 2007;28:118–21.

Yamamoto N, Minami S, Kidoguchi M, Shindo A, Tokumaru Y, Fujii M. Large cell carcinoma of the submandibular gland: case report and literature review. Auris Nasus Larynx. 2014;41:105–8.

Xu B, Chetty R, Perez-Ordonez B. Neuroendocrine neoplasms of the head and neck: some suggestions for the new WHO classification of head and neck tumors. Head Neck Pathol. 2014;8:24–32.

28 Warthin's Tumor

Warthin's tumor affects primarily adults and presents at a mean age of approximately 60 years. Women are involved less than men. The majority of cases involve the parotid gland, presenting as single or multiple masses. Warthin's tumor may be circumscribed or multi-nodular, comprised of multiple cell types (columnar and cuboidal), and exhibit a variety of architectural patterns (solid, cystic, and papillary) (Figs. 28.1–28.19).

J. J. García, *Atlas of Salivary Gland Pathology*, https://doi.org/10.1007/978-3-319-09021-4_28

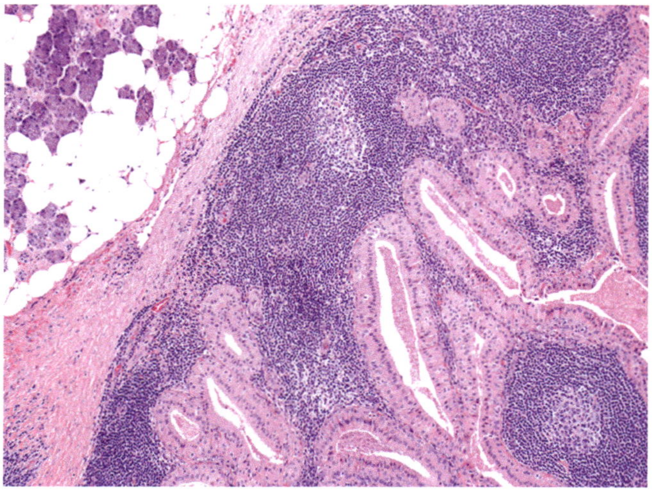

Fig. 28.1 (H&E, 100×) Warthin's tumor, circumscribed

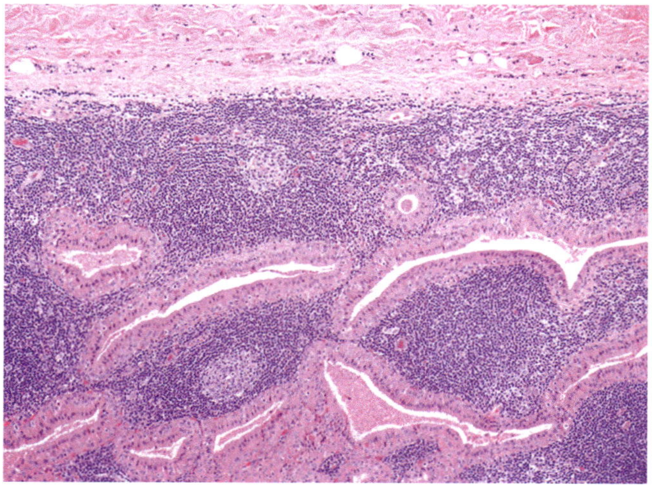

Fig. 28.2 (H&E, 100×) Warthin's tumor, circumscribed

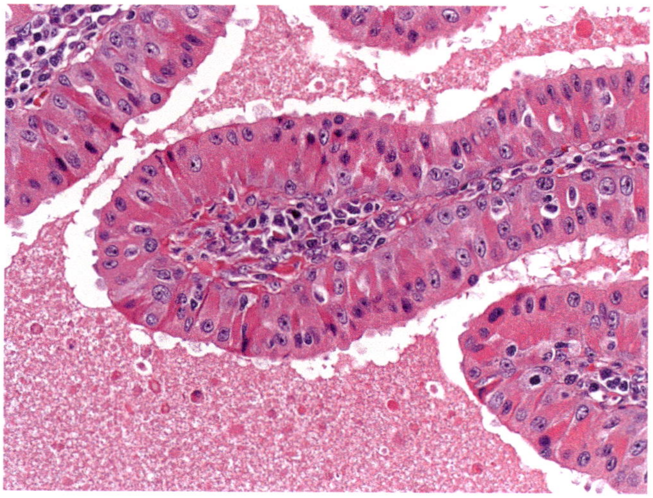

Fig. 28.3 (H&E, 400×) Warthin's tumor, biphasic

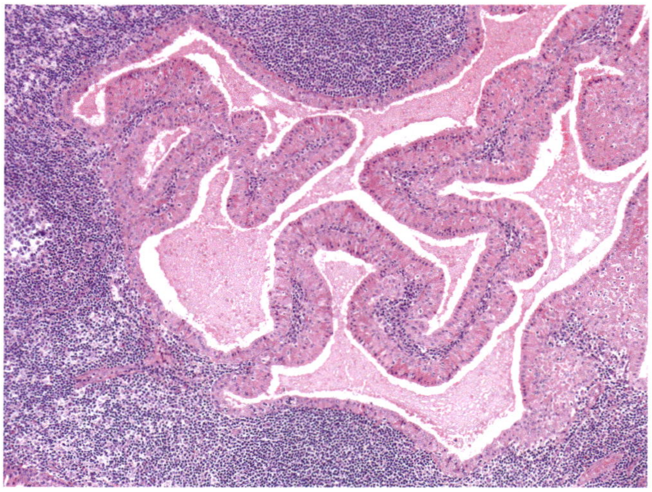

Fig. 28.4 (H&E, 100×) Warthin's tumor, cystic

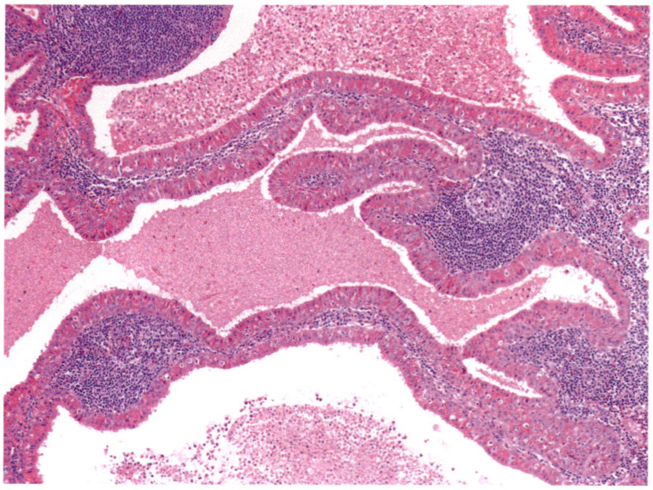

Fig. 28.5 (H&E, 100×) Warthin's tumor, cystic

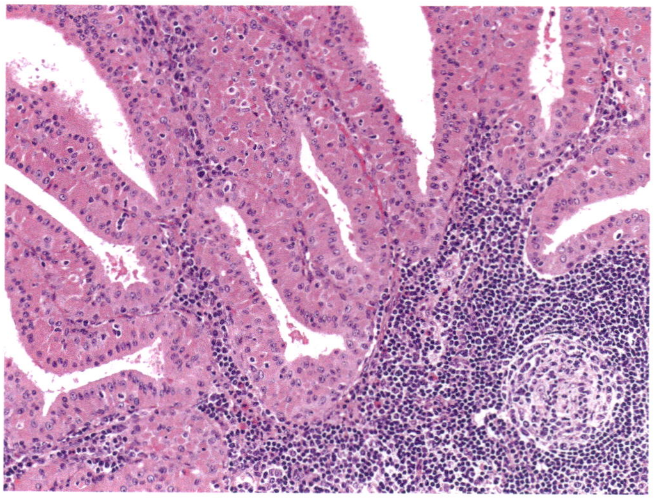

Fig. 28.6 (H&E, 200×) Warthin's tumor, papillary

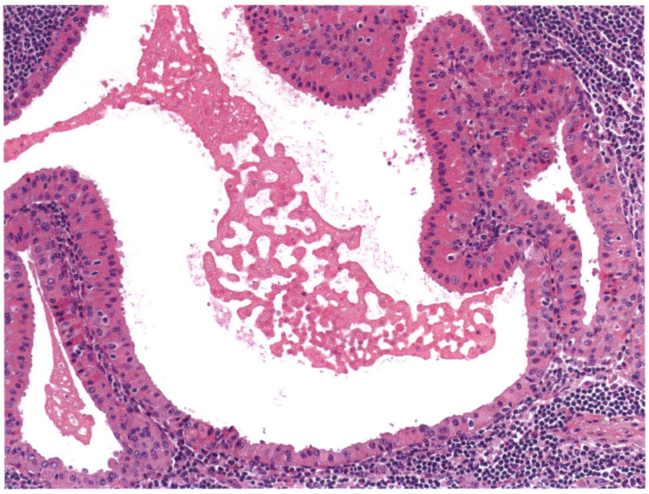

Fig. 28.7 (H&E, 200×) Warthin's tumor, papillary

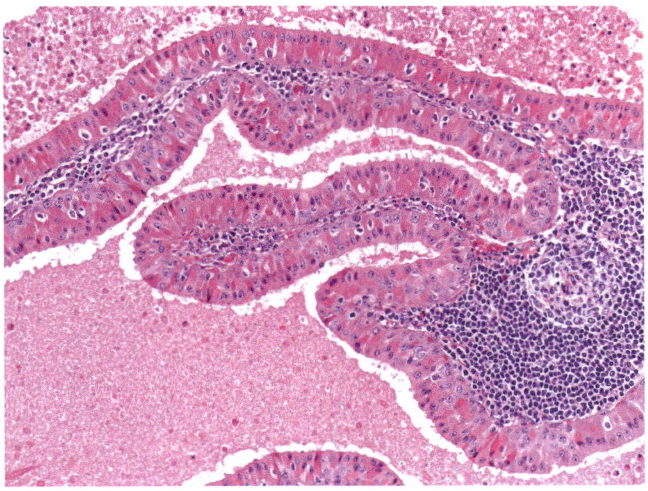

Fig. 28.8 (H&E, 200×) Warthin's tumor, lymphoid stroma

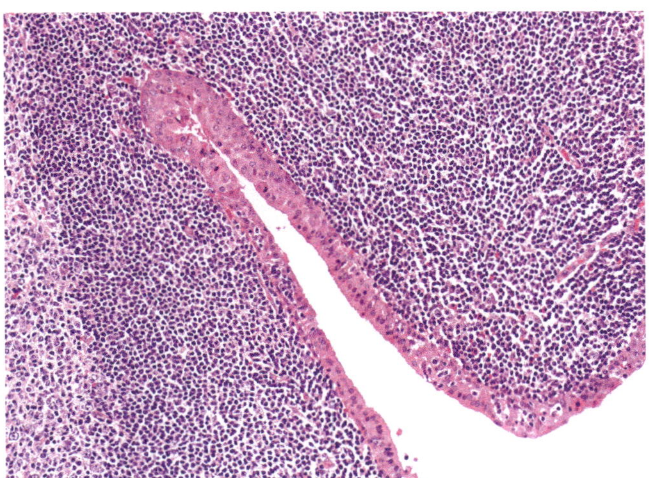

Fig. 28.9 (H&E, 200×) Warthin's tumor, lymphoid stroma

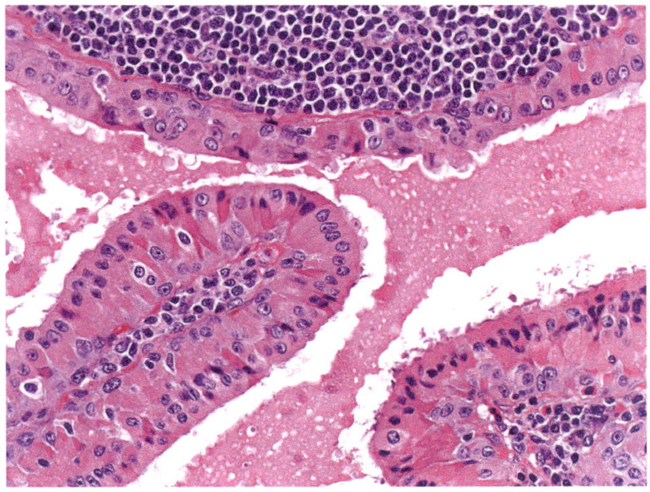

Fig. 28.10 (H&E, 400×) Warthin's tumor, oncocytes

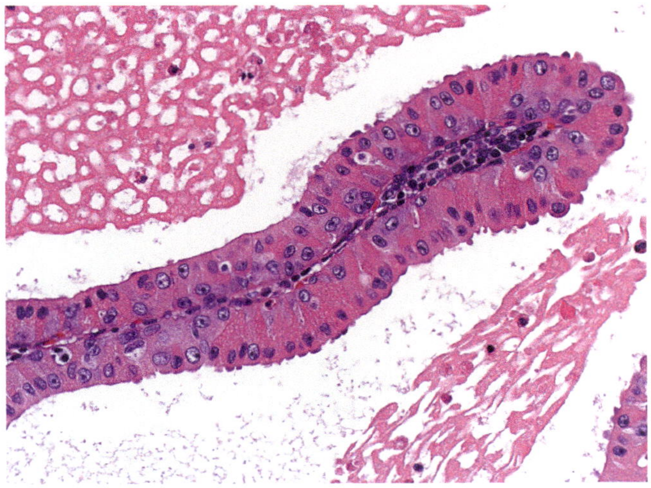

Fig. 28.11 (H&E, 400×) Warthin's tumor, oncocytes

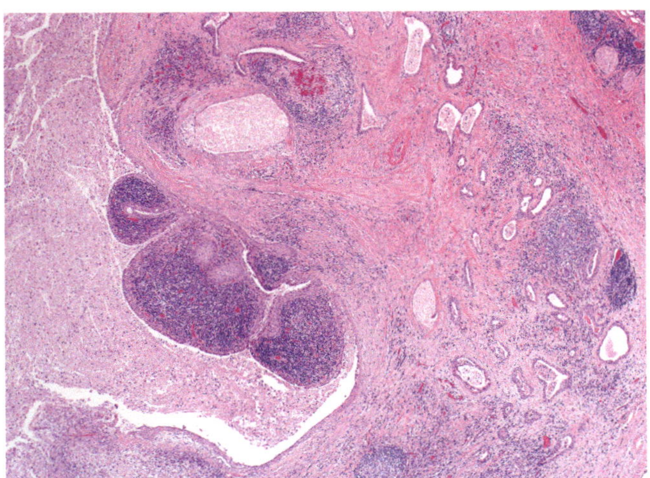

Fig. 28.12 (H&E, 40×) Warthin's tumor, necrosis (biopsy-related)

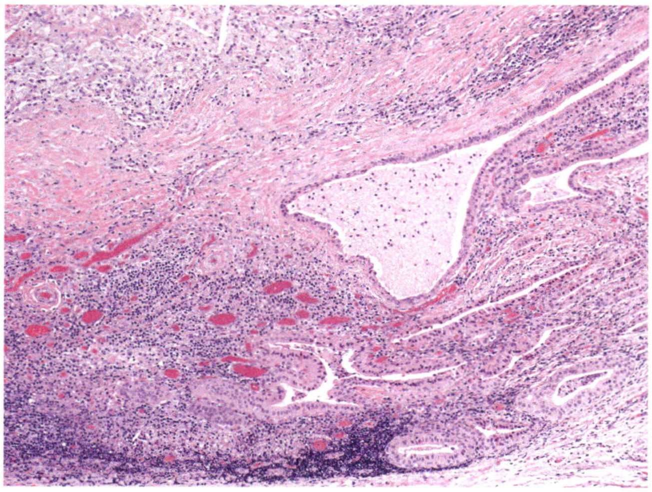

Fig. 28.13 (H&E, 100×) Warthin's tumor, necrosis (biopsy-related)

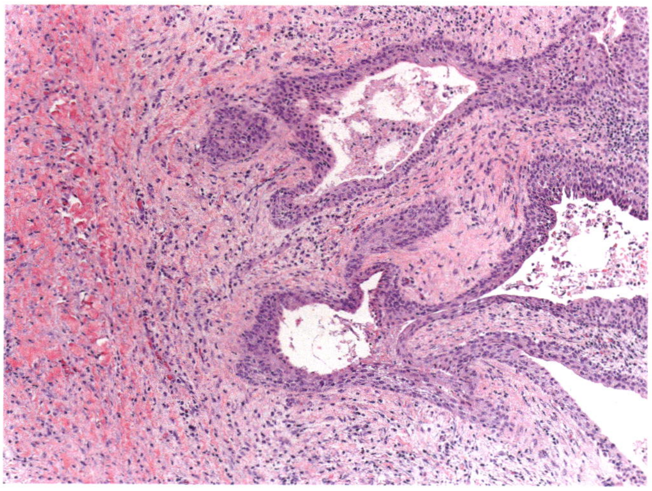

Fig. 28.14 (H&E, 100×) Warthin's tumor, squamous metaplasia (biopsy-related)

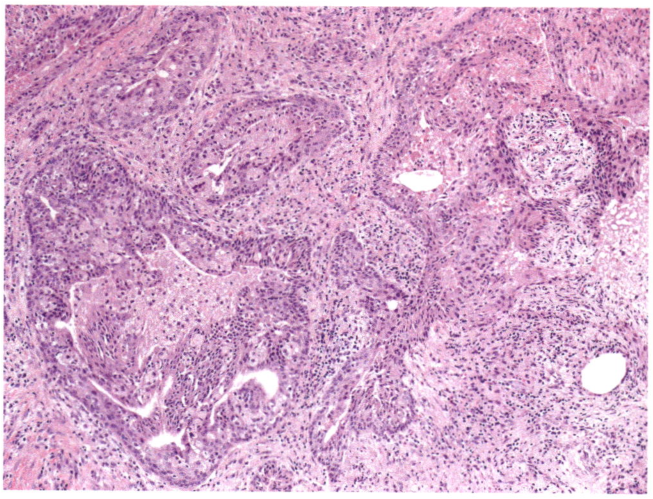

Fig. 28.15 (H&E, 100×) Warthin's tumor, squamous metaplasia (biopsy-related)

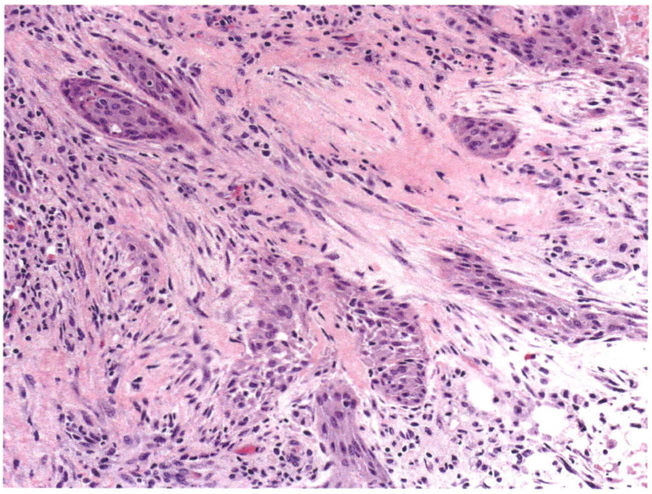

Fig. 28.16 (H&E, 200×) Warthin's tumor, cytomorphologic atypia (biopsy-related)

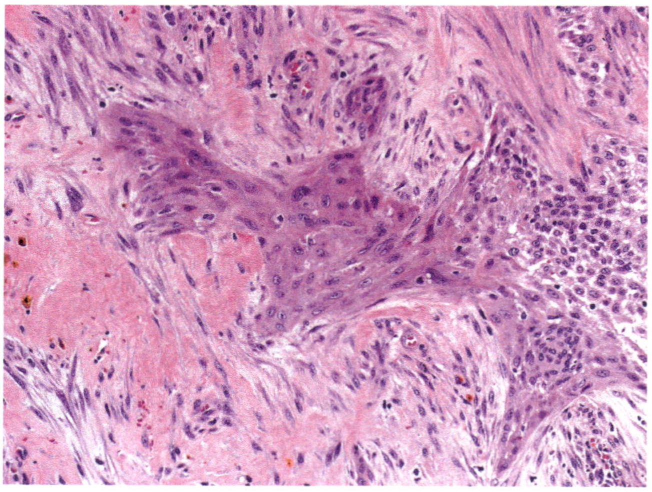

Fig. 28.17 (H&E, 200×) Warthin's tumor, cytomorphologic atypia (biopsy-related)

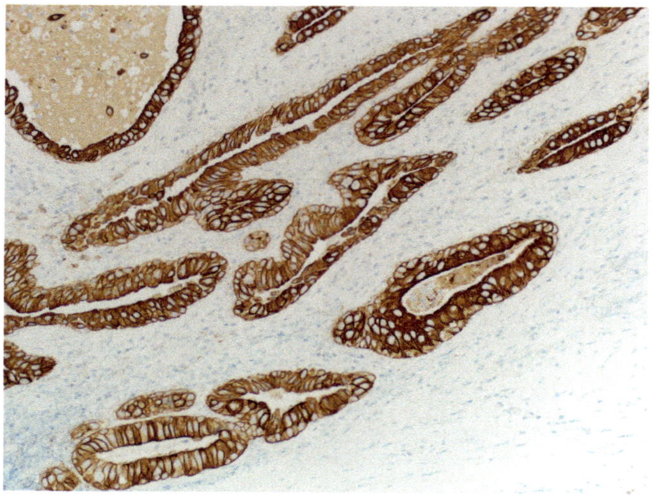

Fig. 28.18 (AE1/AE3, 200×) Warthin's tumor, diffuse immunoreactivity

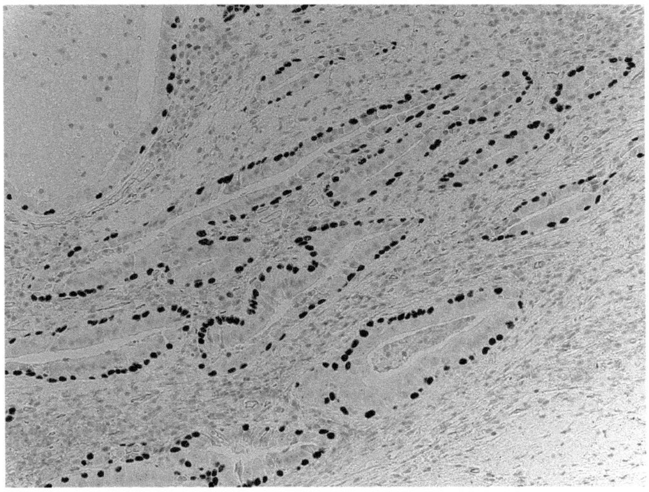

Fig. 28.19 (p63, 200×) Warthin's tumor, basal immunoreactivity

Suggested Reading

Ballo MS, Shin HJ, Sneige N. Sources of diagnostic error in the fine-needle aspiration diagnosis of Warthin's tumor and clues to a correct diagnosis. Diagn Cytopathol. 1997;17(3):230–4.

Di Palma S, Simpson RH, Skalova A, Michal M. Metaplastic (infarcted) Warthin's tumor of the parotid gland: a possible consequence of fine needle aspiration biopsy. Histopathology. 1999;35:432–8.

Ellies M, Laskawi R, Arglebe C. Extraglandular Warthin's tumors: clinical evaluation and long-term follow-up. Br J Oral Maxillofac Surg. 1998;36:52–3.

Ethunandan M, Pratt CA, Higgins B, Morrison A, Umar T, Macpherson DW, et al. Factors influencing the occurrence of multicentric and "recurrent" Warthin's tumor: a cross sectional study. Int J Oral Maxillofac Surg. 2008;37:831–4.

Eveson JW, Cawson RA. Warthin's tumor (cystadenolymphoma) of salivary glands. A clinicopathologic investigation of 278 cases. Oral Surg Oral Med Oral Pathol. 1986;61:256–62.

Flezar M, Pogacnik A. Warthin's tumor: unusual vs. common morphological findings in fine needle aspiration biopsies. Cytopathology. 2002;13:232–41.

Gallo O, Bocciolini C. Warthin's tumor associated with autoimmune diseases and tobacco use. Acta Otolaryngol. 1997;117:623–7.

Goonewardene SA, Nasuti JF. Value of mucin detection in distinguishing mucoepidermoid carcinoma from Warthin's tumor on fine needle aspiration. Acta Cytol. 2002;46(4):704–8.

Lam KH, Ho HC, Ho CM, Wei WI. Multifocal nature of adenolymphoma of the parotid. Br J Surg. 1994;81:1612–4.

Maiorano E, Lo Muzio L, Favia G, Piattelli A. Warthin's tumor: a study of 78 cases with emphasis on bilaterality, multifocality and association with other malignancies. Oral Oncol. 2002;38:35–40.

Pinkston JA, Cole P. Cigarette smoking and Warthin's tumor. Am J Epidemiol. 1996;144(2):183–7.

Sadetzki S, Oberman B, Mandelzweig L, Chetrit A, Ben-Tai T, Jarus-Hakak A, et al. Smoking and risk of parotid gland tumors: a nationwide case-control study. Cancer. 2008;112:1974–82.

Seifert G, Bull HG, Donath K. Histologic subclassification of the cystadenolymphoma of the parotid gland. Analysis of 275 cases. Virchows Arch A Pathol Anat Histol. 1980;388:13–38.

Skalova A, Vanecek T, Simpson RH, Vazmitsel MA, Majewska H, Mukensnabi P, et al. CRTC1-MAML2 fusions were not detected in metaplastic Warthin tumor and metaplastic ploeomrphic adenoma of salivary glands. Am J Surg Pathol. 2013;37:1743–50.

Veder LL, Kerrebijn JD, Smedts FM, den Bakker MA. Diagnostic accuracy of fine-needle aspiration cytology in Warthin tumors. Head Neck. 2010;32:1635–40.

Verma K, Kapila K. Salivary gland tumors with a prominent oncocytic component. Cytologic findings and differential diagnosis of oncocytomas and Warthin's tumor on fine needle aspirates. Acta Cytol. 2003;47(2):221–6.

Index

J. J. García, *Atlas of Salivary Gland Pathology*, https://doi.org/10.1007/978-3-319-09021-4